PHARMACOEPIDEMIOLOGY AND PHARMACOECONOMICS

CONCEPTS AND PRACTICE

PHARMACOEPIDEMIOLOGY AND PHARMACOECONOMICS

CONCEPTS AND PRACTICE

K. G. Revikumar
B.Sc., D.J., D.Ger., LLB, M.Pharm, (Hosp. Pharm) Ph.D.

Principal,
Nirmala College of Health Science (Pharmacy),
Meloor, Kunnappilly, Chalakudy, Thrissur, Kerala.

(Formerly, Chief & Head Dept. of Hosp. & Clinical Pharmacy,
Govt. Medical College, Trivendrum)

PharmaMed Press
An imprint of Pharma Book Syndicate

A unit of BSP Books Pvt. Ltd.

4-4-309/316, Giriraj Lane,
Sultan Bazar, Hyderabad - 500 095.

Pharmacoepidemiology and Pharmacoeconomics: ***Concepts and Practice by*** **K.G. Revikumar**

Published by

PharmaMed Press
An imprint of Pharma Book Syndicate
A unit of BSP Books Pvt. Ltd.
4-4-309/316, Giriraj Lane, Sultan Bazar, Hyderabad - 500 095.
Phone: 040-23445605, 23445688; Fax: 91+40-23445611
E-mail: info@pharmamedpress.com

ISBN: 978-93-5230-132-4 (HB)

Dedication to,

This book is dedicated to my teacher, mentor and professor at Delhi University Dr. B.D. Miglani, the living legend of Indian hospital pharmacy. His constant support, inspiration and motivation helped me to achieve many positions in my professional life.

K. G. Revikumar

Preface

In the late 1990s while working as the head of the Department of Hospital and Clinical Pharmacy, Government Medical College, Trivandrum, the author of this book made an earnest effort to start the Doctor of Pharmacy (PharmD) program in Trivandrum Medical College with the objective of moulding a battalion of teachers of Pharmacy Practice in the Country. Though the initial formalities and related works were completed and the University of Kerala, to which the Medical College was affiliated, accepted the proposal at its Board of Studies and Faculty levels, the program could not be started as the author was transferred to Calicut Medical College in the early 2000.

Later the PharmD was introduced as a professional pharmacy degree program in 2008 in India with a rigid syllabus framed by the Pharmacy Council of India and published through a gazette notification. It was in this background that along with my mentor and Professor Dr. B.D. Miglani, we published the Textbook of Pharmacy Practice in 2009. One chapter each on Pharmacoepidemiology and Pharmacoeconomics were included in the Textbook of Pharmacy Practice. Since then, pharmacy practice students and their teachers in India were demanding a detailed book on Pharmacoepidemiology and Pharmacoeconomics. It is this demand and request from the students and their teachers that empowered me to write this book.

The present book entitled "Pharmacoepidemiology and Pharmacoeconomics – Concepts and Practice" through its 28 chapters tries to discuss the concepts, principles, practice, and applications of Pharmacoepidemiology and Pharmacoeconomics in Indian context. Within the limitations of the subject matters, sincere efforts were made to make the presentations and the structure of the book as simple as possible. Illustrations and case studies are incorporated with the objective of making the learning process easy for the beginners. Though the book is written from the perspective of Indian students of Pharm.D, M.Pharm Pharmacy Practice and research, I hope and believe that it is useful for all those who are interested in Pharmacoepidemiology and Pharmacoeconomics. All types of suggestions, feed back and critical evaluations are welcomed.

April, 2016
K. G. Revikumar

Contents

PART I

PHARMACOEPIDEMIOLOGY

PART I

PHARMACOEPIDEMIOLOGY

Pharmacoepidemiology and Pharmacoeconomics

Concepts and Practice

Pharmacoepidemiology is the application of epidemiological methodologies for the study of drugs focusing on their use and effects in a large number of people. It is drug epidemiology.

Chapter 1

Background and Introduction of Pharmacoepidemiology

Chapter Mission

After learning this chapter you may be able to know:

- Background, definition, concepts and scope of *epidemiology*.
- Background, definition, concepts and scope of *clinical epidemiology*.
- Definition, concepts and scope of *pharmacoepidemiology*.
- Relationship between *epidemiology*, *clinical epidemiology* and *pharmacoepidemiology*.

Background and Introduction

In 1900 AD, there was only one potent analgesic - Morphine, three analgesic antipyretics- Aspirin, Acetanilide and Antipyrin, one antispasmodic- Belladonna, one antimalarial - Quinine and only one heart drug - Digitalis. Anticancer drugs, antibacterials, anti-TB drugs, anti-hypertensive drugs, psychopharmacological agents, antidiabetic medicines, sulpha drugs etc., were not at all available. There were only limited number of medicines and most of them were processed from natural sources. During the second half of the twentieth century we got a large number of medicines which helped the doctors to treat and manage the diseases that were earlier untreated.

Today modern medicine is blessed with pharmaceutical armamentarium that is much more powerful than the past. We can see that the volume, potency and complexity of modern medicines are increasing day by day and medicines are becoming highly sophisticated and potential items. As medicines became potential, they became more and more toxic and started to harbor with them lot of hazards if not prudently used. If the patients are not made aware of the medicines prescribed to them, they may not be able use them safely. Knowledge of the benefits and risks of medicine use in human population is essential to make the practice of pharmacotherapy safe and effective. There is a paramount need to compare the therapeutic efficacy or benefits of medicines with their potential to cause harm or risks .

However our understanding about the efficacy, safety and risks of the medicines relies heavily on the studies conducted during the developmental process and approval of the drug product. Only after the drug product is introduced for marketing, it will be used widely by the general and ordinary population. Such a wide use will help to identify many additional risks and sometimes some additional benefits. These risks and benefits may range from minor or trivial to major or serious effects. There are number of medicines that were once accepted as highly useful but became dangerous subsequently as earlier unknown risks were subsequently identified when used in large population. Penicillin is a classical example. We could also identify newer uses to the existing medicines and Aspirin is a classical example. German apothecary Felix Hoffman in 1898 gave acetyl salicylic acid to his father who was suffering from both arthritis and the bad effects of salicylic acid used to treat arthritis. When the drug was found highly effective, the Bayer Pharmaceuticals started marketing it under the trade name 'Aspirin' which later became its generic name. By the time Aspirin celebrated its hundred years of its use as an analgesic and anti-inflammatory drug, it was found very much useful as a cardiac protective agent (Anti platelet).

Chemie Grunenthal, the German firm started marketing 'thalidomide' in October 1957 under the name 'countergan'. Thalidomide was synthesized in the Company in 1956 by Dr Muckter and his colleagues. On 16th December 1961,

Lancet published first report in Medical Press indicating that thalidomide might be a human teratogen (Mc Bride 1984). Thousands of deformed babies were born to mothers who were given thalidomide to cure their 'morning sickness' during early periods of pregnancy. Epidemiologic studies established its cause to be in utero exposure to thalidomide and the drug was withdrawn from the world market. The adverse effects on human fetus can be estimated only through observational methods, not through experimental methods. In 1996, a relation between appetite suppressant drugs and the risks of primary pulmonary hypertension was reported (Abenhaim L 1996). In the next year another report came out showing the relationship between the drug and valvular heart disease (Connolly HM 1997). These are only some examples of serious adverse effects discovered after the drugs were put in wide use. Such cases help us to remind about the inherent limitations of the drug development process and the need to study populations receiving medications through routine prescriptions of doctors. Today we have subjects like Epidemiology, Clinical Epidemiology and Pharmacoepidemiology in health sciences helping the authorities to frame effective policies in health care including drug usage, surveillance and other medicine related aspects.

Epidemiology

Epidemiology is the rigorous and scientific study of occurrence, patterns, causes, distribution and determinants of diseases in defined human populations. Epidemiology helps to shape policy decisions and evidence based practice by identifying the risk factors for the diseases. Epidemiology has two major areas - one is the study of infectious diseases in large populations called epidemics and the second is the study of chronic diseases. Epidemiological studies help diagnose such health problems and provide a basis for the care of people. During its progress and development, epidemiology has made available precise and strict methodologies for the study of diseases.

The objectives of Epidemiology include application of the information or findings to improve the structure, activities, programs and the outcomes of public health care and for that purpose develop health policies rooted in evidence. Epidemiology helped to develop methodologies that can be used in clinical research, public health and also basic research in health and biological sciences. Major areas of epidemiology include surveillance and screening of diseases, disease etiology and transmission, outbreak related studies, management and monitoring and comparison of treatment effects including clinical trials. Application of scientific principles of biology helps to understand the disease process better. Application of statistics helps to make efficient and effective use of data and arrive at appropriate conclusions. Application of principles of social science helps to understand the proximate and distal causes and engineering for exposure assessment.

Box 1.1 Selected Milestones in the History of Epidemiology

1849-54	John Snow formed and tested hypothesis on the origin of cholera in London - one of the first studies in analytic epidemiology
1920	Goldberger published a descriptive study report showing the dietary origin of pellagra
1940's	Fluoride supplements added to public water supplies in randomized community trials
1949	Initiation of the Framingham study of risk factors for cardiovascular disease
1950	Epidemiological studies link cigarette smoking and lung cancer, demonstrating the power of case-control study design
1954	Field trial of the polio vaccine (Salk), the largest formal human experiment
1959	Mantel and Haenszel developed a statistical procedure for stratified analysis of case-control studies
1960	Mac Mahon published first epidemiologic text with a systematic focus on study design
1964	US Surgeon General's Report on Smoking and Health establish criteria for evaluation of causality
1970's	Large community based trials implemented for worldwide eradication of smallpox
1980's	Chronic disease, injury and occupational epidemiology; HIV epidemic
2000's	Genetic and molecular epidemiology; health disparities; racialism;
2002	bioterrorism; anthrax and smallpox threat and vaccinations
2003	SARS quarantines and public health law; and world-wide epidemiology; BSE in Canada
2004	SARS recurrence; BSE in USA; flu epidemic
2009	2009 H1N1 pandemic

Epidemiological studies can be divided into two main types:

Descriptive Epidemiology

Descriptive epidemiology deals with disease and/or exposure and may consist of calculating rates like incidence and prevalence. Such descriptive studies help to generate hypotheses, but not test them. Studies of drug use would generally fall under descriptive studies.

Analytic Epidemiology

Analytic epidemiology includes two types of studies: observational studies, such as case-control and cohort studies, and experimental studies which include clinical trials or randomized clinical trials (RCT). The analytic studies compare an exposed group with a control group and usually designed as hypothesis testing by studies. Only during the second half of 20th century that the discipline drifted apart, with separate schools, training, journals, and opportunities for employment.

Clinical Epidemiology

'Clinical epidemiology' is the application of epidemiologic principles and methods to problems and issues encountered in clinical medicine. It studies the determinants and effects of clinical decisions. Clinical epidemiology guides clinical decision-making based on quantitative analyses of previous research findings. The term clinical epidemiology originated from two parent disciplines - clinical medicine and epidemiology. It is "clinical" because it seeks to answer clinical questions and to guide clinical decision making with the best available evidence and is "epidemiologic" because many of the methods used to answer these questions have been developed by epidemiologists.

The International Clinical Epidemiology Network (INCLEN) was established in 1980 as a project of The Rockefeller Foundation registered in USA. It is converted into and independent non profit organization in 1988. It is helping clinicians and other health care scientists obtain knowledge and tools to improve health of people in developing countries. Today INCLEN is spread over to 34 countries in the world and membership includes 89 institutes, 59 Clinical Epidemiology Units and 31 Clinical Epidemiology Research and Training Centers (CERTCs). It promotes research and training in clinical epidemiology and biostatistics and carry out multidisciplinary collaborative research works. IndiaCLEN is one of the seven regional networks of INCLEN established in 1991 at Trivandrum Medical College. Its units are established in selected medical colleges in India.

Definition and Scope of Pharmacoepidemiology

Patients and health care providers increasingly rely on pharmacists to appropriately evaluate the benefits and risks of drug therapy. It indicated a need for pharmacoepidemiology training and education in pharmacy schools and colleges. Although epidemiologic terms and statistics often appear in the clinical literature, pharmacy students were not accurately understood such terms till 1980s even in US where PharmD was in existence since 1950s.

Pharmacoepidemiology developed as speciality sometime in the late 1970s at a time when it became increasingly evident, that factors affecting drug use by the community played a critical role in the success or failure of drug therapy. However it was first described and defined in 1984 when it was proposed that a new discipline was necessary to integrate epidemiology and drug-related events. Since then, pharmacoepidemiology research has evolved into an important discipline that analyses information pertaining to areas such as adverse drug events, drug utilization patterns, drug efficacy, and post-marketing surveillance research. The World Health Organization (WHO) started to promote research in pharmacoepidemiology by conducting workshops, publishing manuals, training investigators and encouraging research by funding projects as they identified it as a 'research tool of global importance'.

The term Pharmacoepidemiology has with it two components, namely 'pharmacon' and epidemiology which makes it clear that it is the epidemiology of drugs or medicines. Pharmaco-epidemiology is the amalgamation of the terms 'Pharmacology' and 'Epidemiology'. Some authors state that Pharmacoepidemiology is the child obtained after the 'marriage' of clinical epidemiology and clinical pharmacology.

Most of the initial works related to Pharmacoepidemiology were done by Professors and Researchers of Medicine who were trained in Epidemiology and Biostatistics. Founders of epidemiology and early authors of Pharmacoepidemiology were from the field of medicine, mostly clinicians.

Definition of Pharmacoepidemiology

Pharmacoepidemiology is the epidemiological study of the uses and effects of drugs or medicines in a defined human population. Pharmacoepidemiology uses all the techniques of epidemiology to study the use of and the effects of medicines. It is one of the most useful non-experimental methods of research in drug usage and related aspects. It helped to generate a number of product liability suits against pharmaceutical manufacturers.

Pharmacoepidemiology gives the health care professionals significant information about the health care and cost outcomes of medicines and similar items used in health care after their approval for clinical use. Pharmacoepidemiology is drug epidemiology and applies epidemiological methodologies for the study of drugs focusing on their use and effects in a large number of people. It aims at studying the effects of drugs in people.

The field of Pharmacoepidemiology uses the techniques of chronic disease epidemiology to study the use of and effects of drugs. It helps to get an estimate of probability of beneficial effects as well as probability of adverse effects on populations. It applies all the principles of biological sciences, clinical pharmacology, clinical epidemiology, biostatistics and social sciences. The pharmacoepidemiological studies principally concentrate on the period after the drug enters the market known as post marketing surveillance (PMS) period. Traditionally the Pharmacoepidemiological studies were concerned with the study of adverse effects of drugs. The growing concern related to adverse effects of medicines and their increasing cost helped considerably for the popularization of pharmacoepidemiological studies in recent times.

Pharmacoepidemiology can contributes body of knowledge that promotes the optimal use of medications. It also helps clinicians to take better-informed drug therapy decisions. Pharmacoepidemiology today plays in important role in the drug-approval process in many countries including the United States, Canada, Australia and France with regard to drug safety. Withdrawals of marketed medications during the last few decades were primarily due to findings from pharmacoepidemiological studies. The significance of pharmacoepidemiology is also demonstrated by its inclusion in one of the objectives of US Health Policies. Healthy People 2010 published by the US Department of Health and Human Resources highlights pharmacoepidemiological databases as resources that can be used by health care organizations to monitor and report adverse events related to medical therapies.

The US Accreditation Council for Pharmacy Education (ACPE) later took a decision that education in US pharmacy programs should provide students with the sufficient background in understanding bio-statistical and clinical epidemiological concepts. The 2006 ACPE standards and guidelines recommended the inclusion of pharmacoepidemiology in the social, behavioural, and administrative sciences component of the pharmacy curriculum. While the ACPE has adopted new standards for pharmacoepidemiology curricula taught in US colleges of pharmacy, they have only provided general guidelines for incorporating pharmacoepidemiology topics into pharmacy curriculum. It subsequently increased the extent of Pharmacoepidemiology in pharmacy education.

Education and Training facilities Global Vs India

Pharmacoepidemiology is emerging as an important component of pharmacy education throughout the world, particularly when Doctor of Pharmacy (PharmD) evolved as the global program in pharmacy education, replacing B.S (Pharmacy) and B.Pharm. Since the M.Pharm Pharmacy Practice and the Doctor of Pharmacy (PharmD) programs in India have incorporated Pharmacoepidemiology as a topic or subject in the syllabus it is important to provide didactic and practical training on Pharmacoepidemiology in global versus national situations during their courses and promote research in the areas. Pharmacoepidemiology is an important component of pharmacist education and training as the pharmacists' role in drug therapy decision-making and monitoring is expanding in India in recent times.

Pharmacoepidemiology topics include:

- Application of principles of epidemiology to the study of drug use and outcomes in large populations
- Studies that provide an estimate of the probability of beneficial effects in populations, or the probability of adverse effects in populations, and other parameters relating to drug use benefit
- Methods for continual monitoring for unwanted effects and other safety-related aspects of drugs.

At the global level, training programme in field of epidemiology are conducted by more than 40 countries, mostly of two-year duration. Three member states of South East Asia Region of WHO namely India, Indonesia and Thailand are conducting the two year training programme in Field Epidemiology. In India two year's training programme in field epidemiology (MPH) is being conducted by National NICD, Delhi and NIE, Chennai, each having an enrolment capacity of 15 students per year. The goal of the course is to strengthen public health services by developing a cadre of professional field epidemiologists.

Some of the topics or areas given for advanced course work in Pharmacoepidemiology for PharmD students and researchers in Pharmacy Practice in Hospital and community pharmacies in certain Universities are noted in Box 1.2.

Box 1.2 Topics or areas for advanced studies

- Introduction to Pharmacoepidemiology
- Fundamentals of Epidemiology
- Pharmacoepidemiology and Risk Management
- Epidemiology Research Methods
- Epidemiology of Infectious Disease
- Epidemiology, Prevention, and Control of Chronic Diseases
- Epidemiology of Aging
- Measurement in Epidemiology & Outcomes Research
- Epidemiology cribic, Literaturer Review & Critique
- Design & Conduct of Clinical Trials
- Cancer Epidemiology, Prevention, Early Detection, and Control
- Grant Writing Skills in Epidemiology and Clinical Research
- Molecular and Genetic Epidemiology
- Cardiovascular Disease Epidemiology
- Paediatric Epidemiology
- Epidemiology, Prevention, and Control of Infectious Diseases
- Management for Epidemiologic & Clinical Research

The National Institute of Communicable Diseases (NICD) is situated in New Delhi and is now renamed as National Center for Disease Control. It was established in July 1963, by Government of India to expand and reorganize the activities of the Malaria Institute of India (MII). The reorganized Institute was established to develop a national centre for teaching and research in various disciplines of epidemiology and control of communicable diseases. The Institute is affiliated to Guru Govind Singh Indraprastha University Delhi. The Institute was also entrusted with the task of developing reliable rapid economic epidemiological tools which could be effectively applied in the field for the control of communicable diseases. The objectives of the Institute broadly cover three activities viz., training, service and operational research in the field of communicable diseases and their prevention and control in the country.

National Institute of Epidemiology (NIE) was established in 1999 July at Chennai under the control of ICMR. The main objectives of the NIC include development of human resources in epidemiology and biostatistics, networking of the various ICMR and non-ICMR institutes at the national level for epidemiological purposes and Consultancy services. The Institute offers 2-year Post Graduate course (M.Sc.) in Epidemiology and Doctorate programme (Ph.D.). Post graduate course in Epidemiology was started in the year 2001 for graduates in Medicine / Dental / Indian

Medicine / Allied Health Sciences. The courses are affiliated to DR. MGR University, Chennai. Today NIE is under the control of Department of Health Research (DHR), Government of India.

The Indian Institute of Public Health – Delhi (IIPH-D) commenced its operations in November 2008 with the launch of the Post Graduate Diploma in Health Economics, Financing and Policy. Since then, the institute has expanded its activities and launched Post Graduate Diploma in Public Health Management and Post Graduate Diploma in Clinical Research. IIPH Delhi has successfully conducted many short-term training Programmes and workshops in various fields related to public health and is still conducting such programs regularly. The activities get funding support from the Ministry of Health and Family Welfare, Department of AYUSH, Indian Council of Medical Research, Central Council for Research in Unani Medicine, Department of Science and Technology, Medical Council of India and similar agencies.

The INCLEN centres in India conduct courses and training programs on various aspects of clinical epidemiology in about 17 Medical Colleges. However the Indian Universities are yet to start specialised programs like masters in Pharmaco-epidemiology or Pharmacoeconomics. However research studies at PhD and M.Phil levels are undertaken by scholars in many Indian Universities. At the global level, many Universities currently offer specialised programs and training in Pharmacoepidemiology. Many American Universities including Johns Hopkins and Harvard took Pharmacoepidemiology at post graduate/ masters and PhD levels in recent decades.

Pharmacoepidemiology is the application of epidemiological methodologies for the study of drugs focusing on their use and effects in a large number of people. It is drug epidemiology.

CHAPTER 2

Genesis and Development of Pharmacoepidemiology

Chapter Mission

After learning this chapter you may be able to know:

- Origin and evolution of *pharmacoepidemiology*.
- Reasons for withdrawal of drugs after marketing.
- Working of International Society for Pharmacoepidemiology (ISPE).

Hippocrates, the father of modern medicine was the first person who examined the relationship between the occurrence of disease and environmental factors influencing the disease. He coined the term 'endemic' for diseases generally found in some places, but not in other places and the term ' epidemic' for diseases that are found only in sometimes and absent in other times. In the 16th century a doctor from Verona named Girolamo Fracastoro highlighted the importance of personal and environmental hygiene to prevent diseases. The discovery of microscope by Leeuwenhoek in 1675 helped to identify germs responsible for diseases.

John Snow who investigated the cause of cholera epidemics in 19th century and used chlorine to clean water is considered as the father of modern epidemiology. In 1865 British surgeon Joseph Lister discovered antiseptics in the light of works of Louis Pasteur. During the early part of 20th century Ronald Ross and his team members introduced mathematical methods into epidemiology. In the later part of 20th century molecular epidemiology focusing on relationship between biomarkers and diseases evolved. Genetic epidemiology also emerged during the period focusing on genetic variations.

Today Pharmacoepidemiology has emerged as a discipline due to various reasons and factors emerged during the twentieth century. The traditional clinical pharmacology was focusing its attention on pharmacokinetics and pharmacodynamics of drugs covering absorption, distribution, metabolism and excretion of drugs. Such studies usually involved small number of persons, often ranging from 6 to 25 and were conducted mainly for determining the dose and frequency of new drugs in the treatment of patients. Such findings were solely aimed at the approval process of new drugs. However such studies are of limited use in giving information regarding the new medicine after their marketing.

Many times the drug products are recalled immediately after their marketing or little later. The main reason for such recalls is the identification or reporting of certain uncommon harmful drug effects which may occur only one in 25000 persons or so. In the pre-marketing studies typically 3000 to 4000 patients may be treated with the drug. Once marketed, the same drug reaches millions of patients and rare events can become manifested.

In 1906, the US law - *the Pure Food & Drugs Act* - was passed in response to excessive adulteration and misbranding of the food and drugs available in those days. In 1937 over 100 children died in the US due to renal failure as a result of the use of sulfanilamide syrup marketed by Massengill Company. It was in response to this incident that the Food, Drug and Cosmetics Act 1938 was passed in the US (Geiling EMK 1938). Even then, much attention was not seen paid to the adverse reactions of drugs until the early 1950s, when it was found that Chloramphenicol could cause aplastic anemia.

In 1952, the American Medical Association Council on Pharmacy and Chemistry started the first official registry of adverse drug effects with the objective of collecting data on incidents of drug-induced blood dyscrasias. The FDA itself got involved in collecting reports of ADR and sponsored hospital-oriented drug monitoring programs. Johns Hopkins Hospital and the Boston Collaborative Drug Surveillance program developed the use of in-hospital monitors to perform cohort studies to explore the short- term effects of drug used in hospitals.

In 1956, Dr. Muckter and his colleagues working for the German company, Chemie Grunenthal, synthesized a drug called 'thalidomide'. It showed considerable promise as a sleeping pill and had the great advantage of not having the serious side effects of barbiturates. Chemie Grunenthal started selling thalidomide in Germany in October 1957 under the name "Countergan" and in England the Distillers Company started to sell it under license as "Distaval". In the early 1960s the world experienced the so called 'thalidomide tragedy'. This disaster caused birth of thousands of deformed babies-monsters, that were without limbs. All those unfortunate babies were called "thalidomide babies".

On 16 December 1961 Lancet published the first report in the British Medical Press indicating that thalidomide might be a human teratogen [Mc Bride 1961, Mc Bride 1984]. Epidemiologic studies established its cause to be *in utero* exposure to thalidomide. It is to be noted that before the thalidomide, many other drugs were involved in the issue of producing serious adverse drug reactions (ADR) in human beings. However the manner in which the ADRs of thalidomide were exposed and the birth of hundreds of babies without hands, without legs or without both hands and legs attracted the attention of world population and created a dramatic impact in health care in all countries. Spontaneous reporting of ADRs were initiated in some countries while in a large number of countries other methods of ADR surveillance activities were started during 1960s.

The FDA in US had never permitted the marketing of thalidomide. The US was spared of the thalidomide epidemic as new drugs take longer time to penetrate their regulatory screen. However inspired by the tragedy, the Kefauver Harris Amendments were passed in the USA in 1962 to strengthen the requirements for proof of drug safety. As a result of this amendment, extensive pre-clinical pharmacological and toxicological testing become essential before a drug could be tested in man and the data were required to be submitted to FDA in Investigational New Drug (IND) Application. Requiring "substantial evidence that the drug will have the effects it purports or is represented to have" resulted in the establishment of the randomized clinical trial (RCT) as the "gold standard" for proof of efficacy. The 1962 amendments also required manufacturers to report adverse drug events detected in the post marketing setting to the FDA. The area of Pharmacotherapy got developed during the twentieth century which helped for the growth of areas of Pharmacovigilance, Pharmacogenomics and Pharmacoeconomics.

Inspired by the thalidomide disaster, the Committee on Safety of Drugs (CSD) was established in the UK in the early 1960s. Sir Derrick Dunlop was the chairman of the CSD and Dr. Bill Inman, the author of the book, "*Don't Tell the Patient*", was associated with the committee right from its beginning. The "yellow card system" was started by the CSD in 1964. It was Bill Inman who introduced the concept of Adverse Reactions Profile in CSD system in 1964. The Medicine Act was implemented in the UK in 1968. With all these developments, the 1960s marked the beginning of the discipline of pharmacoepidemiology. **Table 1** gives the names of selected drugs that were withdrawn from the market due to the establishment of serious ADRs.

Table 2.1 List of selected drugs withdrawn from market due to ADR

Drug name	Withdrawn	Country	Remarks
Thenalidine	1960	Canada, UK, US	Neutropenia
Thalidomide	1961	Germany and many other countries	Because of risk of teratogenicity.
Triparanol	1962	France, US	Cataracts, alopecia, ichthyosis.
Bunamiodyl	1963	Canada, UK, US	Nephropathy.
Dantron	1963	Canada, UK, US	Genotoxicity.
Ethyl carbamate	1963	Canada, UK, US,	Carcinogenicity.
Benziodarone	1964	France, UK	Jaundice.
Butamben (Efocaine) (Butoforme)	1964	US	Dermatologic toxicity; psychiatric Reactions.
Xenazoic acid	1965	France	Hepatotoxicity.
Ibufenac	1968	UK	Hepatotoxicity, jaundice.
Chlorphentermine	1969	Germany	Cardiovascular Toxicity.
Diethylstilbestrol	1970s		Risk of teratogenicity.
Clioquinol	1973	France, Germany, UK, US	Neurotoxicity.
Nialamide	1974	UK, US	Hepatotoxicity.
Dipyrone(Metamizole)	1975	UK, US, Others	Agranulocytosis, anaphylactic reactions.
Phenacetin	1975	Canada	An ingredient in "A.P.C." tablet; withdrawn because of risk of cancer and kidney disease. Germany Denmark, UK, US, others Reason: nephropathy.

Table 2.1 ***Contd...***

Drug name	Withdrawn	Country	Remarks
Phenformin and Buformin	1977	France, Germany, US	Severe lactic acidosis.
Buformin	1978	Germany	Metabolic toxicity.
Alclofenac	1979	UK	Vasculitis, Rash.
Ticrynafen (Tienilic acid)	1980	Germany, France, UK, US others	Liver toxicity and death.
Benoxaprofen	1982	Germany, Spain, UK, US	Liver and kidney failure; gastrointestinal bleeding; ulcers.
Clomacron	1982	UK	Hepatotoxicity.
Isoxicam	1983	France, Germany, Spain, others	Stevens johns syndrome.
Propanidid	1983	UK	Allergy.
Zimelidine	1983	Worldwide	Risk of Guillain-Barré syndrome, hypersensitivity reaction, hepatotoxicity banned worldwide.
Methaqualone	1984	South Africa (1971), India (1984), United Nations (1971-1988)	Withdrawn because of risk of addiction and overdose.
Nitrefazole	1984)	Germany	Hepatic and hematologic toxicity.
Oxyphenbutazone	1984-1985	UK, US, Germany, France, Canada	Bone marrow suppression, Steven Johnson Syndrome.
Cianidanol	1985	France, Germany, Spain, Sweden	Hemolytic Anemia.
Phenylbutazone	1985	Germany toxicity.	Off-label abuse, hematologic
Suloctidyl	1985	Germany, France, Spain	Hepatotoxicity.
Nomifensine	1981-1986	France, Germany, Spain, UK, US, others	Hemolytic Anemia, hepatotoxicity, serious hypersensitive reactions.
Prenylamine	1988	Canada,France, Germany, UK, US, others	Cardiac arrhythmia and death.
Sulfacarbamide	1988	Germany	Dermatologic, hematologic and hepatic reactions.
Proglumide	1989	Germany	Respiratory reaction.
Dilevalol	1990	UK	Hepatotoxicity.

Table 2.1 *Contd...*

Drug name	Withdrawn	Country	Remarks
Terodiline (Micturin)	1991	Germany, UK, Spain, others	Prolonged QT interval, ventricular tachycardia and arrhythmia.
Ketorolac	1993	France, Germany, others	Hemorrhage, renal Failure.
Remoxipride	1993	UK, others	Aplastic anemia.
Alpidem (Ananxyl)	1995	Worldwide	Not approved in the US, withdrawn in France in 1994 and the rest of the market in 1995 because of rare but serious hepatotoxicity.
Chlormezanone (Trancopal)	1996 Japan	European Union, US, South Africa, ecrolysis.	Hepatotoxicity; Steven-Johnson Syndrome; Toxic Epidermal N
Fenfluramine	1997	European Union, UK, US, India, South Africa, others	Cardiac valvular disease, pulmonary hypertension, cardiac fibrosis.
Phenolphthalein	1997	US	Carcinogenicity.
Terfenadine (Seldane, Triludan)	1997-1998	France, South Africa, Oman, others, US	Prolonged QT interval; ventricular tachycardia
Bromfenac	1998	US	Severe hepatitis and liver failure (some requiring transplantation).
Ebrotidine	1998	Spain	Hepatotoxicity.
Sertindole	1998	European Union	Arrhythmia and sudden cardiac death
Tolcapone (Tasmar)	1998	European Union, Canada, Australia	Hepatotoxicity
Aminopyrine	1999	France, Thailand	Risk of agranulocytosis; severe acne.
Astemizole (Hismanal)	1999	US, Malaysia, Multiple Non-specified Markets	Fatal arrhythmia
Grepafloxacin (Raxar)	1999	Withdrawn from Germany,UK, US others	Cardiac repolarization; QT interval prolongation.
Alosetron (Lotronex)	2000	US	Serious gastrointestinal adverse events; ischemic colitis; severe constipation. Reintroduced 2002 on a restricted basis.

Table 2.1 ***Contd...***

Drug name	Withdrawn	Country	Remarks
Cisapride (Propulsid)	2000	US	Risk of fatal cardiac arrhythmias
Troglitazone (Rezulin)	2000	US, Germany	Hepatotoxicity
Trovafloxacin (Trovan)	1999-2001	European Union, US	Withdrawn because of risk of liver failure
Ardeparin (Normiflo)	2001	US	Not for reasons of safety or efficacy.
Cerivastatin (Baycol, Lipobay)	2001	US	Risk of rhabdomyolysis
Sparfloxacin	2001	US phototoxicity.	QT prolongation and
Kava Kava	2002	Germany	Hepatotoxicity.
Levomethadyl acetate	2003	US	Cardiac arrhythmias and cardiac arrest.
Rofecoxib (Vioxx)	2004	US	Risk of myocardial infarction and stroke
Valdecoxib (Bextra)	2004	US	Risk of heart attack and stroke
Thioridazine (Melleril)	2005	Germany, UK	Withdrawn worldwide due to severe cardiac arrhythmias
Gatifloxacin	2006	US	Increased risk of dysglycemia.
Ximelagatran (Exanta)	2006	Germany	Hepatotoxicity
Clobutinol	2007	Germany	Ventricular arrhythmia, QT-prolongation.
Aprotinin (Trasylol)	2008	US	Increased risk of death
Rimonabant (Acomplia)	2008	Worldwide	Risk of severe depression and suicide.
Propoxyphene (Darvocet/Darvon)	2010	Worldwide	Increased risk of heart attacks and stroke.
Rosiglitazone (Avandia)	2010	Europe	Risk of heart attacks and death. This drug continues to be available in the US
Sitaxentan	2010	Germany	Hepatotoxicity.
Tetrazepam	2013	European Union	Serious cutaneous reactions.
Oxyphenisatin (Phenisatin)		Australia, France, Germany, UK, US	Hepatotoxicity.

It may also be noted that the Clinical Pharmacy as a super specialty of Hospital Pharmacy originated in USA during the 1930s and 40s which culminated in the starting of the worlds first doctor of pharmacy (Pharm D) program in pharmacy education in 1950 at University of Southern California (USC) followed by University of California at San Francisco in 1955. Various clinical pharmacy programs at BS/ B.Pharm and MS/M.Pharm levels were also introduced in USA in the 1950s and 60s and such programs necessitated the involvement of pharmacists in various studies related to prescriptions, medicine usage and medication errors.

Parallel to the developments in Pharmacy Practice and education in US, Clinical Pharmacology was evolved in the medical education and research as a super specialty of medical Pharmacology which was adopted by pharmacy and nursing education in some countries. All such developments contributed for the development and evolvement of Pharmacoepidemiology as an independent study area in the 1960s and started establishing in the 70s and popularizing in the 1980s throughout the world with the support of programs like International Conference on Pharmacoepidemiology.

International Society for Pharmacoepidemiology

The International Society for Pharmacoepidemiology (ISPE) was launched officially by Stanley A. Edlavitch, David E. Lilienfeld, and Hugh A. Tilson in 1989 during the Fifth International Conference on Pharmacoepidemiology (ICPE) in Minneapolis in USA. The ISPE is a professional non-profit international organization dedicated to advancing the health of the public. ISPE is committed to provide an unbiased scientific forum to the views and opinions of all parties with interests in drug development, drug delivery, drug use, drug costs, and drug effects. It provides a forum for the exchange of scientific information and the development of education policies in the field of pharmacoepidemiology taking up activities related to pharmacovigilance, drug utilization research, outcomes research, comparative effectiveness research, and therapeutic risk management.

Many experts in drug safety and pharmacovigilance have served as its Presidents, and its Officers and Trustees since 1991. Members of the Society come from over 50 countries including India who are mostly from academia, industry, clinical research organisations and government agencies like FDA. The official journal of the society is *Pharmacoepidemiology and Drug Safety* which is indexed in ' Medline'. The newsletter *Scribe* is available on the website of ISPE. Another organisation named 'International Society for Pharmacoeconomics and Outcomes Research' (ISPOR) take up activities related to outcomes research epidemiology.

Some prestigious Universities **(See Box 2.1)** in the world are associated with the International Society for Pharmacoepidemiology for promoting research, education and consultancy in the area of Pharmacoepidemiology.

Box 2.1 Some of the leading Universities or schools in the world engaged in specialised education and research in Pharmacoepidemiology

Center for Drug Safety & Effectiveness, Department of Epidemiology, Johns Hopkins School of Public Health

Center for Drug Safety & Pharmaceutical Health Services Research Graduate Program, University of Maryland School of Pharmacy

Center for Pharmacoepidemiology Research and Training (CPeRT), Perelman School of Medicine at the University of Pennsylvania

Department of Pharmaceutical Outcomes & Policy, College of Pharmacy, University of Florida

Division of Pharmacoepidemiology & Pharmacoeconomics, Brigham and Women's Hospital & Harvard Medical School

Drug Safety Research Unit, Associated Department, School of Pharmacy, Portsmouth University

Harvard School of Public Health

London School of Hygiene and Tropical Medicine

McGill Pharmacoepidemiology Research Unit, McGill University

Pharmacoepidemiology Program, Department of Epidemiology, Gillings School of Global Public Health, University of North Carolina at Chapel Hill

Russian National Society of Evidence-Based Pharmacotherapy

Rutgers, The State University of New Jersey.

The members of ISPE represent various scientific disciplines like the pharmaceutical industry, academic institutions, government agencies, private organizations etc., engaged in areas of drug related aspects. ISPE members have degrees in a number of fields, including epidemiology, biostatistics, medicine, nursing, pharmacology, pharmacy, law, health economics, and journalism. With members in more than 50 countries and national chapters in countries like Argentina, Belgium, Denmark, and the Netherlands, ISPE provides an international forum for sharing knowledge and scientific approaches to foster the science of pharmacoepidemiology. It also sponsors conferences and seminars. Students of Pharmacy and Pharmacy Practice can start student chapters in their institutions in India with the help of senior faculty member who are eligible and financially capable to become its members or Fellows. The details of the membership and other activities of ISPE can be obtained from its web site http://www.pharmacoepi.org/. In 1996, ISPE developed Good Epidemic Practices for Drug, Devices and Vaccine Research in USA and updated the same in 1998.

Role of Strom in Popularizing Pharmacoeconomics

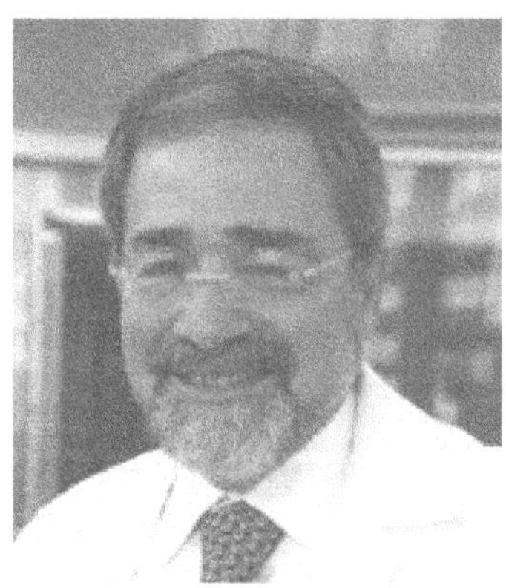

Brian L Strom, Philadelphia, USA has contributed very much for the development, popularization and promotion of pharmacoepidemiology in the world. His Text books and reference books on the subject of Pharmacoepidemiology are exhaustive, illustrative and authoritative for the students, researchers and teachers on all aspects of the subject.

B.L Strom has taken his B.S. degree (Molecular Biophysics and Biochemistry) from Yale University in 1971, M.D (Medicine) from Johns Hopkins University in 1975 and M.P.H (Epidemiology) from University of California, Berkeley in 1980. In 1985 he became Elected Fellow of American College of Epidemiology and in 2003 became Elected Fellow of International Society of Pharmacoepidemiology.

In 1995 B L Strom became the Director, Division of Epidemiology, Department of Biostatistics and Epidemiology of University of Pennsylvania and in 2012 took the charge as Executive Vice Dean for Institutional affairs at Perelman School of Medicine, University of Pennsylvania. He is serving as editorial consultant and referee of more than 30 international journals. He serves as a consultant in pharmacoepidemiology to many large pharmaceutical corporations and many governmental bodies at global level. Currently Brian L Strom is Emeritus Professor of Biostatistics and Epidemiology at Philadelphia.

Pharmacoepidemiology is the application of epidemiological methodologies for the study of drugs focusing on their use and effects in a large number of people. It is drug epidemiology.

CHAPTER 3

Need and Applications of Pharmacoepidemiology

Chapter Mission

After learning this chapter you may be able to know:

- Need of pharmacoepidemiology in India.
- Aims and applications of pharmacoepidemiology in health care and pharmacy practice in India.

Need of Pharmacoepidemiology

The volume, potency and complexity of modern medicines are increasing. Knowledge of the benefits and risks of medicine use in human population is essential to make the practice of pharmacotherapy safe and effective. There is a paramount need to compare the therapeutic efficacy (benefits) of medicines with their potential to cause harm (risks). However, our understanding about the efficacy, safety and risks of the medicines relies heavily on the studies conducted during the developmental process and approval of the drug product.

Only after the drug product is introduced for marketing, will it be used widely by the people. Such a wide use will help to identify many additional risks and sometimes some additional benefits. These risks and benefits may range from minor or trivial to major or serious effects.

When new drugs are approved by the licensing authorities and introduced into the market, they are having only limited safety study information with them. Less than five thousand humans, often between 3000 and 4000, may have been exposed to the drug. Serious adverse reactions occurring less frequently, may be difficult to identify through such studies. Post marketing safety mainly relies on spontaneous reporting of adverse reactions. Such reporting is often incomplete also. Observational epidemiological studies can be used to investigate drug risk hypotheses, but they are expensive, time consuming and dangerous if the hypothesis is correct.

If we analyze the history of drug regulations in the world, we can see that most of them have a connection with some adverse drug reaction "disasters". In 1996, a relation between appetite suppressant drugs and the risks of primary pulmonary hypertension was reported (Abenhaim L, 1996). In 1997 another report came out showing the relationship between the use of anorectic agents (appetite depressants for purpose of weight loss) dexfenfluramine and fenfluramine and valvular heart disease. Fenfluramine was introduced in the US market in 1973 as Pondimin and dexfenfluramine (marketed under the name Redux) was approved by FDA in 1996. Both dexfenfluramine and fenfluramine were withdrawn by the US FDA in 1997. The manufacturers later agreed to withdraw the products worldwide.

Troglitazone, an oral anti-hyperglycemic agent was introduced in United States in 1997 for treatment of type 2 diabetes as Rezulin. It was soon marketed in other countries as Resulin and Rezulin. After the introduction into the open market, cases of liver toxicity were reported from various centers. The drug was withdrawn from the US market because of its hepatocellular injury in 2000. Afterwards it was pulled out in other global markets.

Carisoprodol was developed in the late 1950s and marketed under the brand names Soma and Vanadom. It was first marketed as a centrally acting muscle relaxant for muscle pain, lower back pain, tension, headache, spondilosis and rheumatoid arthritis. This drug having a market standing for more than 45 years was recommended for suspension of all its uses in Europe by the European Medicines Association in November 2007 based on the adverse reactions identified through pharmaco-epidemiological studies. (Revikumar K G 2009).

These are only some examples of serious adverse effects discovered after the drugs were put to wide use. Some other examples are also cited in other chapters of this book. The adverse effects on human fetus can be estimated only through observational methods, not through experimental methods. Such cases help us to remind about the inherent limitations of the drug development process and the need to study populations receiving medications through routine prescriptions of doctors. A concise list of drugs withdrawn after marketing and the reasons are listed earlier in Table 2.1 of Chapter 2 of this book.

Pharmacoepidemiological studies provide certain effective approaches to the evaluation of drug effects. They are non-experimental or observational studies and can be retrospective also which helps to take advantage of various available sources of data. In the pre-clinical studies populations like children, old aged, and pregnant are not included and a single indication is investigated.

Who are in need of Pharmacoepidemiology?

If pharmacoepidemiology is considered as a science of understanding of medicine safety issues, and not as a science of manipulation, it can serve the ailing humanity in many ways. All those who use, prescribe, study, monitor or deal with medicines at academic, research or regulatory levels need pharmacoepidemiology.

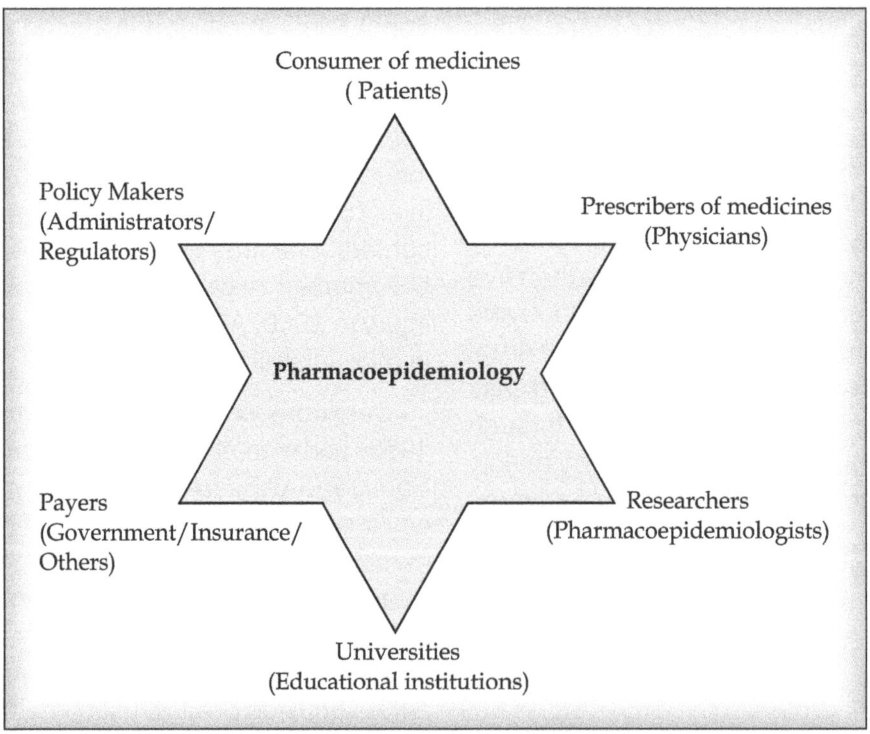

Aims and Applications of Pharmacoepidemiology

Aims of Pharmacoepidemiology

Pharmacoepidemiology as a discipline in health care gives significant information about the safety, efficacy, and cost estimates of medicines and related items used in patient care after their approval for clinical use. Pharmacoepidemiology is the application of epidemiological methodologies for the study of drugs focusing on their use and effects on a large number of people. The pharmacoepidemiological studies concentrate on the period after the drug enters the market known as post marketing surveillance (PMS) period. Pharmacoepidemiological studies are concerned with two main aspects:

(i) the study of adverse effects of drugs

(ii) the appropriate use of medicines.

Signal Generation

The terms 'signal', 'signal generator' and 'signal detector' are widely used in electronics for many years. It was coined in ADR reporting and Pharmacovigilance in recent times with the evolvement of ADR monitoring system at global level with the support of WHO. It is used as an early warning sign in the case of ADRs.

Signal is a reported information on a possible causal relationship between an adverse event and a drug or medicine provided such a relationship was either not known or not recorded previously. Signal generation often helps to identify new or severe type of ADRs. It can also help to identify new applications for existing drugs. Aspirin was first indicated for pain and inflammation. When it was found through case reports that its use can cause thinning of blood delaying clotting time helped to identify uses in cardiac diseases. Today low dose aspirin is used as a cardio protective throughout the world. Another example is Minoxidil which was originally used as a drug for hypertension. Signals generated out of its use found that it can cause hypertrichosis in women. Analysis of the signal and further studies led to the use of Minoxidil to stimulate hair growth and is found useful in cases hair loss after chemotherapy or radiation therapy.

In Pharmacovigilance signals are often generated when reports or informations are obtained from reliable sources. Spontaneous Reporting is the most widely used method in generating signals in pharmacovigilance. Other methods like prescription event monitoring, case control surveillance, follow up studies, automated data resources etc., are also used in generating signals. We had seen that Pharmacoepidemiology is an effective tool in generating signals useful for the identification of ADRs in Pharmacovigilance.

Spontaneous Reporting System

Spontaneous reporting system (SRS) an important aspect of Pharmacovigilance. We know that an important purpose of pharmacoepidemiology is drug safety. Hence there is a close relationship between spontaneous reporting and pharmacoepidemiology. Spontaneous Reporting System is one of the most popular methods for signal identification and ADR reporting. A spontaneous report is an unsolicited, voluntary, communication from the side of users of medicine (patients) or health care professionals who happen to be known or informed about the adverse event of a drug. Experts are of opinion that 'Individual Case Safety Report' is more appropriate than 'Spontaneous Report', though the latter is more popular. The emphasis of spontaneous reporting is on identification of new findings, but often encourages reporting any reactions suspected to be an ADR. It helps for promoting a culture for reporting useful pharmacovigilance studies.

Risk Quantification

Risk quantification is the process of evaluating the risks that have been identified and developing the data for other purposes like making decisions on other occasions. If it is certain that an event cannot occur, it is given a probability of '0' and if it is certain that it will occur, it is given a probability of '1'. Uncertain risks are assigned between 0 and 1. Maximum risk at maximum uncertainty occurs when its probability is 0.5.

Various measures of risk are used in pharmacoepidemiology to quantify the probability of experiencing an adverse outcome and capture the relative increases in risk between treated and untreated populations. Cumulative incidence, incidence rate, absolute risk reduction, relative risk, odds ratio, incidence rate ratio, and time to event outcomes are examples.

Risk quantification of ADR rates generally require a large sample size. If an adverse event occurs in one of every five thousand population (1/5000), that may require 15000 (three times of five thousand) people to ensure 95% certain that the sample would include one case. Even that one case may not be exhibited with clinically significant sign of severity. But pharmaco-epidemiological methods can be applied in such cases.

Hypothesis Testing

A statistical hypothesis is a hypothesis that is testable on the basis of observing a process that is modelled via a set of random variables. A statistical hypothesis test is a method of statistical inference. Hypothesis testing is the use of statistics to determine the probability that a given hypothesis is true. The usual process of hypothesis testing consists of four steps

1. Formulate the 'Null Hypothesis' H_0 (commonly, that the observations are the result of pure chance) and the 'Alternative Hypothesis' H_a (commonly, that the observations show a real effect combined with a component of chance variation).
2. Identify a Test Statistic that can be used to assess the truth of the Null Hypothesis.
3. Compute the P-value, which is the probability that a test statistic at least as significant as the one observed would be obtained assuming that the Null Hypothesis were true. The smaller the P- value, the stronger the evidence against the Null Hypothesis.

4. Compare the P-value to an acceptable significance value α (sometimes called an Alpha Value). If $p < \alpha$, that the observed effect is statistically significant, the null hypothesis is ruled out, and the alternative hypothesis is valid.

In Pharmacoepidemiology Hypothesis testing involves the use of comparison groups of population to find out whether there are differences variables like drug characteristics, risk factors, adverse events, clinical effects etc. With the support of statistical methods it can be found whether the noted or observed variations could have occurred by chance or not. The relationship between exposure to a drug and the clinical outcome (event) can be endorsed or rejected based on the ability to reject or accept the Null Hypothesis.

Applications of Pharmacoepidemiology

Pharmacoepidemiology is having a number of applications in health care and drug therapy as it provides both qualitative and quantitative information about medicines. The information can be grouped into categories like Descriptive Data and Analytical Data. The findings of pharmacoepidemiology helps to generate a bank of information that can improve therapeutic decisions. Hence pharmacoepidemiology can influence policy decisions and administrative activities in health care.

Post Marketing Surveillance

All drugs have adverse effects either to a limited or to a large extent. Pharmacoepidemiological studies cannot prevent them, but surely help to identify or detect them in an early stage. They permit better evaluation of the risk benefit assessment of any particular drug. Pharmacoepidemiological studies have many advantages over the pre-marketing studies. The principles of Pharmacoepidemiology would help to ensure safety of drug use at all levels and its major application is after drug marketing which is known as post marketing surveillance (PMS) of drugs.

Post marketing surveillance (PMS) (also known as post market surveillance) is the practice of monitoring the safety of a pharmaceutical drug or medical device after it has been released on the market and is an important part of the science of pharmacovigilance. Other important post marketing surveillance components include unapproved or off-label drug use, problems with orphan drugs, and lack of paediatric formulations, as well as issues concerning international clinical trials in paediatric population A PMS system ideally must be able to detect a rare event, determine its incidence, and validate the causality.

New Drugs are approved on the basis of data generated based on clinical trials. Clinical trials involve relatively small numbers of people who have been selected for that purpose. The people selected for clinical trials are normally not having other medical conditions which may exist in the general population. Post marketing surveillance can confirm or deny the safety of a drug after it is used in the general population by large numbers of people who have a wide variety of medical conditions.

Post marketing surveillance uses a number of approaches to monitor the safety of licensed drugs, including spontaneous reporting databases, prescription event monitoring, health records (both electronic and other wise), patient registers and case sheets, and data link with health databases.

Post marketing surveillance will continue to benefit from spontaneous reporting of ADEs by clinicians (like literature reports, reports to manufacturers and national regulatory agencies) to detect rare events and will be complemented by the selective use of formal PMS methods in appropriate circumstances.

In United States, Post marketing surveillance is overseen by the Food and Drug Administration (FDA), which operates a system of passive surveillance called MedWatch. Health professionals or the general public can voluntarily report adverse reactions of drugs to MedWatch. FDA also conducts active surveillance of certain regulated products. FDA may monitor safety and effectiveness of medical devices through either a Post-Approval Study, or through a Post market Surveillance Study.

Health Canada is the regulatory body of Canada which approves drugs, and it has a division called "Marketed Health Products Directorate" (MHPD) which coordinates Canadian post marketing surveillance. In European Union a manufacturer of medical devices is required to report incidents (serious adverse events) to the national competent authority of the member state the company resides in.

In United Kingdom The Medicines and Healthcare Products Regulatory Agency (MHRA) and the Commission on Human Medicines (CHM) jointly operate the Yellow Card Scheme for post marketing surveillance. It is to noted that Yellow card scheme is one of the first projects in the world aimed at reducing ADRs.

Pharmacoepidemiological studies are useful in providing information about the beneficial and harmful effects of a drug. In recent years the area of application of pharmacoepidemiology has broadened extensively and is used in performing the clinical trials of drugs. The pharmacoepidemiology got its focus of inquiry from clinical pharmacology and the methods of inquiry from epidemiology.

Pharmacoepidemiology can contribute for supplementing the information available from pre-marketing studies. It will help for better quantization of the incidence of known adverse and beneficial effects. After marketing, non-experimental epidemiological studies can be performed evaluating the effects of drugs administered as part of the ongoing medical care. Pre-marketing studies are generally more artificial in nature. Many important sub groups are not included for ethical reasons in the pre-marketing studies. Pharmacoepidemiological studies help to establish the effectiveness of the medicine in the real practical settings.

Pharmacoepidemiological studies can cover patient groups like elderly, children and pregnant women who are not usually included in the pre-marketing studies. They will help to understand the effect of drugs on special groups like children, pregnant women etc. In pre-marketing clinical studies, for statistical efficacy, subjects who are as homogenous as possible are selected and patients with other illness or who are using other drugs are excluded. The drug under study is not studied as modified by other drugs and illnesses in such studies. Similarly in pre-marketing studies, there is no scope for study of the drug in relation to other drugs used for the same indication. All such issues can be attended in pharmacoepidemiological studies.

The pre-marketing studies will not help to detect uncommon and delayed types of adverse and beneficial effects, but pharmacoepidemiological studies will help to detect them. The pharmacoepidemiological studies also help to identify the drug utilization pattern and the effects of drug overdoses. The economic implications of the drug use are not studied in the pre-marketing studies but are covered in the pharmacoepidemiological studies. For getting approval for a drug, the manufacturer has to evaluate the overall safety and efficacy, but need not evaluate its safety and efficacy in relation to other drugs available for the same indication.

Through the pharmacoepidemiological studies there will be a re-assurance of the drug safety and compliance of ethical and legal obligations (Storm BL 2000). In pharmacoepidemiological studies, conclusions are based on comparisons and observations and are oriented towards groups / populations. Events are described based on time, place and person. The results of pharmacoepidemiological studies will useful for industry, academia and public health. It can minimize adverse effects of medicines to the society and improve the use of drugs that have genuine and safe uses.

Efficacy and Effectiveness

Efficacy and effectiveness are two terms widely used in clinical studies including pharmacoepidemiology. Whether or not a drug achieves its desired effect is referred to as its effectiveness, not efficacy. What is the difference between efficacy and effectiveness? Fletcher and associates suggested a distinction between the two terms based on two questions. Does the treatment work? – "efficacy". Does the benefits of the treatment outweighs its liabilities for those to whom it is offered for treatment?- "effectiveness" (Fletcher RH 1996).

In an efficacy study, patients (population) are selected using narrowly defined eligibility criteria and are monitored closely for compliance as defined in the study protocol. In normal clinical practice, patients are not selected, and the manner in which they use the drug may vary considerably from the intended use for which it was approved. Many factors can affect the patient compliance. It has been reported that clinical outcome is better among patients in RCT than in normal trials patients (Fayers PM 1997). Trials to evaluate therapeutic effectiveness in clinical practice are difficult and expensive for researchers.

Studies of drug effectiveness are mostly conducted with the help of observational study designs, although the RCTs play a significant role in determining drug effectiveness. Results from an RCT offer the best evidence that a drug will be effective under ideal conditions. It is likely that the well controlled designs of RCT will continue to be required for new drug applications (NDA) to the Drugs Control authority for license and / approval. But the circumstances related to the design and implementation of an RCT do not necessarily extrapolate to the individual patient.

Positive and Negative Outcomes

Positive outcomes of drug use refers to the efficacy and effectiveness of the drug used. Efficacy can be studied through RCTs and the effectiveness through pharmaco-epidemiological studies. Negative outcomes are the damages or the adverse events of the use of the drugs. The adverse events involve a relationship between the drug use and the resultant negative outcome, but the causation cannot be established. When the causation is established, the adverse event becomes an adverse drug reaction (ADR).

Pharmacovigilance

Monitoring of ADRs are essential factors in any pharmacoepidemiological study. The monitoring of adverse drug reactions will also receive a boost through such pharmacoepidemiological studies. ADR programs that highlight the incidence of ADR and define the risk/ benefit ratio taking account of the pathophysiological variations of patients will be of immense benefit in the long-term usage of drugs. It can also help in preventing or reducing adverse effects resulting from inappropriate, excessive, or therapeutically incompatible drug use.

Drug Usage Analysis

Pharmacoepidemiological studies help to identify the medicine usage pattern in the institution levels or location levels. It will also help to identify over use and under use and non-use of medicines. The study report can serve as a barometer for the future studies and help to predict changes in the usage. Different methods are available to measure drug utilization.

Descriptive data obtained from dug utilisation studies, drug utilisation reviews, drug utilisation evaluations and prescription audits/ analysis are very much useful for promoting rational drug use and framing policies to that effect.

Drug Surveillance

Pharmacoepidemiology is very much useful in promoting Drug Surveillance in all health care set ups. Prescription data available from hospital pharmacies and community pharmacies can be used as an instrument in improving prescribing behaviour. This aspect is discussed in other chapters in detail.

Pharmacoeconomic Analysis

There is always a "Win- Win" relationship between Pharmacoeconomics and Pharmacoepidemiology. Both were evolved during the same period. If Epidemiologists played a key role in the development of Pharmacoepidemiology, the Clinical Pharmacists and Health Economists joined hand to evolve Pharmacoeconomics. If Pharmacoepidemiology focus on safety and economy of drug use, Pharmacoeconomics focus on economy and safety drug therapy. Data from Pharmacoepidemiology can be used to measure the effects of drugs on overall health cost and the resource consumption. Moderate and serious adverse drug reactions often necessitate hospital admission and increase the financial burden and consumption of resources. Quite often they belong to the preventable type of ADRs.

Framing of Health and Drug Policies

Pharmacoepidemiology has an application or use in framing Policies in the area of health care like Medicine Policy, Antibiotic Policy or Health Policy. It helps to identify the issues, merits and demerits of the existing system and it functioning in health care programs. Pharmacoepidemiological studies help the authorities in drafting policies and guidelines by providing evidence related to the existing practice activities and usage of medicines. If the data shows that there is an increased practice of irrational prescriptions among the prescribers, administration and regulatory agencies can take effective steps to reduce it. Data from pharmacoepidemiology help the policy makers to draft policies based on scientific evidence.

Empowering Pharmacogenomic Studies

Pharmacogenomics look after variations in response to drugs at individual levels focussing on their genetic features. Data from Pharmacoepidemiological studies will help to identify the focus areas of pharmacogenomics in the society.

Evaluation of Formulary Systems

With the support of Pharmacoepidemiological studies, we can evaluate the effects of Formularies like Hospital Formulary, State formulary or National Formulary in promoting rational prescription and usage pattern in the country. Formularies play an important role in promoting generic prescriptions cost effective use of medicines.

Evaluation of Hospital Committees

Pharmacoepidemiological studies will help to identify the strengths and weaknesses of the various hospital committees like Drug and Therapeutic Committees (Pharmacy and Therapeutic Committees), Antibiotic Committee, Therapeutic Committee etc., playing an important role in the determination of drug utilization by patients in hospitals. It is useful to study the functioning of such Committees in order to ensure optimal drug utilization.

Drug Information and Patient Counselling

Strengthening the professional pharmacy service activities like *Drug Information* and *Patient Counselling*. The pharmacist can effectively use the data from Pharmacoepidemiology in giving information, advice and education to the patients. Analysis of data from pharmacoepidemiological studies will help to make the pharmacists more competent and powerful in providing their services related to pharmaceutical care and medication safety.

Age based Medicine use and its Analysis

Pharmacoepidemiological studies can produce data related to the use of medicines in various groups like children and geriatric population. It will also help to identify the medicine use in specified age groups. Studies like use of antidiabetic medicines, cholesterol lowering medicines, oral contraceptives etc., can be conducted and the data will be useful in framing health and drug policies.

Other Applications of Pharmacoepidemiology

- Generation of Data bases for other studies, evaluations and analysis.
- Framing of Protocols and Guidelines for usage of medicine including Standard Treatment Guidelines, Identification and quantification of less common adverse effects of medicines
- Evaluation of efficiency and toxicity of drugs in specific patient groups like children, elderly, pregnant and lactating women.
- Pharmacoepidemiological studies like Cohort a and Case Control are useful to identify unanticipated adverse effects of drugs.
- With the help of Cohort / Case Series or Experimental Studies we can conduct studies on anticipated adverse effects of medicines.
- Cohort Studies are useful to identify beneficial effects of drugs.
- Randomised clinical trials will help to identify efficacy of medicines.

Pharmacoepidemiology is the application of epidemiological methodologies for the study of drugs focusing on their use and effects in a large number of people. It is drug epidemiology.

CHAPTER 4

Pharmacoepidemiology in Pharmacy Practice

Chapter Mission

After learning this chapter you may be able to know:

- Scope and potential of pharmacy practice.
- Role of pharmacoepidemiology in pharmacy practice in India.

Pharmacy Practice

Pharmacy practice refers to the area of pharmacy where the practicing professionals namely pharmacists maintain a close face to face contact and relationship with the patients who are the consumers of medicines. The pharmacists engaged in the pharmacy practice area constitute the group of practicing pharmacists. Apart from dispensing medicines to patients they also provide services like drug information, patient counselling, medication therapy management and other aspects of pharmaceutical care to patients and the society with the objective of ensuring medication safety.

Of all the working pharmacists, about 50 percent are in the community set ups (community pharmacies and community based clinical pharmacies) and 30 percent are in the hospital set ups (hospital pharmacies and hospital based clinical pharmacies). It seems that 75 to 85 percent of all working pharmacists in all parts of the world are engaged in the community and hospital pharmacies (on an average 80 percent). This huge majority of working pharmacists constitute the category of practicing pharmacists, representing community, hospital and clinical pharmacy areas of the profession of pharmacy or pharmaceutical sciences. These days highly qualified pharmacists like Pharm.D, B.Pharm, M.Pharm and PhD qualified pharmacists are working in the area of pharmacy practice ensuring pharmaceutical care to the society. Being highly educated and professionally competent, they engage in many aspects of research including pharmacoepidemiology and pharmacoeconomics.

Pharmacy Practice Education in India

Pharmacy Practice oriented specialized educational program was introduced in India by Dr. B.D. Miglani who is known as *father of hospital pharmacy education in India* in 1984 at Delhi University. He could start India's first M.Pharm Hospital Pharmacy program incorporating Community and Clinical Pharmacy aspects at the Delhi College of Pharmacy, Saketh, New Delhi. It was a Government College which later became Delhi Institute of Pharmaceutical Sciences and Research (DIPSAR).

In 1996 CMC Vellore started a post graduate diploma course in Clinical Pharmacy. It was initiated by one of Dr.B.D.Miglani's students and a colleague of the author of this book, Ms. Chandra. She was sent by CMC to UK for training in clinical pharmacy. During those days Ms. Chandra was the chief pharmacist in the hospital pharmacy services of CMC Vellore. In 1997 J.S.S Hospital & College of Pharmacy Mysore started a post graduate Program (M.Pharm) in Pharmacy Practice giving special importance to Clinical Pharmacy with the help of an Australian University.

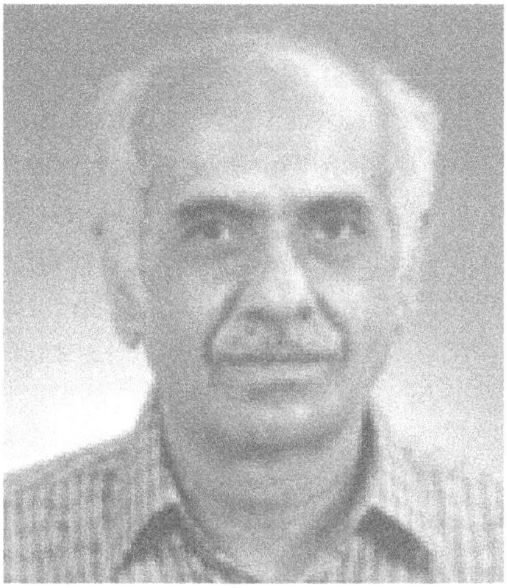

Dr. B.D Miglani

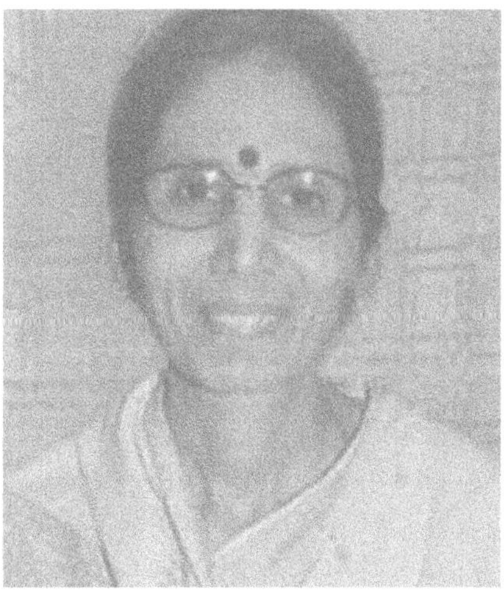

Ms Chandra

Many institutions in India, majority of them being in the south, started post graduate educational program in Pharmacy Practice in the subsequent years. Institutions like K.M.College of Pharmacy, Madurai; Periyar College of Pharmacy, Trichy; SRIPMS, Coimbatore; JSS College of Pharmacy Ooty; Department of Hospital and Clinical Pharmacy, Govt. Medical College, Trivandrum; Annamalai University, Chidambaram, College of Pharmacy, Manipal, KLE's College of Pharmacy, Belgaum; Al-Ameen College of Pharmacy, Bangalore, are examples that started M.Pharm Pharmacy Practice in the late 1990s or early 2000 period in the southern states of India. Institutions like the Hamdard College of Pharmacy, Delhi and National Institute of Pharmaceutical Education and Research (NIPER), Chandigarh also initiated similar program in the northern side of India. Later many Pharmacy Colleges started M.Pharm Pharmacy Practice covering Hospital Pharmacy, Clinical Pharmacy and Community Pharmacy. (Revikumar KG, Miglani BD 2009).

Doctor of Pharmacy (Pharm. D)

The Doctor of Pharmacy degree, abbreviated as Pharm.D. is a professional doctor degree in Pharmacy. It is very much similar to professional degrees like Doctor of Medicine (MD) or Doctor of Dental Surgery (DDS) in USA or equal qualifications in other countries. Today Pharm.D became a global program available in all most all countries in the world. The duration of the program varies from five years (eg. USA, Pakistan) to eight or nine years (eg. Ghana, France) of academic education at the University/ College levels. In some countries like Hungry, Netherland, Portugal etc., it is a post graduate program while in other countries Pharm.D is considered as superior to masters qualification and post graduates are admitted to the program. During the last few years, Pharm.D became popular even in the Middle East countries (Revikumar K G 2014).

The Pharmacy council of India (PCI) introduced six year regular Pharm.D and the three year post baccalaureate Pharm.D in 2008 in the country through a Gazette notification of Government of India dated 16th May 2008. By 2013 the PCI had given approval to over 140 institutions which increased to more than 170 by 2015..

Through the Pharm.D programs the pharmacists are trained to become active and integral members of the patient care team. Increasing emphasis on improving quality of medication use and enhancing medication safety have dramatically increased the demand for clinical pharmacy and the Pharm.D program in all parts of the world. The ward rounds, clinical postings, clerkship and the residency are the core components of the Pharm.D program. It is through this, the students get accustomed to real hospital practice situation and oriented to the evidence based therapy concepts.

Scope of Pharmacoepidemiology in pharmacy practice

The Pharmacoepidemiology falls under the academic and research activities of Pharmacy Practice in pharmaceutical sciences and Clinical Pharmacology in medicine. In the case of Pharmacy Practice, all categories of practicing pharmacists like community pharmacists, hospital pharmacists and clinical pharmacists can conduct or involve in the studies as they are all in direct contact with the patients or consumers of medicines. This advantage is lacking in the case of clinical pharmacologists and certain other categories of professionals. It is to be noted that prior to the popularization of clinical pharmacy and pharmacy practice drug utilization studies were mainly conducted for marketing purposes and were not made available for use by researchers, academicians and health care authorities.

The focus of the study can vary from individual patients to specific groups of patients like diabetic population or epileptic population and can even extend to all patients in a location or area who are using medicines for their ailments. From a single patient researcher or study person can get a specific case report having significant application in the areas of Pharmaco-vigilance or Pharmacogenomics. Similarly we can obtain useful information from the groups- small or large- related to the causes of certain problems or issues related to the use of medicines. Both prospective and retrospective type of studies can be conducted. The information gathered or collected from the population can be analyzed to find the possible causes and other related aspects. Such findings can be applied to other clinical practice situations.

The practicing pharmacists can initiate pharmacoepidemiological studies either independently or jointly with other health care professionals like clinicians or nurses. They can conduct various type of studies like studies of efficacy / effectiveness of individual drugs (positive clinical outcomes), adverse effects / toxic effects (pharma-covigilance) at individual levels or group levels. At the group levels they can study aspects like Drug utilization, prescription analysis, economic evaluations including cost effectiveness and cost benefits. Pharmacoepidemiological studies are integral components of pharmacovigilance studies and pharmacoeconomic studies and are interrelated in certain aspects. Pharmacoepidemiology will also help to quantify certain qualitative aspects of drugs like drug safety, drug toxicity, risks in usage and benefits. As part of Pharmaceutical care community pharmacists and hospital pharmacists including clinical pharmacists can play a vital role in Pharmaco-epidemiological studies and through that process help to develop health policies based on evidence and common sense. Pharmacy Practice professionals and students are capable and competent to carry out the various applications mentioned in **Chapter 3** - Need and Applications of Pharmacoepidemiology.

Pharmacoepidemiology is the application of epidemiological methodologies for the study of drugs focusing on their use and effects in a large number of people. It is drug epidemiology.

CHAPTER 5

Relevance of Pharmacoepidemiology in India

Chapter Mission

After learning this chapter you may be able to know:

- Situation related to drug use in India.
- Limitations of Indian health care.
- Relevance of pharmacoepidemiology in India.

Indian Drug use Situation

India is a country with about hundred and thirty crore (1.30 billion) people spread across 29 states and 7 Union territories with different socio-economic backgrounds. About 70 per cent of population live in rural settings and follow various systems of culture and customs. Though the pharmaceutical industry in India started only in 1900, by 2010 it became one of the leading industry in the world with 4th position in terms of quantity of medicine produced. At the time of independence in 1947, the total production of drugs were worth rupees 10 crores which became one lakh crores by 2015. There are about 20000 manufacturing units and about 8 lakh pharmacy outlets including community and hospital pharmacies.

The people of India utilize various systems of medicine like Modern medicine (Allopathy), Homeopathy, Ayurveda, Siddha, naturopathy etc., which still complicates the matter. In such a scenario, the discipline of pharmacoepidemiology which promises to maintain a close watch over the use of drugs and their effects on people, is of great relevance. In the absence of an effective monitoring and reviewing system, the pharmacological effects of drugs, their adverse effects, interactions and misuse can play havoc with the health system in the country.

We know that in modern times, each person has to take certain medicines at one time or the other in their life period. Often one has to take more than one drug simultaneously, that too for a period of time. The easy availability of drugs in India leads to misuse, irrational use, under use or over use. In many cases, this practice leads to undesired consequences. Aggressive pharmaceutical promotion has led to disease mongering wherein common ailments are turned into medical problems which create huge profits for the industry but an economic burden at individual and community level. Number of drug-related issues and problems such as overuse of antibiotics, analgesics, injectable medicines, increased cost of drug therapy, polypharmacy, medication errors, and adverse drug reactions (ADRs) are prevalent in the healthcare settings of India.

The presence of sound-alike medicines, look-alike medicines, use of brand names for prescription writing of medicines, usage non-accepted abbreviations, improper selection of administration devices etc., are common issues in India. The drug Regulatory agencies in India are under pressure to identify and respond to post approval drug safety issues.

If we analyse the drug situation in the recent decades, it can be seen that many drugs having good market shares, were either withdrawn from the market or banned in India for reasons of adverse effects. Each of these withdrawals was preceded by severe or fatal adverse effects that had been unrecognized or underappreciated at the time of approval and after marketing. Therefore, there is a great need to conduct appropriate pharmacoepidemiological studies that involve multiple regions and in various groups of the population of India, to collect unbiased and reliable information on drug use.

Data obtained from pharmacoepidemiological studies may highlight ways to reduce certain drug-related problems and provide reliable information on the safety profile of drugs. Moreover, clinicians and regulatory authorities can use the data to make drug therapy decisions, drug regulation and policy development. It will help the Drug Control wing in taking decisions regarding marketed drugs at regular intervals.

Prescription Dispensing Situation in India

In many countries drug usage is strictly prescription based, but in India it is yet to be followed in its true spirit. Almost all prescription drugs (scheduled/ legendary drugs) are often freely available over the counter. Prescription filling and registering system is very poor. The Pharmacy Practice Regulations 2015 introduced in early 2015 through a gazette notification of the Government of India is expected to change the situation in the near future.

Drug usage studies in a general population constitute an important aspect of pharmacoepidemiology. It has to be conducted in urban and rural population, at periodic intervals. Once done, it will serve as a barometer for the future health model. Characteristics predicting change in use of prescription and non-prescription drugs over a period of time needs to be considered on a regular basis. Medical professionals and health policy makers whose aim is to improve medication use, require information as to how to integrate strategies and interventions that have been shown to be effective. Analyses of the overall system of events that are implemented to improve medication use are also needed.

Pharmacoepidemiology is useful in providing information about the beneficial and harmful effects of any drug. It permits a better assessment of the risk/benefit balance for the use of any particular patient. Adverse effects of drug products are commonly observed after marketing. Therefore drug surveillance programs are important ways for drug regulatory agencies to keep their fingers on the pulse of adverse drug experiences of countries.

The potential of pharmacoepidemiology for addressing these problems in India is very clear. There should be an organized effort to conduct such studies in various regions of the country. In spite of all the above issues, hardly any major problem with drugs have been identified, registered or recognized in the country! We are forced to believe that it is mainly due to the lack of pharmacoepidemiological studies. In the absence of such studies, issues go un notices.

Key Areas of Drug Therapy

There are certain key areas that need special attention of researchers in the area of pharmacoepidemiology. The surveillance of advanced and controlled drug delivery systems is one of such areas as it is required to monitor the use, efficacy and reliability of these systems in a country like India which is financially strapped. In the Indian context, the economics of drug utilization becomes more and more relevant. Analysis of cost effectiveness, cost benefit and cost utility require special attention. There is a need to incorporate such aspects in pharmacoepidemiological research in India. Pharmacoeconomics has a close association with discipline of pharmaco-epidemiology as it focus on the epidemio-logy of outcomes.

The discipline of pharmacoepidemiology can contribute positively for promoting knowledge and information in the area of medicines. Continuous professional development programs like risk-benefit discussions, prescription behaviour related studies etc., have to be arranged at various levels among health care professionals. India being a country flooded with tens of thousands of medicines, such studies will be of much use, service and utility to the society.

Pharmacoeconomics

Pharmacoeconomics has a close relationship with the field of pharmaco-epidemiology. In the Indian context, the economics of drug utilization becomes even more relevant. Analysis of cost effectiveness, cost benefit and cost utility are gaining importance. Studies on cost of illness is the need of situation in India. Such studies need to be regularly incorporated in pharmacoepidemiological research. It need to be mentioned that the validity of using economic analysis of pharmaceutical sales data as a proxy for prescribing data is being explored in prescribing research.

In this era of information technology, it is important for all health care professionals to keep up with the latest knowledge. This is very true as regards drugs that flood into the market at a rapid pace. However there is acute shortage of computer based data regarding medicine use in India. Researchers have to depend of registers and books for getting the data.

Role of Drug Manufacturers in Pharmacoepidemiology

Pharmaceutical companies are increasingly involved in pharmacoepidemiological studies at global levels. These companies often form alliances with doctors and patient groups and fund studies which exaggerate disease prevalence estimates to show a condition as severe and widespread and requiring treatment. This has been seen in conditions of erectile dysfunction and bipolar disorder in children.

Manufacturers often suppress ADRs of their drug products, while exaggerate ADRs of their competitors. Clinical trials with the involvement of pharmaceutical companies often present the therapeutic benefit of a drug positively and fail to mention risks. Publication of such studies may contribute for promotion of expensive new drugs whose efficacy is overestimated and risks underestimated.

Pharmacoepidemiology provides the best available evidence supporting or refuting a hypothesis, otherwise linking data so that health policy can be written.

In the West, scheduled drug usage is strictly prescription based, they are freely available in India.

Drug Information and Patient Counselling Centers in India

Drug Information centers and Patient Counselling set ups at community and hospital levels are established in all parts of the world for the purpose of ensuring drug safety and promoting prudent use of medicines. They provide wonderful services to educate the patients about the medicines they have to take and empower them for safe and rational use of medicines.

In India the drug information centers originated in the 1960s and the Patient counselling originated in the 1990s. However the service of such centres were limited to certain limited number of hospitals till 2010. After the introduction of PharmD program in 2008, they became popular and the 2015 Pharmacy Practice Regulations make such services essential in Indian community and hospital pharmacy set ups. Studies in the areas of pharmaco-epidemiology and Pharmacoecomics can play an active role in supporting 'medicine information' and patient counselling activities.

Computer based Data Collection and Net-Working

Unlike other developed countries, computerization and its net working is yet to be introduced in health care and related aspects including the drug usage. It is estimated that there are about 8 lakh licensed community and hospital pharmacies in India. Majority of them are not utilizing the potentials of computers in their professional activities. Same is the case with primary health care centers. Insurance in health care is getting popularized during the post 2000 AD period and it is expected that by 2020 about 60 percent of Indian population will have some or other form of health Insurance coverage.

Good Medical Record System

Computers are widely used in India and the achievements of information technology are advantageously used in many areas including railways, telecommunications and a number of service centers. However in the area of health sciences, the situation is very poor and deplorable in the case of drug registries. The researchers have to collect data from the book registers kept in primary care hospitals and pharmacy services at community and hospital levels.

The presence of computerised databases that link the data on the use of medicines and patient medical outcomes are lacking in India. Even there is not networking among major hospitals with respect to medicine use. Researchers have to rely on paper medical records.

One argument for the use of computers in health care registries is that in a country with huge population, people have to use very large amount of medicines. Manual documentation and data analysis become difficult and cumbersome. Pharmaco-epidemiologists in association with software personnel can develop appropriate software programs as tools for pharmaco-therapy audits. Software programs can be used as a means of collecting large amounts of data for a quick, but thorough analysis. This is essential in areas like pharmacoepidemiology since drug usage is constantly changing. Software programs that can determine trends in usage, compliance, areas of misuse, adverse reaction and drug interaction monitoring as well as drug use in specific conditions such as pregnancy, lactation, liver and kidney failure have to be developed. Such systems are in existence in many countries.

Epidemiologic study designs are essential for the evaluation of safety and efficacy of medicines in situations where it is not feasible or is unethical to randomly assign patients to the medicines or placebos. Randomized controlled blinded trial (RCT) is a standard against which other similar study designs are measured, but not suitable for the questions within the discipline of pharmacoepidemiology. Randomized trials cannot contribute for our understanding of the long term or rare adverse effects associated with therapies. Epidemiologic studies of the prescription pattern and drug use are essential to assess the usefulness of a drug (Collett JP 1991).

Computerised Data Management System for Community and Hospital Pharmacies

In a large number of countries there exist systems to register the prescriptions and their dispensing which is monitored by competent authorities. It helps to identify how many prescriptions are dispensed during a period and what are the medicines prescribed and used. However such a system is yet to be implemented in India. Although the hospital pharmacies attached to medium and large hospital use software that provides data on drug use, they keep the information as their private documents. In the case of community pharmacies, majority of them are not using computers for dispensing purposes, though some are using for the business accounting purposes.

Pharmacoepidemiological Guidelines for India

Pharmacoepidemiology is a powerful methodology which will help to assess medicine use related issues like drug safety in various sections of society like paediatric, geriatric and pregnant groups as well as in various groups like people with diabetes, asthma, hypertension etc. Data obtained from pharmacoepidemiological studies can provide information about drug use patterns and ADRs in health institutions and the community. Such processes will promote the rational use of medicines and framing of policies to promote safe and rational use of medicines based on evidence based medicine practices. It also helps to measure the quality of pharmaceutical services at hospital and community levels. The prescriptions can be evaluated and the practices of the prescribers can be studied.

The future of pharmacoepidemiology in India will be determined by the actions taken by experts in the field of Pharmacoepidemiology, Pharmacoeconomics, Clinical Epidemiology and Clinical Pharmacology as well as those interested in the combined subject. A great deal of work needs to be done in the areas of drug toxicity, drug interactions, indigenous drugs, and pharmacogenomics among others. The genetic variations among the population of India are likely to produce more distinct effects than those observed among people involved in the clinical trials in other countries.

The gulf between the rich and the poor is ever widening and many drugs will soon be out of reach for the poor. Studies need to be done to find out cost effective alternatives. Countless other areas in pharmacoepidemiology are waiting for the researchers in India.

Pharmacoepidemiology will help to link exposure and outcome in term of therapeutic gain, length and quality of life or adverse effects for any appropriate sub-groups of population in India in relation to selected drug or drugs. Like other developing countries, India lacks efficient networking between hospitals, and awareness among the general public regarding pharmaco-vigilance. However country has qualified people to look after such aspects.

It is essential that pharmacoepidemiology being a relatively new field in India, a group of experts or those interested come together to formulate guidelines for the set up and follow up of pharmacoepidemiological studies in the country. A group of experts or those interested have to join together and develop suitable guidelines for setting up pharmacoepidemiological studies. The practicing pharmacists, pharmacologists, epidemiologists, bio-statisticians, clinicians of various fields and management personnel related to the drug and medical fields are the important interest groups who can initiate the activities in the country. The guidelines can also incorporate the responsibility of the teams, structures involved in the study, the necessary stages, and the working norms to ensure smooth running from the drafting of the protocol to the final use of the data. Committees for framing guidelines in research in pharmaco-epidemiology have been constituted in other countries even in the 1990s (De Tricornot B 1997).

CHAPTER 6

Data Sources and Data Collection for Pharmacoepidemiological Studies

Chapter Mission

After learning this chapter you may be able to know:

- Health insurance schemes in selected developed countries.
- Health insurance schemes in India.
- Sources of data for pharmacoepidemiological studies.
- Different classes of data.
- Extraction and analysis of data.
- Advantages and limitations of automated data.
- Advantages and disadvantages of Ad hoc data.
- Global Vs Indian scenario of data collection process.

Introduction

In order to understand the sources of data in drug uses (including the computerized network databases) in a country, it is useful to know about the health policies and drug dispensing systems in that country. We can see that during the post 1960s, the concept of health insurance and the networking of health related data including drug uses got popularized in the developed countries and also in some other developing countries.

Since pharmacoepidemiology was originally evolved in USA and got soon popularized in countries like Canada, UK, Sweden, Australia and other developed nations, it is natural that most of the pharmacoepidemiological studies were conducted in such countries. They were naturally analyzing the policies existing in that country. If such data are used for studies in another country where the situation and set ups are totally different, it may be difficult to get correct results.

The health insurance programs and the pharmacovigilance programs of various countries have effectively contributed for data collection for pharmacoepidemiological studies in those countries. In this background we will see how the health insurance system works in selected countries including India and then will go to the data sources for pharmacoepidemiology.

Health Insurance Schemes in the World

Medicaid and Medicare in USA

On July 30, 1965, President Johnson signed the Social Security Amendments of 1965 which established Medicare and Medicaid, promising that they would improve a wide range of health and medical services for Americans of all ages. Under the program, the federal government provides matching funds to states to enable them to provide medical assistance to residents who meet certain eligibility requirements. The objective is to help states provide medical assistance to residents whose incomes and resources are insufficient to meet the costs of necessary medical services. Medicaid serves as the nation's primary source of health insurance coverage for low-income populations.

Medicaid in the US is a social health care program for families and individuals with low income and limited resources. The Health Insurance Association of America describes Medicaid as a "government insurance program for persons of all ages whose income and resources are insufficient to pay for health care". It is jointly funded by the state and federal governments and managed by the states, with each state currently having broad leeway to determine who is eligible for its implementation of the program. Medicaid recipients must be US citizens or legal permanent residents, and may include low-income adults, their children, and people with certain disabilities.

Poverty alone does not necessarily qualify someone for Medicaid. About 50 per cent of American population are covered under the benefit of government owned Medicaid and Medicare program while others are rich enough to have their own coverage.

Omnibus Budget Reconciliation Act 1990 popularly known as OBRA 90 introduced Medicaid Drug Rebate Program and Health Insurance Premium Payment Program (HIPP) as part of the Medicaid and Medicare program in USA in 1990. The Medicaid Drug Rebate Program requires that drug manufacturers shall have a national rebate agreement with the Government represented by its Secretary of the Department of Health and Human Services (HHS) for getting Medicaid coverage for their products. About, 500 pharmaceutical firms participate in the Medicaid Drug Rebate Program.

National Health Services (NHS) IN UK

The National Health Service (NHS) is government funded health care system for UK. It was introduced through the National Health Service Act 1946 which came into existence on 5th July 1948. It is the largest and the oldest single –payer health care system in the world and was launched in 1948. Primarily funded through the general taxation system and overseen by the department of Health., the system provides healthcare to every legal resident in the United Kingdom, with most services free at the point of use. In practice, "free at the point of use" normally means that anyone legitimately fully registered with the system (i.e., in possession of an NHS Number), including UK citizens and legal immigrants, can access the full breadth of critical and non-critical medical care without any out-of-pocket payment. Some services, such as emergency treatment and treatment of infectious diseases are free for everyone, including visitors.

The NHS provides the majority of healthcare in England, including primary care, in-patient care, long term health cares, dentistry and eye care. Some specific NHS services do however require a financial contribution from the patient, for example eye tests, dental care, prescriptions, and aspects of long term care. However, these charges are often free to vulnerable or low income groups, and when not free, often lower than equivalent services provided by private sector.

Private health care has continued parallel to the NHS, paid for largely by private insurance: it is used by about 8% of the population, generally as an add-on to NHS services. During the post 2000 AD period the private sector started to be increasingly used by the NHS to increase capacity, though a section of the public opposed the move.

Healthcare System of CANADA

Health care in Canada is delivered through a government funded public Healthcare System, established through the Canada Health Act of 1984. Most of the services are free at the point of use. Most services are provided by private entities. Canada's health care system is a group of socialized health insurance plans that provides coverage to all Canadian citizens. It is publicly funded and administered on a provincial or territorial basis, within guidelines set by the federal government.

Under the health care system, individual citizens are provided preventative care and medical treatments from primary care physicians as well as access to hospitals, dental surgery and additional medical services. With a few exceptions, all citizens qualify for health coverage regardless of medical history, personal income, or standard of living.

Canada's health care system is the subject of much political controversy and debate in the country. Some question the efficiencies of the current system to deliver treatments in a timely fashion, and advocate adopting a private system similar to the United States. Conversely, there are worries that privatization would lead to inequalities in the health system with only the wealthy being able to afford certain treatments. Regardless of the political debate, Canada does boast one of the highest life expectancies (about 80 years) and lowest infant morality rates of industrialized countries, which many attribute to Canada's health.

Medicare AUSTRALIA

Medicare administered by the federal government of Australia is the publicly funded universal health care system in Australia which was established in 1984. It coexists with a private health system. Medicare is funded partly by a 2% Medicare tax from which the low income and poor sections are exempted. The balance for the Medicare is provided by government from general revenue. An additional tax of 1 percentage is imposed on high-income earners. There is also a separate Pharmaceutical Benefit Scheme in Australia which is also funded by the federal government which considerably subsidises a range of prescription medications.

Health care in Australia is provided by both private and government institutions. The federal Health Ministry is looking after National Health Policy. The state and territory governments administer elements of health care within their jurisdictions, such as the operation of hospitals.

Universal Health Coverage Scheme in JAPAN

Japan introduced Universal Health Coverage program in 1961. It provides all access to preventive, curative and rehabilitative services at an affordable cost. All residents of Japan are required by the law to have health insurance coverage. People without insurance through employers can participate in a national health insurance program administered by local governments. Patients are free to select physicians or facilities of their choice and cannot be denied coverage. Hospitals, by law, must be run as non-profit and be managed by physicians. Business corporations are not allowed to own or operate hospitals. Clinics must be owned and operated by physicians.

Medical fees are strictly regulated by the government to keep them affordable. Depending on the family income and the age of the insured, patients are responsible for paying 10%, 20% or 30% of medical fees with the government paying the remaining fee. Also, monthly thresholds are set for each household, again, depending on income and age, and medical fees exceeding the threshold are waived or reimbursed by the government. Uninsured patients are responsible for paying 100% of their medical fees, but fees are waived for low-income households receiving government subsidy. Fees are also waived for homeless people when they are brought to the hospital by ambulance.

Statutory Health Insurance Plan of GERMANY

Germany has the world's oldest national social health insurance system, with origins dating back to Otto von Bismarck's social legislation, which included the 'Health Insurance Bill of 1883', 'Accident Insurance Bill of 1884' and 'Old Age and Disability Insurance Bill of 1889.' Bismarck stressed the importance of three key principles solidarity, subsidiarity and corporatism. Solidarity means the government is responsible to ensure access by those who are in need. Subsidiarity shows that the policies are implemented without political and administrative influence. Corporatism means the government representative bodies in health care professions deems feasible procedures.

Mandatory health insurance originally applied only to low-income workers and certain government employees, but has gradually expanded to cover the great majority of the population. The system is decentralized with private practice physicians providing ambulatory care, and independent, mostly non-profit hospitals providing the majority of inpatient care.

About 92 percent of the German population is covered by a 'Statutory Health Insurance' plan, which provides a standardized level of coverage through one of their public or private sickness funds. It is estimated that there are over one thousand such funds in the country. Standard insurance is funded by a combination of employee contributions, employer contributions and government subsidies on a scale determined by income level. Higher income workers sometimes choose to pay a tax and opt out of the standard plan, in favour of 'private' insurance. The latter's premiums are not linked to income level but instead to health status. Historically, the level of provider reimbursement for specific services is determined through negotiations between regional physician's associations and sickness funds.

In the 1970s, the government introduced the scheme of an Annual Commission, consisting of representatives of business, labour, physicians, hospitals, and insurance and pharmaceutical industries. The Commission takes into account government policies and makes recommendations to regional associations with respect to overall expenditure targets. In 1986 expenditure caps were implemented and were tied to the age of the local population as well as the overall wage increases. Although reimbursement of providers is on a fee-for-service basis the amount to be reimbursed for each service is determined retrospectively to ensure that spending targets are not exceeded.

Mediclaim in INDIA

Mediclaim policy is a health insurance policy that is designed to take care of one's healthcare expenses up to the sum assured, in case the person faces any sort of medical emergency, be it an illness or an accident that has led to hospitalization. A mediclaim policy in India is issued for a defined time period. Once the renewal date nears, the person needs to pay the premium before the due date so as to continue enjoying its benefits.

Basically there are two types of mediclaim - individual and family floater. Under individual mediclaim policy, only a single person can be covered. The premium to be paid is based on the age of the person, who is being offered with health cover. The insured person can claim the entire sum insured, when needed. Under family floater mediclaim policy, one gets coverage for his or her family as well. The family comprises of self, spouse, dependent children and in some policies even dependent parents. The premium for this type of policy is based upon the family member who has highest age. Furthermore, the entire sum assured can be used by both the entire family jointly or by a single member alone.

Health insurance was launched in India in 1986 and has grown significantly in the subsequent period mainly due to liberalization of economy and general awareness. The first health policies in India were Mediclaim Policies. In 2000 government of India liberalized insurance and allowed private players into the insurance sector.

The advent of private insurers in India saw the introduction of many innovative products like

- Family Floater Health Insurance Plans,
- Senior Citizens Health Insurance Plans
- Health Insurance Top- up Plans
- Critical Illness Insurance Plans.
- Cashless Mediclaim Policies
- Hospital Cash and Top up Policies.
- Group/Corporate Health Insurance Plans.

In the Cashless Mediclaim, health insurance companies tie up with different hospitals after checking quality of their medical services and negotiating rates for different procedures. These hospitals are known as network hospitals and when you get hospitalized in any one of them, you do not have to settle the bill with the hospital. Your insurance company that is represented by TPA (third party administrator) will coordinate and settle the bill with the hospital.

There are standalone health insurers along with government sponsored health insurance providers. But the growth and popularisation of health insurance in the country is slow. The World Bank in the 1990s estimated a health insurance coverage of 25 per cent of population by 2010 and 50 per cent by 2015. However in 2015 it was only 21 per cent of the population got covered under some or other of health insurance in India. A further analysis shows that 14 per cent are covered under government sponsored health insurance schemes, 4 per cent under non-government group cover schemes and 3 percent on individual insurance cover. (Table 6.1)

Table 6.1 Government sponsored health insurance schemes in India

RSBY	Rashtiya Swasthiya Bima Yojana. Introduced in 2001. Covers up to Rs 30,000 INR. Beneficiaries have to pay 30INR while the premium is paid by central and state governments.
ESIS	Employment State Insurance Scheme. It is applicable for the employees of the commercial establishments and for their dependents.
CGHS	Central Government Health Scheme which is applicable for the central government employees and pensioners and their dependents.
AABY	Aam Aadmi Bima Yojana. It is a social security scheme for poor in rural areas and for about 45 occupational employees and their dependents.
UHIS	Universal Health Insurance Scheme for poor families which is implemented by public sector general insurance companies.

Health insurance in India typically pays for only inpatient hospitalization and for treatment at hospitals in India. Outpatient services were not payable under health policies in India. One of the main reasons for the low penetration and coverage of health insurance was the lack of competition in the sector. The Insurance Regulatory Authority of India (IRDA) which is responsible for insurance policies in India is in the process of taking steps to promote health insurance in the country.

Data for Pharmaco-epidemiological Studies

Epidemiological studies include Experimental and Observational studies and Observational studies include both Descriptive and Analytic studies. Descriptive studies estimate the natural history of disease and exposure and Incidence and Prevalence rates are examples of Descriptive epidemiologic data. Inferential studies provide measures of association between exposure and out comes and include measures such as odd ratios, rate ratios or relative risk ratios and hazard ratios.

Pharmacoepidemiology studies involving data analysis use large health care databases to address research questions. Research questions addressed in pharmacoepidemiological studies can be broadly divided into those of drug use (like duration of use of analgesics), drug effects (like development of diabetes among users of certain antihypertensive medicines), and the effects of programmatic efforts to improve drug use (formulary system, generic dispensing, antibiotic policies etc.) .

Sources of Data

Data required to conduct the pharmacoepidemiological studies come from a variety of sources like

(i) Medical Records and Patient registries. They include all data entered by clinicians, hospitals and other health care institutions and include registers like surveillance epidemiology registers and end result registries. It may be available in paper files, register books or computers (including networking)

(ii) Administrative databases. These include data from various medical or health insurance schemes or similar heath care programs existing in the country. It may come in the form of administrative reports or computer data bases.

(iii) Clinical Study data. These include data from ad hoc and regular general studies being carried out. In countries where the regulatory agencies or other bodies supervise the clinical studies and clinical trials through online registries, it is easy to get such data. Otherwise we have to depend on publications and reports.

(iv) Data from large studies including meta-analysis.

Classification of Data

There are two types of data - Primary data and Secondary data. Primary data include data collected prospectively for the purpose of the study. Secondary data are such data that were already collected for some other purpose. Data from prescription dispensing databases or chart reviews (case sheet or prescription reviews) are examples of secondary data.

Primary Data

Primary data are gathered for certain specific objectives or purposes. They are collected prospectively and are also known as *de novo* data. They represent details not previously made available in a consolidated format. The primary data can be collected in different ways like using

Questionnaires,

Conducting interviews

Direct face to face talk

Phone calls

Electronic means like Email, WhatsApp etc.

Primary data are more informative compared to secondary data. If you need information about how people take paracetamol tablets for headache, you can ask that to participate in the study and find the answer. Such information may be difficult to get from secondary data. Often such information may not be available and if available, may be time consuming and expensive to make it from the huge databases. Conducting interviews are also time consuming and expensive. The limitations of using primary data are the high expenses and the time consuming activities for gathering or collecting them.

Secondary Data

Secondary data are pre-existing data collected for some other purposes as in the case of medical records database or medical administrative databases (examples- Medicaid, NHS, etc.) They include data obtained from hospitals or clinics, pharmacies or from other studies like randomized controlled trial (RCT) . The secondary data are easy to get and less expensive compared to primary data and may offer advantages in terms of increased sample size and applicability. Secondary data are useful to study topics like prescription analysis, drug utilization, ADR, drug effects and many other policy issues.

An important de-merit of secondary data is that they are principally collected for some other purposes and typically not for the present purpose or objective. In the case of administrative databases, their owners maintain physical control of data for privacy and security reasons. Academic or research people may find difficult to get them for studies or analysis.

Medical Records

Generally medical record databases are registered or recorded as part of the process of clinical care. Medical record reflect the clinicians view points. In the case of administrative databases medical record information is only a by-product of their financial, economic or other related evaluations. However the information recorded in the two types of databases (medical record or administrative databases) are similar in nature and are dated entries related to prescription drugs and medical diagnoses.

Electronic Medical Records

A number of countries have computer supported national or regional medical records, known as Electronic Medical Records. If administrative databases are created for billing purposes, electronic medical records are created as part of the clinical patient care activities. These type of databases usually contain data entered by general practitioners (GP) into their practice computers and are maintained primarily for documenting the patients' conditions and treatments. Compared to administrative databases, medical records databases include much more detailed information on their patient files.

In US, General Practice Research Database (GPRD) and Mediplus are in existence and clinicians even at the primary care level register the medical records in computer systems. GPRD created in June

1987 as a value added medical products (VAMP) research databank is considered to be the largest medical records database. It is comprehensive in nature and collects information on demographics, medical diagnosis, prescriptions, referrals to hospitals, smoking status, immunization details, weight and height and laboratory details. GPRD is derived from medical records while a number of other medical records in US are derived from pharmacy dispensing records.

In Europe medical records databases, derived from the electronic clinical records maintained by practising physicians and clinicians in the course of providing health care are largely available. The physicians or their office staff register information obtained from the patients including past medical history, life style parameters including alcohol use and smoking history, body mass index, out-patient conditions diagnosed by the general practitioner, hospital admissions including hospital diagnosis, prescribed drugs and procedures performed by them. Where ever computerised registries are maintained for health care activities, authored agencies link, co-ordinate and manage such data bases.

Some medical record databases are also including laboratory results. All information related to medications prescribed are entered in medical records. Prescription drug information usually refers to prescribed drugs rather than those dispensed. Some prescriptions written by doctors or physicians are never filled at the pharmacy. Hence dispensing records may be more closely reflecting actual drug use compared to prescribing records. It is also true that not all doses that are dispensed are actually taken by the patients. Medical records databases being the product of data entered by the primary care physician's office, medications prescribed by specialist physicians may be incomplete in such records.

The Health Improvement Network (THIN) of UK

Created in 2002, THIN is a large electronic medical record (EMR) research database of United Kingdom (UK). Anonymized patient records are downloaded directly from participating general practitioners' (GPs') offices, providing medical information for research purposes. Variables collected include: practice and patient registration details, demographics, including age and sex of patient; medical diagnosis; prescriptions, including repeats; limited notation on events leading to withdrawal of a drug or treatment; referrals to specialists and hospitals; treatment outcomes including hospital discharge reports; smoking status, height, weight, immunizations, and lab results. The data are organized in files by individual practice and provide a longitudinal medical record for each patient. The patient population represented in THIN is broadly representative of the UK population.

PHARMO in Netherlands

PHARMO is an automated pharmacy record data linkage in Netherlands established in the early 1990s. It is a population based data system that includes the drug dispensing records from community pharmacies. The records include information on diagnoses and symptoms, laboratory test results, referrals to specialists and healthcare product/drug prescriptions. The prescription records include information on type of product, date, strength, dosage regimen, quantity and route of administration. Drug prescriptions are coded according to the WHO Anatomical Therapeutic Chemical (ATC) Classification System (WHO Anatomical Therapeutic Chemical Classification System [www.whocc.no]). Diagnoses and symptoms are coded according to the International Classification of Primary Care (ICPC) (International Classification of Primary Care [www.nhg.org]), which can be mapped to ICD codes, but can also be entered as free text. GP data cover a catchment area representing 2.5 million residents.

IMS Health

'IMS Health' is an American company that provides information, services and technology for the health care industry. It is the largest vendor of U.S. physician prescribing data. IMS Health was founded in 1954 by Bill Frohlich and David Dubow. IMS Health Customers include pharmaceutical, consumer health and medical device manufacturers and distributors, providers, payers, government agencies, policymakers, researchers and the financial community.

Medical Records in India

In India we are yet to have a computerised database or Electronic Medical Record system like those available in developed countries. Prescriptions are not registered at the level of clinicians or dispensing pharmacists (community and hospital levels) in a computer system in India. Such databases can generally be obtained from paper files of prescriptions or from hospital medical records in India. The physicians (GP) are not maintaining medical records either as paper files or on computers in their private practices. Though certain individual hospitals and health insurance agencies have their own electronic data bases, it is difficult to obtain them for pharmacoepidemiological studies and analysis as there is no supervising government authority for them in the country.

Even prescription drugs are dispensed without prescriptions in Indian community pharmacies as there is no effective system for the prescription filing and preservation of the data. Computer or internet based, coordinated registry for health care related activities are yet to be established in India.

Many hospitals at public and private set ups have established their own computerised management information systems (MIS) for data registry, but are maintained as their own private documents. The situation at primary health care levels are still deplorable in the country.

Administrative Databases

Administrative data refers to information collected primarily for certain administrative purposes and not for research or study purposes. Administrative purposes include claims for reimbursement from insurance companies and government departments.

Generally government departments and other organisations like insurance firms or professional bodies establish such systems for the purpose of registration, record keeping and other transactions during the delivery of services. The data sets are used to produce official statistics and for policy making. Education and health are the extensive users of this type of data. The administrative data extracts can be linked with other data sources for creating more comprehensive and effective data sets for analysis. For example individual level administrative data can be linked with cross-sectional or longitudinal survey data.

Administrative data collection is the set of activities involved in the collection, processing, storage and dissemination of statistical data from one or more administrative sources. The process of collection of administrative data is very much similar to a data collection through survey. The only difference is that if data is collected on direct contact with respondents in survey, the administrative records are the source for administrative data collection.

Administrative data is generated through the routine administration of the health care program for which the system or scheme was established. Administrative databases are primarily used for payment, accounting, and other fiscal functions related to the provision of patient care. The use of such data for pharmacoepidemiological purposes is a secondary use. An automated administrative data system can manage a large data files and can establish interaction levels for centralised and regional activities. In the US, there are two kinds of healthcare data - clinical data in Electronic Health Records (EHRs) and administrative billing data that is used by payers, researchers, and the government. Billing data is imprecise and lack exactness. But it is a starting point to describe the care given by a doctor or hospital. In US administrative databases record drugs prescribed by any physician, as they are dispensed by pharmacies which are part of the net work. The pharmacies also submit bills to the administrative system. Hospital admissions are recorded automatically in administrative databases.

Routine administrative databases are increasingly being used for performance monitoring in healthcare in various countries. Administrative databases of hospital admissions are increasingly being used, mostly without validation, for epidemiological and clinical outcomes studies. Clinical databases, run by various bodies including professional societies, could potentially record more detailed clinical information and might permit better adjustment for case mix.

Administrative datasets are typically huge and large not otherwise normally (or financially or logistically) achievable through survey methods. The research component is lacking in this method and there may not be well established theory and methods to guide the data collection. The Table 6.2 summarises some of the general advantages and disadvantages of using administrative data.

Table 6. 2 Advantages and disadvantages of administrative data

Advantages of administrative data	Disadvantages of administrative data
Collected for operational purposes. No additional costs of collection. Only expenses for extraction and cleaning.	Information collected is restricted to data required for administrative purposes. Limited to users of services and administrative definitions.
Collection process not intrusive to target population.	Lack of researcher control over content.
Regularly or continuously updated.	Proxy indicators sometimes have to be used.
Can provide historical information and allow consistent time-series to be built up.	May lack contextual /background information.
Often collected in a consistent way.	Changes to administrative procedures could change definitions and make comparison over time problematic.
Subject to rigorous quality checks.	Missing or erroneous data.
Almost r 100% coverage of population interest.	Quality issues with variables less important to the administrator e.g., address details may not be updated.
Reliable at the small area level.	Metadata issues may be lacking or of poor quality.
Counterfactuals and controls can be selected subsequently	Data protection issues.
Captures individuals who may not respond to surveys.	Access for researchers is dependent on support of data providers.

Administrative Databases

While discussing the health insurance schemes in various countries we had seen some of the health insurance companies in certain countries. All those firms have their own automated administrative databases. They are examples of leading databases available for pharmacoepidemiology. We will see some other administrative databases here.

OptumInsight of USA

OptumInsight is clinically-rich healthcare database comprised of billing claims from a US commercially-insured population. Enrolment data, medical claims, and prescription claims are available from 2000 and clinical laboratory results from 2001. The completeness of Optum data allows the investigation of any number of patient, physician, treatment, and clinical attributes.

Geographic diversity, combined with the longitudinal nature of these data and the ability to see treatments in many settings, affords a unique perspective to the researcher. Subjects can be studied longitudinally, as individuals who dis-enrol and re-enrol can be identified. This is considered to be a significant advantage of Optum data over most commercially-available databases that erroneously count multiple enrolments as distinct members.

LHAD of Canada

The number of studies that use secondary data for population health and health services research is rapidly increasing in Canada, as are the variety of data sources being used. For example, Statistics Canada, through its Longitudinal Health and Administrative Data (LHAD) Initiative, links provincial / territorial administrative health databases with national population based health survey, vital events, and cancer registry data to better understand the relationships between the determinants of health and health outcomes. Electronic medical records are used for research and surveillance through initiatives such as the Canadian Primary Care Sentinel Surveillance Network. The Canadian Network of Observational Drug Effect Studies (CNODES), which relies primarily on provincial prescription drug administrative databases for post-marketing surveillance of drug exposures and outcomes, and the 'Canadian Chronic Disease Surveillance System', which uses hospital and physician billing claims databases to produce prevalence and incidence estimates for diabetes and hypertension are examples of secondary data.

Selected Administrative data sources in India are shown in Box 6.6.

Box 6.1 Public Health Insurance Schemes in India

RSBY	Rashtiya Swasthiya Bima Yojana (RSBY) - for beneficiaries enrolled .
ESIS	Employment State Insurance Scheme. (ESIS) - for the employees of the commercial establishments.
CGHS	Central Government Health Scheme (CGHS) - for the central government employees and pensioners.
AABY	Aam Aadmi Bima Yojana (AABY) - for beneficiaries enrolled (working class) .
UHIS	Universal Health Insurance Scheme (UHIS) - for enrolled poor families.

Clinical Study Data

The clinical study data include data from clinical studies including Trials and Bio-availability and Bio-equivalence studies. Though they can be generated from both ad hoc and regular general studies being carried out, most of the clinical data are originated from clinical trials conducted as regular studies with the support of approved protocols and ethical committee clearances. Ad hoc studies are conducted mainly for publication purposes and as pilot studies for general research projects. In countries where the regulatory agencies or other bodies supervise the clinical studies and clinical trials through online registries, it is easy to get such data. Otherwise we have to depend on publications and reports.

Clinical studies including Clinical trials hold enormous potential for benefiting patients, improving therapeutic regimens and ensuring advancement in medical practice that is evidence based. The data and reports of various trials are often difficult to find. People will not publish the data if the study was abandoned. Need has been felt on the imperative for transparency, accountability and accessibility in order to re-establish public trust in clinical trial data, which is feasible only if all clinical trials conducted are registered in a centralized clinical trials registry. Registration of trials will ensure transparency, accountability and accessibility of clinical trials.

Indian Situation with Respect to Clinical Trials

The Clinical Trials Registry- India (CTRI) hosted at the ICMR's National Institute of Medical Statistics (http://nims-icmr.nic.in), is a free and online public record system for registration of clinical trials conducted in India. It was launched in 2007 as a voluntary initiative which became mandatory in June 2009. Editors of certain major Biomedical Journals of India declared that only registered trials would be considered for publication.

Today, any researcher in India, who plans to conduct a trial involving human participants, of any intervention such as drugs, surgical procedures, preventive measures, lifestyle modifications, devices, educational or behavioural treatment, rehabilitation strategies is expected to register the trial in the CTRI before enrolment of the first participant. Trial registration involves public declaration and identification of trial investigators, sponsors, interventions, patient population etc., before the enrolment of the first patient. Trials related to herbals preparations and Ayurveda studies should also be registered with the CTRI.

Submission of Ethics approval and DCGI approval (if applicable) is essential for trial registration in the CTRI. Multi-country trials, where India is a participating country, which have been registered in an international registry, are also expected to be registered in the CTRI. In the CTRI, details of Indian investigators, trial sites, Indian target sample size and date of enrolment are captured. After a trial is registered, trialists are expected to regularly update the trial status or other aspects as the case may be. After a trial is registered, all updates and changes will be recorded and available for public display. Being a Primary Register of the International Clinical Trials Registry Platform (ICTRP) (http://www.who.int/ictrp/search/en/), registered trials are freely searchable both from the WHO's search portal, the ICTRP as well as from the CTRI (www.ctri.nic.in).

Data from Large Studies and Meta-Analysis

Large studies often use computer aided registries and resources from various data bases. Outcomes from a meta-analysis include a more precise estimate of the effect of treatment or risk factor for disease, or other outcomes, than any individual study contributing to the pooled analysis. The benefits of meta-analysis include a consolidated and quantitative review of a large, and often complex, sometimes apparently conflicting, body of literature and data.

Data Analysis

In the case of centralised data warehouse, all those who have access to the data warehouse can conduct analyses. In the case of independent or de-centralised models (distributed model), independent analytical procedures can be conducted which do not require to conform to a common data model. In such distributed model cases, if the data owners publish their date and results independently, they can be combined together at a central coordinating centre for aggregation or meta-analysis.

In the case of data stored in a common data model, either a coordinated or distributed model analytic approach can be used. In such an approach, the common data model is specified and implemented based on a common study protocol. The central study team can create an analytic code based on the protocol and data model which is then distributed to each data owner for execution. Both approaches should include comprehensive data characterisation analyses to evaluate variability across the data partners with respect to overall cohort metrics, such as age and sex distribution, and study-specific metrics, such as exposure and outcome rates by age, sex and year.

Data Extraction

The first step in using multi-purpose database is to extract a specific study population (e.g., all patients over 18 years old with a diagnosis of diabetes) either by request from the data warehouse or by direct access. All predefined study variables for this study population will then be extracted for the final analysis. Much of the investigational work to understand data generation, capture and storage should be carried out prior to developing a data extraction protocol.

Ad hoc Data Sources

Definition and Use of Ad hoc Data Sources

Ad hoc is a Latin term or phrase meaning 'as the occasion requires'. It signifies a specific situation and on the spot of type decisions or solutions to the problem or issue or task under consideration. We come across terms like ad hoc meeting, ad hoc committee, ad hoc commission, ad hoc organisation, ad hoc association, ad hoc research projects etc., in professional and academic/research discussions. Ad hoc represents that it is not actual or planned one and that it may not comply with the required formalities and structure of the actual. Hence ad hoc implies that they are not generalizable and not intended to be adopted for other purposes.

Ad hoc data sources are those specific and particular data sources that are not having a wider, long standing or generalizable application as in the case of planned actual data sources. They are non-standard, semi-structured / non-structured data sources and processing tools (transformation tools) and libraries may not be available to handle them. Ad hoc data refers to a data at hand without consideration for wider planned applications. The data that constitutes a single, abstract source may come from different concrete destinations across the internet. The ad hoc data used to fill the gaps left by the static, regular reporting. Ad hoc analysis may be used to create a report that does not already exist, or drill deeper into a static report to get details about accounts, transactions, or records. The process may be also used to get more current data for the existing areas covered by a static report. Although most ad hoc reports and analyses are meant to be run only once, in practice they often end up being reused and run on a regular basis.

Advantages and Disadvantages of Ad hoc Data

Ad hoc data are used in scientific studies and analysis widely in India as actual planned databases are very much limited in health care in India (Box 6.2).

Box 6.2 Advantages of the Ad hoc data and its sources

1. It is easiest and simplest method.
2. Any one can do it.
3. It does not require proper scheduling or planning.
4. There is only limited work load and need of Information Technology (IT) professionals and related works.
5. Not much training or other orientation programs are needed.
6. Financial expenses are less.
7. Ad hoc reports enable easy and quick analysis and flexible reporting of information and performances.
8. Ad hoc reporting allows end users to dynamically modify and drill through report data for powerful information analysis and build their own reports.
9. Ad hoc reporting allows users to modify existing reports with little or no training.
10. It generated reports that meet individual requirements quickly.

Though there are many advantages for the ad hoc data over the actual planned structured data, there are many disadvantages for ad hoc databases, Some of the important disadvantages are shown in Box 6.3.

Box 6.3 Disadvantages of the Ad hoc data and its sources

1. It is not a pure structured data.
2. Generated for a specific purpose.
3. May not comply with the required formalities and structure of the actual.
4. Not generalizable.
5. Generated for one purpose is used for other distinct purposes repeatedly.
6. Reports should be reviewed periodically for efficiencies to determine whether they continue to be relevant and scientific.

Sources of Ad hoc Data

We know that the pre-clinical studies are conducted on structured manner based on research protocols. However the post marketing studies (discussed in Chapter 9) are often conducted in an ad hoc manner and hence constitute the sources of ad hoc data bases in pharmacoepidemiology.

The following are some of the important sources for ad hoc data.

1. Spontaneous Reporting (Discussed in Chapter 9)
2. Prescription Event Monitoring (Discussed in chapter 9
3. Ad hoc Cohort Studies
4. Ad hoc Case control studies
5. Existing data collected as part of other ad hoc studies.
6. Computerised collections of data from organised medical care programs.

In Chapter 8, while discussing the analytical methods of observational studies we have discussed the Cohort Studies and Case Control studies. Both the methods can be conducted as ad hoc studies. In the case of ad hoc Case Control, cases can be recruited from whatever source is appropriate for that drug event. Hospitals, clinics, outpatient practice centers, houses or offices can be source for data. In **Chapter 11** a case study on ad hoc cohort study was mentioned.

Automated Data Systems

Automated data is a creation and implementation of technology that automatically process data. The technology include computers and other electronic communications that can gather, store, process, prepare and distribute data. The purpose of automated data processing is to quickly and efficiently process large amounts of information with minimum human interaction. Automated or semi-automated data analysis represents an important feature of large-scale public health surveillance systems.

During the last three decades computerised so called automated databases have been increasingly used as a potential data sources for pharmacoepidemiology studies. In the beginning of this Chapter we saw the health insurance schemes of various countries including India. All such agencies are having their own administrative databases which are automated. Various automated data sources are used world-wide for conducting pharmacoepidemiological research. Some of them are shown in the Box 6.4.

Box 6.4 Selected examples of automated global data bases used in pharmacoepidemiology

Group Health Cooperative	-	for HMO members
Health Maintenance Organisation (HMO) Research Network	-	for beneficiaries of member organisations
Medicaid (US)	-	for Low income individuals and family members
United Kingdom General Practice Research Dataset	-	for persons who receive care in general practice settings in the UK
WHO program for international Drug Monitoring	-	for global monitoring.

Developed countries like USA, UK, Canada, Australia, France, Germany and Japan have electronic drug claims databases that accurately record information about health care details. Prescription drug utilization studies began in Canada in the late 1970s, with development of population-based drug insurance claims databases. Automated databases have been used for pharmacoepidemiological studies in USA since 1980s. In USA, and Canada details regarding prescriptions dispensed in retail pharmacies like dispensation date, name and quantity of the drug dispensed are available at region and country wise. They have a system of registry based on a unique patient identifier number.

To meet the needs of pharmacoepidemiology, an ideal data base shall contain records from inpatient and out patient care, emergency care, laboratory tests and other investigations and all prescription and non-prescription drugs. The population covered by the database should be large enough to identify rare events for the drug in question. The patients shall have a unique identifier and the records have to be updated regularly

The automate databases that are available for use in pharmacoepidemiological studies include

1. Administrative database (Discussed earlier in this chapter)
2. Non-administrative data bases or Electronic health medical records and linkage systems (Discussed earlier in this chapter)

The other types of automated data include Pharmacy dispensing databases and Service information databases. They are widely used in USA and Europe. The administrative databases are often used globally while others are for 'in-house' type of uses.

Advantages and Limitations of Automated Databases

There are a number of clear advantages for using automated data in pharmacoepidemiology. The computerised data bases have a potential for providing very large sample size and getting sufficient sample size a big problem in epidemiological studies. The research can be conducted in a real life setting and permits analysis of populations that are generally excluded in clinical trials like elderly and women. Many of the automated data provide population based data covering entire population of an area and are fully representative in nature. Large sample size like lakhs and millions can be included in the studies that can help to find rare effects in large populations. Cost of the study will be less as data are already collected and stored in computerised format. The data is a by-product of the existing administrative systems. The time required to complete the study will be very less compared to other prospective studies. Databases do not require informed patient consent and less prone to bias from nonresponse. They can demonstrate precise drug dispensing patterns as they avoid patient recall and interviewer bias which is a typical concern with primary data collection.

The limitations of the automated data rest on the fact that they are basically designed for some other purpose and its use is secondary in pharmacoepidemiology. Administrative data bases are typically designed for billing and record keeping purposes and not for research. Electronic medical records are created as part of clinical patient care and not for research. The validity of diagnostic details may not be certain in the case of administrative databases, particularly for out-patients. It may be noted that unlike the insurance cover in India, all health insurances cover both in-patient and out-patient treatments in US and Europe. In India most of the health insurances cover only in-patient treatment. Databases often do not include data on medications obtained without prescriptions like over the counter (OTC) or non-legend or non-scheduled items. The databases may not include items not covered under the insurance or reimbursement scheme. Even the prescription drugs may not come in the databases if the drugs are obtained outside the prescription plan like self-payment or sharing with others in the family.

How to Get the Data for Epidemiological Studies?

In US and the European countries where the automated databases are used for pharmacoepidemiological studies, first the researchers have to submit a protocol to an ethics and review committee constituted specifically for such purposes. Based on the protocol and its hypothesis or research question, the ethics and review committee will recommend for giving the specific data needed for the particular research question. They will charge a fee for the data based on the time needed for extracting from the data base. In India we don't have such systems. However many research organisations in epidemiology get data from the government and other databases based on requests showing the purpose.

Automated Data- Indian Situation

The presence of computerised databases that link the data on the use of medicines and patient medical outcomes are totally lacking in India. Though the data from public health insurance firms operating in the country can be obtained for studies, they are insignificant and sectarian in nature. Networking among major hospitals, public or private, with respect to medicine use is also absent in the country. Researchers have to rely on paper medical records. Although the hospital pharmacies attached to medium and large hospital use software that provides data on drug use, they keep the information as their private documents. In the case of community pharmacies, majority of them are not using computers for dispensing purposes.

How many prescriptions are dispensed in India? No body knows. Why? There is no system in existence in the country to make computer based databases for the community pharmacy services. Bills are generated on paper books in a most of the community pharmacies as computerization is not mandatory for their working. Central drug regulatory agencies like Drugs Controller General of India (DCGI) and Central Drugs Standard Control Organisation (CDSCO) do not have a registry of licensed manufacturers and their products. No system is in existence to make a registry of the medicines manufactured in the country. There is no registry of the licensed hospital pharmacies or community pharmacies. An active movement has initiated in 2015 in India for computerization and networking of the drugs control system in the country aimed at making computerised registry of the medicines and their manufacturers and distributors. The Pharmacy Practice Regulations of 2015 may also help to create a computerised database for Indian hospital and community pharmacies in the coming years.

CHAPTER 7

Study Design in Pharmacoepidemiology

Chapter Mission

After learning this chapter you may be able to know:

- Different classes of epidemiological studies.
- Study design in epidemiology and pharmacoepidemiology.
- Outline of widely used epidemiological methods.
- Various steps in study process.
- Pharmacoepidemiology.
- Errors in epidemiological studies.

The Pharmacoepidemiology helps to collect evidence for Evidence Based Medicine (EBM) through research, which uses a variety of study designs. Pharmacoepidemiological studies are conducted for revealing unbiased relationships between exposures to medicines, surgical items or similar products and health related issues like risks (mortality or morbidity) or benefits (therapeutic effects). The identification of causal relationships between these exposures and outcomes is an important aspect of pharmacoepidemiology as in the case of epidemiology. Different study designs help to provide information of different quality. However we always prefer to use the best possible design. However sometimes this is not practical or ethically acceptable. We cannot do an experiment to expose some people to a harmful substance to see what effect it has. Therefore, we need to understand the strengths and weaknesses of each type of study design, as applied to a particular research purpose.

The purposes considered may include

1. Describing the prevalence of health problems (Example: prevalence of Stevens-Johnson syndrome (SJS) with Sulpha drugs).
2. Identifying causes of health problems (etiological research), and
3. Evaluating therapy, including treatment and prevention.

Types of Study Design in Pharmacoepidemiology

We may follow one classification of grouping Pharmacoepidemiological studies into two major groups or classes as shown in Fig. 7.1 namely:

1. Observational Studies
2. Experimental / Interventional Studies

In Observational studies, as researchers we simply observe and systematically collect the information, but do not try to change the people or animals, or reagents being observed. There is no intervention by the researcher or his team in the Observational studies. Hence they can also be called as Non-Interventional Studies.

In Experimental Studies, the researcher intervenes to change something (for example gives some patients a drug) and then observes what happens. Hence Experimental Studies are also known as Interventional Studies.

A distinguishing characteristic of an intervention study is that the intervention – the preventative or therapeutic measure – being tested is allocated by the investigator to a group of two or more study subjects. Study subjects can be individuals, households, or communities. Subjects are followed prospectively to compare the intervention Vs the control or standard treatment and no treatment/ placebo.

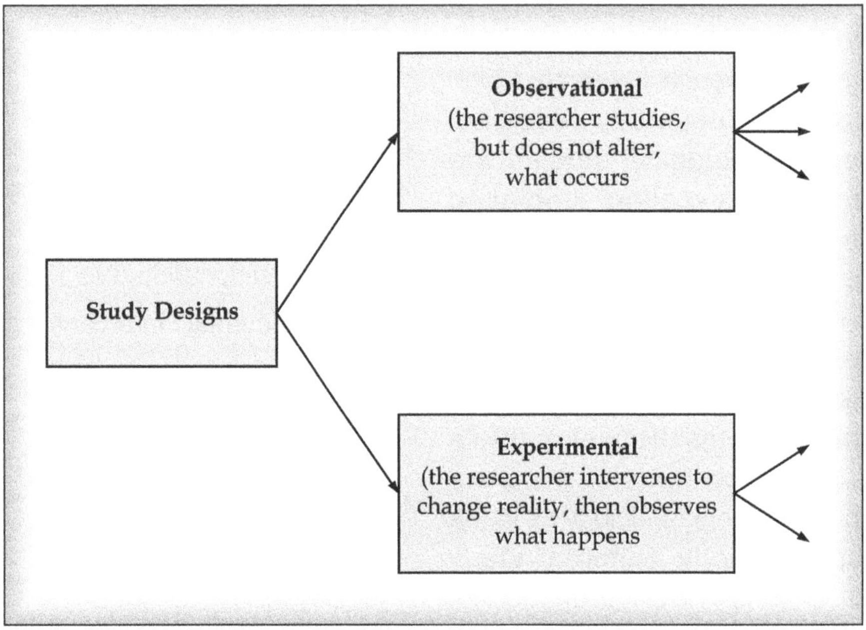

Figure 7.1 Classification of pharmacopidemiological studies.

Method 1. Stage 1: Grouping into observational and experimental studies.

Examples of observational studies:

- A survey of taking iron tonic among pregnant women.
- A researcher who joins a gang of students to study their lifestyle (note, as long as the researcher does not try to change their behaviour, it's an observational study);
- Taking blood samples of a group of workers to measure blood sugar levels during first Monday morning of every alternate months. (Note, you are intervening to take the blood, but you are not trying to change the blood glucose level: it's just a measurement).

Examples of experiments:

- Plying a pregnant women with Ferrous iron tablets to see whether pregnant women perform better when iron tablets are given.
- Encouraging students in one group to stop taking junky foods like Lays to see whether they get better health.
- Warning one group of workers that you are going to take blood sugar levels in the first Monday of next month to test for glucose and comparing their levels to another group that you did not warn.

When do you do an observational study?

- When you merely want to collect descriptive information: "Is the incidence of diabetes rising?"
- When you want to report on the causes of a problem without disturbing the natural setting (I want to find out why patients do not take the prescribed course of antibiotics)
- When you can't do an experiment: "How fast does the earth move around the sun?"
- When it's not acceptable to do an experiment: "How much does not wearing a condom increase the likelihood of HIV infection?"

Observational Study Design

Observational studies have two components, descriptive and analytical. Descriptive observations pertain to the "who, what, where and when of health-related state occurrence". However, analytical observations deal more with the 'how' of a health-related event. Case control, Cohort, Case Cohort and Analytic Cross sectional studies are examples of Analytic Studies. Cross Sectional Studies, Case Reports, Case Series and Correlational studies are included in Descriptive Studies. Though there are many types of observational studies, we at this point of discussing the study design focus on three of them only (Fig. 7.2).

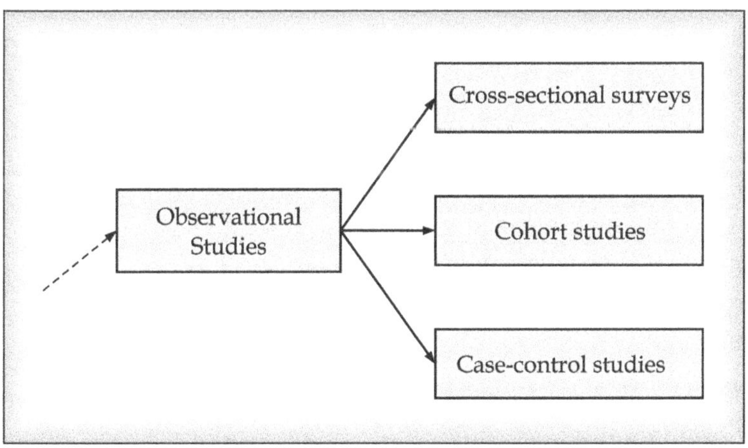

Figure 7.2 Stage 2: Classification of observational studies.

Cross-sectional Surveys

Example: what is the prevalence of diabetes in this community? Here, you draw a random sample of people and record information about their health in a systematic manner. You can also compare people with, and without, diabetes in terms of characteristics (such as being overweight) that may be associated with the disease. The problem is that you cannot be sure which came first: the diabetes or the weight problem, so this is a very weak design for drawing conclusions about causes.

Cohort, or "Longitudinal", or "Prospective" Studies

These are like surveys, but extend over a time period. This allows you to study changes and to establish the time-sequence in which things occur. Therefore, you can use this to study causes. For example, you could draw a sample of people (Pharmacy practice, for example) who do not have the disease you are interested in, and collect information on the factor you have hypothesized to be a cause of the disease. Maybe you want to see whether smocking is associated with lung cancer.

So, collect information on how many cigarettes each student smoke in a day, week, month or year and collect this information over a *long* time, and then eventually collect information on who gets lung cancer. You could then see whether the cases of lung cancer increased among the people who used cigarettes. In technical terms, you record the incidence of cancer among those who use cigarettes in a pre-determined quantity and compare this to the incidence in the non-smokers and calculate the 'relative risk'.

The advantages of this study design are that it can establish that the smoking predates the lung cancer, and it allows for accurate collection of exposure information ('exposure' = use of cigarettes).

However, there are some problems with this design. Lung cancer is rare, so you will need a very large cohort of students; you will also need to keep in contact with them for a very long time and you will probably get very bored waiting for the results. We need a quicker solution?

The "Case-Control" Study

This is more practical, but suffers from other disadvantages. It is a "retrospective" study. This means that. like a detective in crime investigation or a technocrat in reverse engineering, you begin at the end, that is with the disease, and then work backwards to hunt for possible causes.

In our example, you could identify a group of patients with lung cancer (these would be the cases in "case-control"). Then identify a control group who do not have lung cancer. [Please Note : In fact, great care is needed in choosing the control group: should you select patients with other types of cancer, or healthy people, or both?] Then, collect information on their previous use of cigarettes dating back as far as you can manage. Again, you might be able to collect this "exposure" information from their friends or others. The hypothesis would be that smoking would be significantly higher in the lung cancer group than the control group. After collecting the data you can test how well the data fit this hypothesis using a statistical test.

The advantages are that a case-control study can be done faster and more cheaply than a cohort study. However, it may be difficult to collect the information you require on past exposures, and there may be other ways in which the cases and controls differ, not just the smoking , which could also be causing the lung cancer. Sometimes you also have difficulty in being sure which came first: the disease or the exposure. The law of retrospection says "one cannot tell which way the train went by looking at the rail track".

With a case-control design we cannot calculate 'incidence' of lung cancer (because the cases already had lung cancer when you began) and this weakens the analysis. Similarly we cannot calculate 'prevalence', because it was you who decided how many cases and how many controls to choose, and this determined the apparent prevalence in the study.

Instead of the relative risk, you have to use a calculation called an "odds ratio" to estimate the association between smoking and lung cancer. Since Case-Control studies are much more practical for studying the causes of many chronic diseases, they are used very commonly

Experimental/ Intervention Study Design

The Experimental or Intervention studies are very much similar to laboratory studies. In experimental studies, the researcher is the one in control of all of the factors entering the study, in contrast to observational studies, where nature is allowed to "take its course", as epidemiologists observe from the side lines/ outside.

Types of experimental interventions may include:

Therapeutic agents

Prophylactic agents

Diagnostic agents

Surgical procedures

Health service strategies

Advantages and Disadvantages of Intervention/ Experimental Trials

Intervention trials are the epidemiological studies that most closely resemble the experiments conducted by scientists in the laboratory. The essential and distinguishing feature of such studies lies in the investigator's direct control over the allocation of subjects to study groups. In contrast, in observational studies, the allocation is determined by the subjects themselves and the researchers are just passive observers of what happens.

Intervention trials provide the strongest evidence with which to test hypotheses. However, they are not the most usual study design in epidemiology, mainly because of ethical constraints. It would be unacceptable to allocate people to either be or not be exposed to a substance or to be subjected to a procedure for which there is some suspicion that it may be harmful. It is, however, possible to conduct a trial to test whether removal of such an exposure will decrease subsequent incidence and mortality. Thus, intervention trials in epidemiology are limited to interventions for which there are grounds to believe that there will be a potential benefit to individuals.

Experimental studies can be further classified into Randomised Control Trials (RCT) and Non Randomised Control Trials (NR CT) (Fig. 7.3).

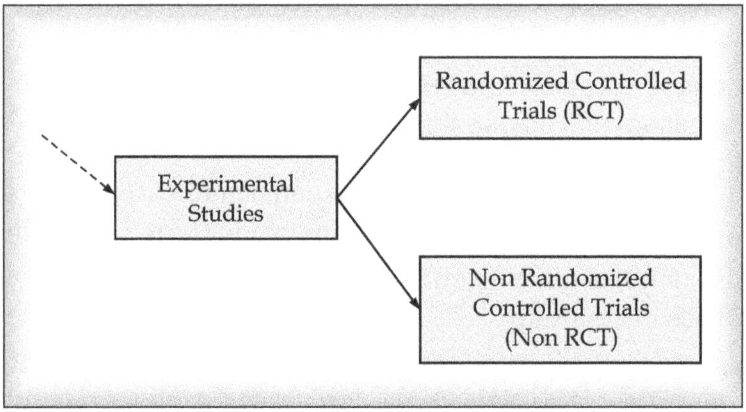

Figure 7.3 Stage 3: Classification of experimental studies.

Randomised Controlled Trial

Randomised Controlled Trial (RCT) is also known as Randomised Clinical Trial. RCT constitute the mainstay of experimental medical studies used in testing new drugs and treatments.

- A sample of patients with the condition, and who meet other selection criteria, are randomly allocated to receive either the experimental treatment, or the control treatment (commonly the standard treatment for the condition).
- Occasionally, a placebo or sham treatment will be used in the control group. Where there is already an accepted treatment, it is unethical to use placebos.
- The experimental and control groups are then followed for a set time, and relevant measurements are taken to indicate the results (or 'outcomes') in each group.

The randomised controlled trial is considered as the most rigorous method of determining whether a cause-effect relationship exists between an intervention and outcome. The strength of the RCT lies in the process of randomisation that is unique to this type of epidemiological study design.

Generally, in a randomised controlled trial, study participants are randomly assigned to one of two groups: the experimental group receiving the intervention that is being tested and a comparison group (controls) which receives a conventional treatment or placebo. These groups are then followed prospectively to assess the effectiveness of the intervention compared with the standard or placebo treatment.

The random allocation of subjects is used to ensure that the intervention and control groups are similar in all respects (distribution of potential confounding factors) with the exception of the therapeutic or preventative measure being tested. The choice of comparison treatments may include an existing standard treatment or a placebo or a sham treatment.

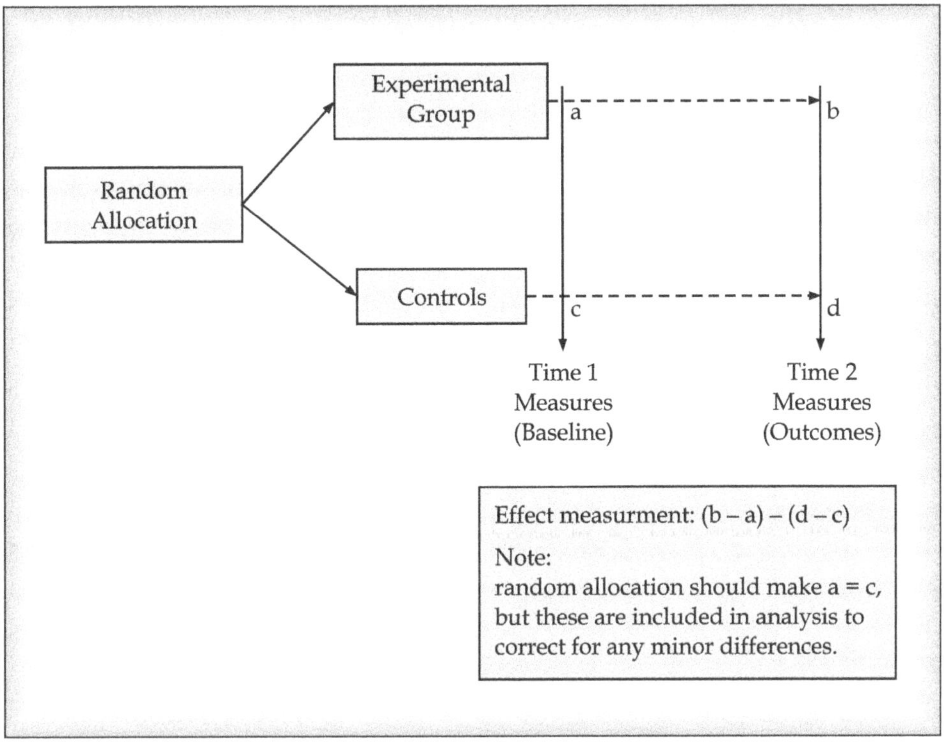

Figure 7.4 Random allocation in RCT.

The term "random" in RCT refers to random allocation to either experimental or control group. It does not refer to random selection or sampling of the patients to include in the trial.

Do not confuse random allocation to experimental and control groups with random selection of a sample. Random selection of a sample ensures that the sample is representative of the broad population. It is typically used in a survey (i.e., an observational study). Random allocation ensures the experimental and control groups are equivalent, but does not ensure they are representative of the broad population. Indeed, they are most likely not, as they all have the disease being studied.

Random allocation means allocating them by chance (toss of a coin or odd and even number). If the groups are relatively large (like 50 or more people in each), the study will help to end up equivalent in terms of factors such as age, sex, and even other things that you do not even know like their response or reaction to the medication.

Random allocation is mainly to avoid confounding. Confounding refers to confusing the effects of two or more variables like the treatment you want to study and some other factor, such as age or sex, on which the two groups may differ.

To make sure that any differences in the final outcome measurements were due to your experimental treatment and not to something else, you want the two groups to be comparable on all other factors. That is, you want to control all other factors. In theory, if randomly allocated groups are sufficiently large, they will be equivalent and hence directly comparable, on any variable you intend to measure.

If we know about a confounder before starting the experiment, we could match the two groups on it (for example ensure equal numbers of males and females in each group). However, matching would not remove the effects of a confounder that we do not know about, such as a biochemical parameter that modifies the action of the drug. Here lies the importance of random allocation. Often randomization helps to protect against all potential confounding factors, both known and unknown.

Because of natural biological variations, the two groups (even though randomly allocated) will not be identical in perfect sense. Hence a statistical test is used to indicate whether any difference we observe in the outcomes for the two groups may just have reflected natural variability or whether it seems to represent a "statistically significant" difference. Examples of statistical tests include a t-test, or analysis of variance (ANOVA).

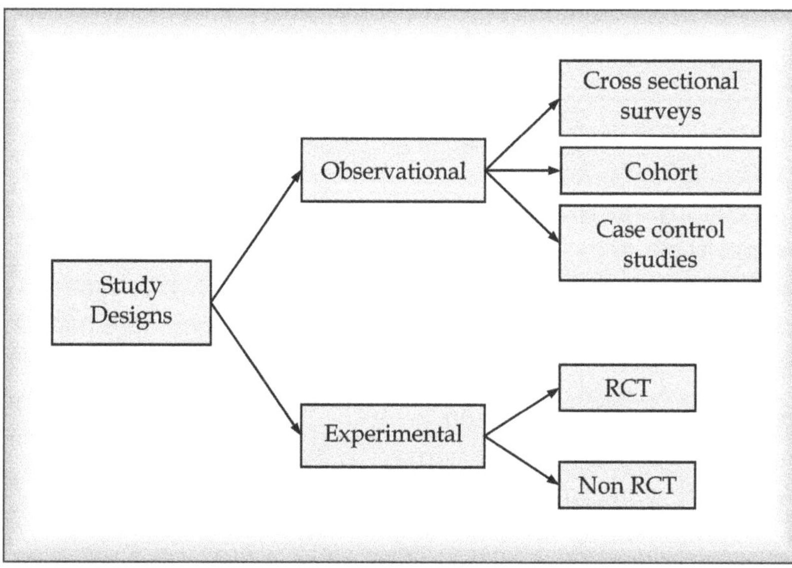

Figure 7.5 Method 2: Classification of pharmacoepidemiology.

Non Randomized Controlled Trials (RCT)

Non RCT can be further grouped into Community Trials and Field Trials. That is, there are three types of Experimental studies in epidemiology, namely

1. Randomized Controlled Trials (RCT). It is often used for new medicine or drug testing.

2. Field Trials . It is conducted on those at a high risk of conducting a disease. and
3. Community Trials (research on social originating diseases)
   (Also see the Intervention studies)

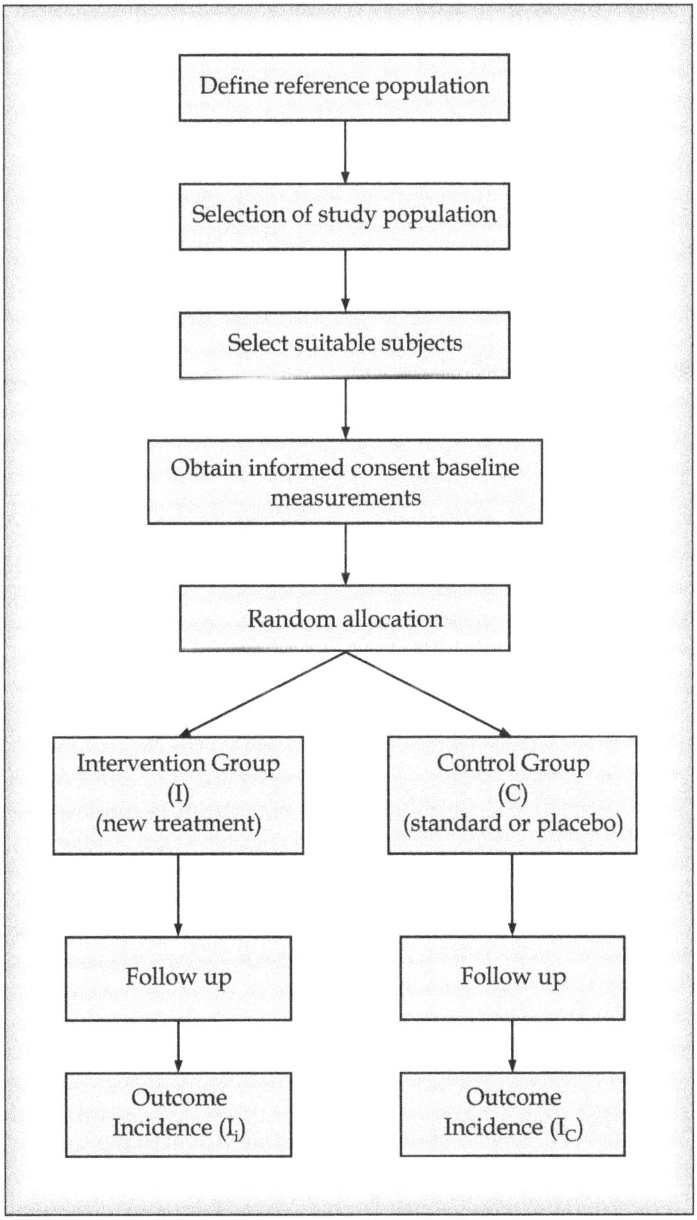

Figure 7.6 Stages of RCT.

Field Trials and Community Trials

Intervention trials consist of trials to prevent disease (field trials) or trials to treat established disease processes (clinical trials). The objective of a clinical trial is to evaluate one or more new treatments for a disease or condition. For instance, a clinical trial may be designed to assess whether a chemotherapeutic agent can prevent recurrence of cancer, increase survival or improve quality of life (Case No 1)

> **Case 1** A total of 474 adult patients with malignant glioma (astrocytoma) grade 3 or 4 were randomized to receive 45 Gy (in 20 fractions over four weeks) or 60 Gy (in 30 fractions over six weeks) of radiotherapy postoperatively. The main objective of the study was to assess whether the higher dose would improve survival (Bleehen & Stenning, 1991).

Since clinical trials involve diseased people, they are often carried out in hospitals or other clinical settings where the subjects are treated and followed up for their condition.

Field Trials

Field trials deal with subjects who are disease-free. A field trial involves evaluation of whether an agent or procedure reduces the risk of developing disease among those free from that condition at enrolment. Because these trials involve healthy rather than diseased people, they tend to be logistically more difficult to carry out than clinical trials. They generally have to be conducted in the 'field' rather than in hospitals or clinics. Moreover, whereas the adverse consequences of a given disease (e.g., disease recurrence, death) may occur with high probability during a relatively short time, typically the risk of contracting a disease among people who are initially free of it is small. This is particularly true for rare diseases such as cancer. Consequently, field trials usually require a greater number of subjects followed up for longer periods than clinical trials. Field trials can be carried out among individuals (Case 2) or groups of people (Case3). In the first case, the unit of allocation to the intervention is the individual, whereas in the second, it is the group. The group may be a household, a block of houses, a school or a whole community.

> **Case 2** A randomized trial was carried out among Whitehall (English) civil servants to measure in middle-aged men the health effects of stopping smoking. A total of 1445 male cigarette smokers aged 40–59 years who were at a high risk of developing cardio-respiratory diseases were randomly allocated to intervention (714 men) or normal care (731 men). Those in the intervention group received individual advice on the relation of smoking to health. Most then expressed their wish to stop smoking and received further support over the next 12 months. The two groups were then followed up for twenty years (Rose & Colwell, 1992)

Community Trials

Field trials in which whole communities are the unit of allocation are called community trials (Case 3) .

> **Case 3** The Community Intervention Trial for Smoking Cessation (COMMIT) was a multicentre project designed to evaluate a community wide smoking cessation programme in the USA. This trial began in 1989 in 11 matched pairs of communities. One community of each pair was randomly assigned to receive the smoking cessation programme with the other acting as a control. The intervention was designed to promote smoking cessation by using a wide range of community resources to affect attitudes and policies towards smoking (COMMIT Research Group, 1991)

There are various reasons for selecting groups rather than individuals as the study unit. Many interventions are impossible to assign at an individual level. Environmental interventions such as water fluoridation or improvement of air quality can be conducted only at a group level. Most health education interventions also fall into this category. For instance, the intervention (i.e., the smoking cessation programme) was aimed primarily at the community rather than the individual; thus, it was appropriate to choose the community as the study unit. It may also be logistically easier to conduct the trial among groups of people than among individuals.

Randomized Clinical Trial (RCT) is the hardest to perform, Cohort Study is less hard, Case Control Study is still less and Case Reports the easiest. The design of Case Report is less convincing while that of RCT is most convincing.

Quasi-Experimental Designs

There is a category of studies that falls between observational and true experimental studies; they are called "*quasi-experimental* studies". In these, there is an intervention, but it is often not completely planned by the person doing the research.

The term 'epidemiologic triad' is used to describe the intersection of 'Host', 'Agent' and 'Environment' in analysing an outbreak. The principles of epidemiological studies as such or with necessary modifications can be followed in pharmacoepidemiology.

Steps in pharmacoepidemiology Study Design

Therapy is always individualized or tailored to the need of specific patient. This individualization of therapy requires the determination of a risk benefit ratio specific to the patient. For example, take the case of a patient who has an impaired liver function and is suffering from a serious infection. Normally gentamicin is having a small probability of causing renal disease. But a patient who is having impaired liver function has a greater risk of ADR of gentamicin (causing renal disease) than one with normal liver function (Moore RD 1986).

The pharmacoepidemiology got its focus of inquiry from clinical pharmacology and the methods of inquiry from epidemiology. Hence in pharmacoepidemiology the methods of epidemiology are applied to the content area of clinical pharmacology.

Three Step Procedure

The scientific method in epidemiology is a three step procedure. In the first step the sample of the study subjects is studied. In the second step the inference from the sample of study subjects is generalized and a general conclusion regarding the population is drawn. In the third step a general conclusion is drawn regarding the scientific theory or causation.

Step 1: Study of Sample

A study is always conducted on a selection of individuals who represent the study subjects. The study subjects theoretically represent a random sample of a defined population. Take the case of a randomized clinical study of efficacy of glibenclamide 5 mg in lowering blood sugar level in diabetes mellitus. Fifty people of age group 60-70 having diabetes were identified and given either glibenclamide 5 mg or placebo (25 in each group) and observed their blood sugar level after two weeks.

We would normally and reasonably expect to see the blood sugar level of the 25 persons who had taken glibenclamide decrease considerably than those who were given the placebo. In this case the 50 study group would represent the study sample of people with diabetes mellitus of age group 60-70. However in reality the group of 50 may not be a true random sample of the target population group as it is logically impossible to identify every one who belongs to the target group and then randomly choose from among them. Still the study sample is treated as if it were a random sample of the target population.

Step 2: Inference from Sample Study

At this stage one can make a generalization that glibenclamide reduces the blood sugar level in the diabetes mellitus patients of age group 60-70. But it is essential to explore whether the findings or observation could have occurred simply by chance, that is due to random variation in the blood sugar level. In order to evaluate this possibility we do the statistical test. Through the statistical test the investigator can quantitate the probability that the difference seen between the two study groups occurred simply due to chance. The science of statistics prescribes rules and procedures for making such decisions. If the results of any study under consideration demonstrate a statistically significant difference, then it is said to have an *association.* The process of assessing whether random variation could have led to a study's findings is known as *statistical inference.* The statistical inference represents the major role for statistical testing in scientific method.

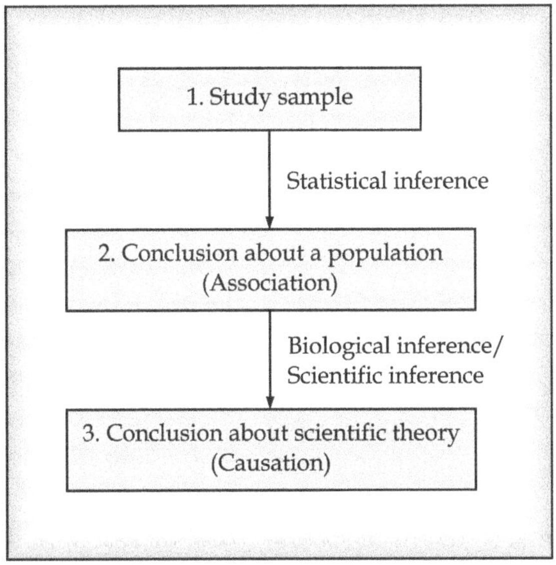

Figure 7.7 Three step procedure.

Step 3: Causation or General Conclusion

If there is no statistically significant difference then the process stops there. If there is an association, then one may even dare to generalize the results of the study even further and state that glibenclamide is an antidiabetic drug in general. This is referred to as *scientific* or *biological inference*. The result is a conclusion about *causation.* The causation in the present example is that the drug glibenclamide really does lowers blood sugar level in diabetes mellitus patients who were administered the drug. To come to such conclusive findings we have to generalize to populations other than that included in the study, including groups of people who were not represented in the study sample like pregnant women, children and elderly. Unlike statistical inference, there is no specific quantitative rules for biological inference. Based on the data obtained and the available scientific literature one has to make a subjective judgment. The criteria for causal nature of an association as discussed below can also be used while making the judgment.

Criteria for the Causal Nature of an Association

Sir Austin Bradford Hill in 1965 suggested the criteria for causal nature of an association (Hill AB 1965). Later many modifications and changes were made in the criteria. None of the criteria is essential for an association to be causal association and none of them is sufficient to consider an association to be a causal association. If more of the criteria are present, that make the chance of an association to be a causal association more. The fewer criteria that are met, the less likely it is that an association is a causal association. The following are some of the important criteria suggested by various authors (Storm BL 2000).

Coherence with Existing Information or Biological Plausibility

This simply means whether the association makes a sense in the light of information and findings available in the literature. Data from other human studies, findings from other related questions, data from animal studies or *in vitro* studies, scientific theory, pathophysiological findings etc., are useful tools in making a decision regarding the association. Take the case of association of cigarette smoking and lung cancer. Based on animal data cigarette smoke is a known carcinogen. In humans it is known to cause cancers of head and neck, pancreas and the bladder. Cigarette smoke goes into the lungs exposing the tissues therein. All this shows that it is biologically plausible that cigarette smoking could cause lung cancer (Experimental carcinogenesis with tobacco smoke 1981).

Consistency of the Association

If a finding is scientific, one should be able to reproduce it in different settings. This could include different study centers, different population, different study designs etc. It is difficult for one to believe a finding reported only once. There is every chance to commit an error in a study which is not apparent to the investigator or the reader. In the case of cigarette smocking and lung cancer the association has been reproduced in many different studies in different geographic locations using different study designs.

Time Sequence

This means that a cause must precede and effect. In some cases it may be difficult to determine the sequence. Take the case of candidates who are contesting an election. If we perform a survey asking each candidate whether he/she currently takes any medicine like diazepam tablet and also whether he or she is anxious, there could be a strong association between the use of medicine (diazepam) and anxiety. However this does not mean that diazepam causes anxiety or tension. One may find it difficult to differentiate from this type of cross-sectional study which variable came first and which came second. In the case of cigarette smoking and lung cancer, cigarette smoking precedes the lung cancer. If the opposite were the case the patient would not survive long enough to smoke much.

Specificity of the Association

This is the analysis of the question whether the cause can occur without the presumed effect and whether the effect can occur without the presumed cause. This criterion is generally not complied in biology and health sciences, though there can be exceptions. In the case of rabies the disease never occurs without the rabies virus. Every one who gets infected with rabies virus develops rabies unless treated early.

Measles never occurs without the measles virus. However in this case every one who is infected with measles virus need not develop clinical measles. Every smoker may not develop lung cancer and every patient with lung cancer may not be a smoker. Some are of opinion that this criterion should not be treated as a criterion for causal nature of an association. It is important to note that whenever this criterion is complied with, it gives a strong support for the conclusion that an association is causal.

Strength of the Association

The strength criterion can be analyzed based on the quantitative strength, dose-response or duration response relationship or the study design. The quantitative strength refers to the size of the study group. A quantitatively large association can be obtained only by a causal association or by a large error that should be apparent in evaluating the study. A quantitatively small association can also be causal, but could be created by a subtle error which could not be apparent in evaluating the study. Epidemiologists generally consider an association with a relative risk (RR) of less than 2.00 as a week association. In the case of studies on cigarette smoking and lung cancer the association show relative risks from 10.00 to 30.00. A dose-response relationship is established when an increase in the intensity of an exposure results in an increased risk of the disease under study. Similarly a duration-response relationship is established when an increase in the duration of the exposure causes an increased risk of the disease under study. In the case of cigarette smoking and lung cancer, it has been found repeatedly that an increase either in the number of cigarettes smoked in a day or in the number of years of smoking cause increase in the risk of developing lung cancer (Biomedical evidence for determining causality 1982). The existence of a dose-response relationship or duration-response relationship is a strong indication of causal association.

Types of Errors in Epidemiological Studies

Pharmacoepidemiology aims to estimate the effects of drugs when they are prescribed after marketing. Since the drug exposure is not a stable process and depends on many factors like indication for prescribing, compliance and disease condition, estimation of the effect of drugs is not an easy task. A major challenge of pharmacoepidemiology is the achievement of an accurate estimate without error. An epidemiologic study is viewed as an exercise in measurement with accuracy as the objective.

Error

There are three types of error that can be produced in a study:

1. Chance error which is also called unsystematic error or random error.
2. Bias or systematic variation and
3. Confounding.

Chance Error

Chance is a random error appearing to cause an association between an exposure and an outcome. An important assumption in epidemiology is that we can draw an inference about the experience of the entire population based on the evaluation of a sample of the population. But a problem with drawing such an inference is that the role of chance can affect the results of an epidemiological study because of the effects of random variation from sample to sample. The effect of random error may produce an estimate that is different from the true underlying value. The effect of random error can result in either an under-estimation or over-estimation of the correct value.

The probability of random error can be quantitated using statistics. Bias has to be prevented by proper designing of the study. Confounding can be controlled in the study design or in the study analysis. If all the three types of error are avoided then one can have a true causal association.

Association that can be observed in a study can be classified into 4 types

(i) None or no association

(ii) Artificial association or spurious association

  (a) Chance or unsystematic or random

  (b) Bias or systematic

(iii) Indirect or confounded association

(iv) Causal association or direct / true association

The first type of association is *no association*. The second one is *artificial association* which also known as *spurious association* or *false association*. This can occur by two means- chance or bias. Chance is unsystematic or random variation. The main aim of statistical testing is to evaluate the probability that the result observed in the study could have happened purely by chance.

Bias

Bias is used in epidemiology in a different sense from the common use. It is a deviation from the truth. Bias is a systematic manner in which the two study groups have been treated differently. The presence of a bias causes a study to yield incorrect results. In epidemiology bias is systematic variation, that is, a consistent manner in which two study groups are treated or evaluated differently. This consistent difference can create an apparent association which does not really exist. Usual practice of classifying bias is grouping them into selection bias, measurement bias and confounding bias.

Selection Bias

Selection bias is a problem in clinical studies which are not randomized. If the groups are not balanced in terms of important characteristics we get lopsided groups for comparison in the study. This will result in giving wrong results. Selection bias is a distortion of the measurement of an estimate of effect, which is due to the selection into the study groups of subjects who have an unusual and unequal relationship between drug exposure and outcome. A classical example of selection bias involves the prescription pattern of doctors after the introduction of new drugs in the market. Referral bias, self selection and prevalence study bias are often found reasons for selection bias.

Measurement Bias

Measurement bias originates when the various groups involved in the study are measured differently. Misclassification of the of the event of interest can be a problem in measurement. In order to reduce the measurement bias it is important to make certain that groups being compared derive from the same population and that the instruments used to measure are the same.

Confounding Bias

Confounding literally means causing surprise or confusion in (someone), especially by not according with their expectations. In epidemiological studies terms like confound, confounder, confounding factor or confounding variable are used in the same sense that it is an extraneous variable that correlates with both dependent and independent variables. Confounding produces incorrect estimates of the association like bias. But one can often adjust for confounding in the analysis in order to remove its distorting effects to obtain a more accurate measure of association.

Confounding occurs when the estimate of a measure of association between drug exposure and health status is distorted by the effect of one or more variables that are also risk factors for the outcome of interest. The indirect association is called the confounded association. Confounding is a form of bias that confuses the results of pharmacoepidemiologic studies. A confounder is a factor that is associated with the outcome of the study. If this factor is not properly considered and adjusted, the result will be changed dramatically leading to erroneous study conclusions.

A confounding variable is a variable other than the risk factor which is related independently to both the risk factor and the outcome variable. In the case of cigarette smocking and lung cancer, one can find a very strong association of having yellow finger tips and development of lung cancer. This is not a causal association. It is an indirect association confounded by cigarette smoking. Cigarette smoking causes both yellow finger tips and lung cancer. The Causal association is the true association. Another example is the relationship between alcohol and cancer. Smoking is known to cause cancer and people who drink alcohol may also smoke. Therefore the relationship between alcohol consumption and cancer is confounded by smoking.

The bias can be of other types like interviewer bias and recall bias or memory bias. Bias cannot be corrected and the only protection against bias is proper study design.

Pharmacoepidemiology is the application of epidemiological methodologies for the study of drugs focusing on their use and effects in a large number of people. It is drug epidemiology.

CHAPTER 8

Methods for Pharmacoepidemiologic Studies

Chapter Mission

After learning this chapter you may be able to know:

- Various study methods in pharmacoepidemiology.
- Comparison of various methods in pharmacoepidemiology.
- Strengths and limitations of various methods.
- Application of the methods in pharmacoepidemiology.

Background

Method is an established or systematic procedure for achieving certain ends with accuracy and efficiency. Methodology is the systematic, theoretical analysis of the methods applied to a field of study. A large number of study methods are used to generate data on the 'use' and 'risk' issues related to both new drugs and old drugs.

Ethical issues, formalities and costs limit the use of experimentation and hence observational methods are used widely in epidemiological studies. The common method to study adverse drug events starts with collection of spontaneous reports of drug related mortality and morbidity issues. Epidemiologic study designs like case control, cohort, and cross sectional studies are used largely. In practice, epidemiologic studies do not use randomization to determine who will receive a particular drug, instead ascertain association between exposures and diseases with the help of observational study designs and statistical analysis.

In recent times in the developed countries, methods like large automated database, meta-analysis, and hybrid designs like nested case- control studies are widely used in pharmacoepidemiological studies. There is growing focus of interest in using computerized data base for pharmacoepidemiologic studies *(Storm BL 1990)*. The database include details on patient demographics, outpatient medicines, discharge details, ambulatory care details etc. Generally patient care data are collected from different registers like pharmacy billing files, admission files, patient discharge files and medical reimbursement services with the help of record linkages. Individual patient based longitudinal files can be created with the help of record linkage on adhoc basis which will be much useful in the pharmaco-epidemiological studies. Some of the merits and demerits of the linked data base for pharmacoepidemiological studies have been discussed by Faich and Shapiro *(Faich GA 1989, Shapiro S 1989)*.

Common Pharmaco-epidemiological Methods

There are a number of methods in Epidemiology and quite a large number of them are used in Pharmacoepidemiology also. It is beyond the scope of this book to discuss all of them. There are also different approaches in the classification of the method used in Pharmacoepidemiology from different concepts or perspectives. (We have discussed one approach in the classification of Pharmacoepidemiological/ Epidemiological research methods in the previous chapter, namely Chapter 7 on Study Design in Pharmacoepidemiology). The discussion in this chapter will focus on such aspects that are not elaborately covered in the previous chapter.

The discussion in this chapter is based on the classification shown in Fig. 8.1.

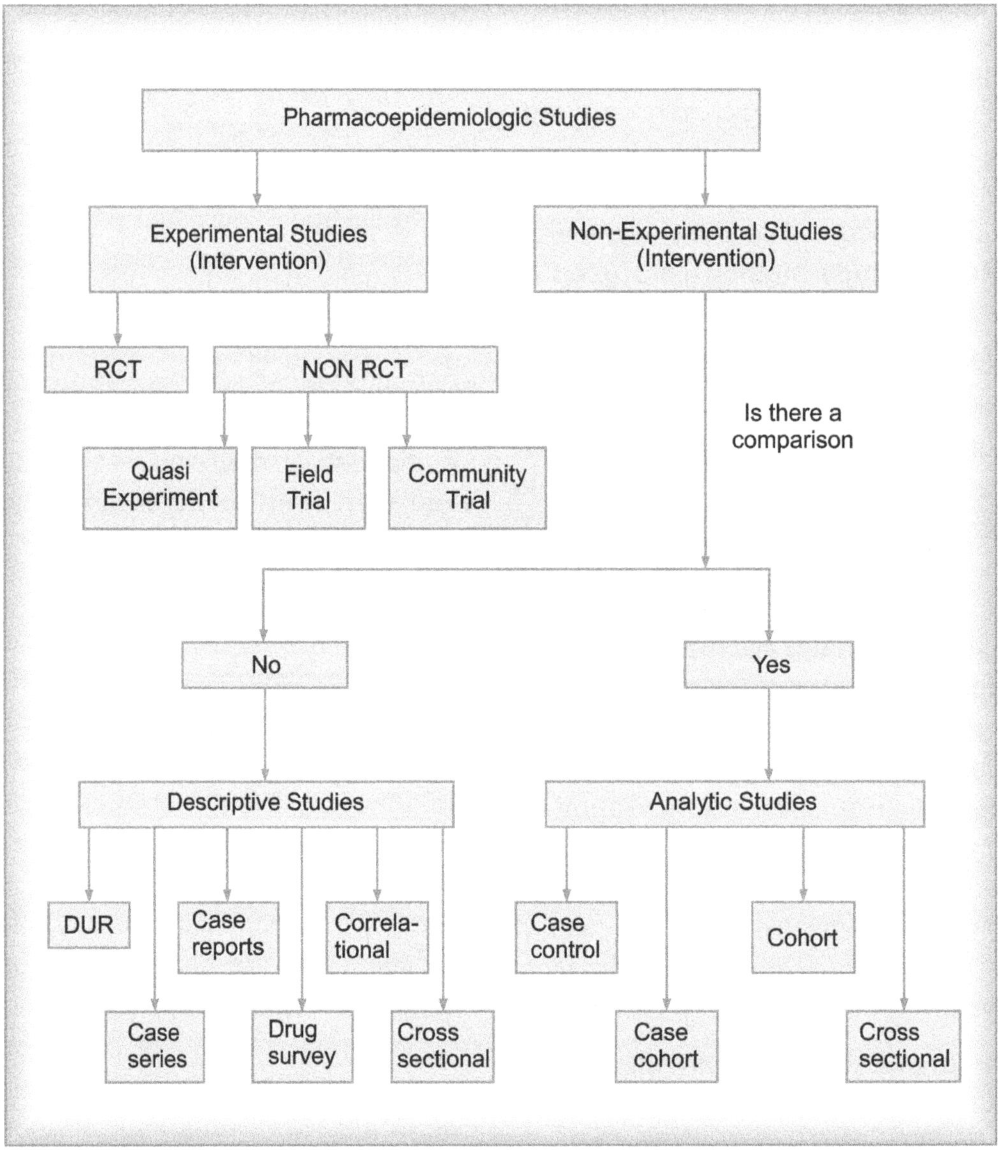

Figure 8.1 Classification of pharmacoepidemiological studies.

Experimental Studies and Non- Experimental Studies

The two fundamental types of studies in pharmacoepidemiology are experimental and non-experimental studies. They are distinguished by the method in which subjects are subjected to the treatment.

Experimental Studies or Interventional Studies

In Experimental Studies, the researcher intervenes to change something (for example gives some patients a drug) and then observes what happens. This is the reason why Experimental Studies are also known as Interventional Studies. A distinguishing characteristic of an intervention study is that the intervention – the preventative or therapeutic measure – being tested is allocated by the investigator to a group of two or more study subjects. Study subjects can be individuals, households, or communities. Subjects are followed prospectively to compare the intervention Vs the control or standard treatment and no treatment/ placebo.

The Experimental or Intervention studies are very much similar to laboratory studies. Experimental analytic studies include clinical trials such as RCT. Though experiment is an important step in establishing causality, it is neither feasible nor ethical to subject human beings to risk factors in studies. Epidemiologists often make use of 'natural experiments' when available. More frequently epidemiological researchers resort to non-experimental studies.

In experimental studies, the researcher is the one in control of all of the factors entering the study, in contrast to observational studies, where nature is allowed to "take its course", as epidemiologists observe from the side lines/ outside. In Pharmacoepidemiological studies, interventions are with respect to the exposure of therapeutic agents, prophylactic agents, diagnostic agents, surgical procedures, health care services or similar aspects.

Experimental studies include the following:

1. Randomized Controlled Trials (RCT). It is often used for new medicine or drug testing.
2. Non RCT Studies

Randomized Controlled Trial (RCT)

Randomized Controlled Trials are also known an Randomized Clinical Trials and is considered as a "gold standard " method for producing reliable data in Pharmacoepidemiology. However it is time consuming, expensive and with many formalities to be complied with. Prospective, blinded, randomized clinical trial is the ideal and most dependable study to determine the beneficial and adverse effects of drugs. Here patients are randomly assigned for the treatments which helps to avoid many bias. Neither the patient nor the physician is able to identify the drug product being studied. Typically RCT is conducted when comparing the efficiency of two drugs or of one drug against a placebo.

In countries like US and UK Randomized clinical trials may cost millions of dollars. They are often unethical for studies of adverse effects of drugs. Patients may not enroll for a study with the only aim of detecting the adverse effects of a drug. In the case of rare events a large number of patients are needed to conduct studies. Because of these reasons other pharmacoepidemiological methods are sometimes preferred for studies of adverse effects of drugs. (Please refer Chapter 7 for further information regarding Experimental studies.)

Non RCT Studies

Non Randomized Controlled Trials have only limited applications in Pharmacoepidemiology, though certain researchers use seriously such methods. Non RCT studies include Quasi Experiments, Field Trials and Community Trials

Quasi-experimental Designs

With the increase in computerization in health care, databases exploring pharmaceutical outcomes are largely used in studies. Often the databases from other departments like health insurance are used for the studies as they are less expensive. Since such studies do not rely on random assignment of subjects, they are described as quasi-experimental designs. It includes a treatment group or exposed group and a control group or non-exposed group.

Field Trial and Community Trial are briefly mentioned in **Chapter 7.** Field Trials and Community Trials are having more applications in health studies .

Non-Experimental Studies

Non-experimental studies are also known as 'observational studies'. In non-experimental studies unlike in experimental studies, the patients are not assigned to treatments by the investigator. Patients who receive medication from the conventional settings of medical care are selected as the subjects for the study. Non-experimental studies can be Descriptive or Analytic (also called Analytical) in nature. Sometimes it may be combination of both. .

Descriptive Studies

Descriptive studies are Qualitative in nature and involves a detailed investigation on individuals for collecting data useful to improve knowledge and understanding. Descriptive Pharmacoepidemiological studies are often aimed at evaluating how medicines and other related items are prescribed by health providers or used by patients. Descriptive studies do not use control groups. Since descriptive studies do not involve comparison of groups, they are unable to test Hypothesis. They are not structured formally as in analytical or experimental studies. Results of descriptive studies help for generating Hypothesis. Descriptive studies help to describe a situation like occurrence of ADRs in patients and give explanation for drug related events including ADRs. Through medical auditing or drug utilization reviews, descriptive studies help to improve rational prescription in health care.

Pharmacoepidemiological Descriptive Studies include the following

- Drug Utilization Review (Survey)
- Case Reports
- Case Series
- Surveys of Drug Use.
- Correlational Studies*
- Cross Sectional Studies*

*Limited, but specialized uses in pharmaco-epidemiological studies.

Analytic Studies

Analytic studies (Analytical Studies) are Quantitative in nature and involve comparison of groups. They are used to test Hypothesis. It is to be noted that the two important qualities studied in pharmaco-epidemiological studies are drug safety and effectiveness of medicines. The ideal model for the study of drug effects is the Double blind RCT which is studied under the experimental studies in pharmaco-epidemiology. We could also see that for various reasons like ethics, expense and the formalities involved, RCT is not often applied in pharmacoepidemiological studies including post marketing surveillance. The important Analytic studies used in pharmacoepidemiology include the following:

- Cohort
- Case Control

Descriptive Studies (Qualitative Models)

Drug Utilization Review (DUR)

Drug Utilization Reviews (DUR) are also referred to as Drug Utilization Evaluations (DUE) or Medication Utilization Evaluations (MUE). DUR is defined as an authorized, structured, on- going review of prescribing, dispensing and use of medication. DUR encompasses a drug review against predetermined criteria that results in changes to drug therapy when these criteria are not met. It has great applications in evaluating the appropriateness of prescription writing and promoting rational use of medicines in the society.

DURs involve a comprehensive review of patients' prescription and medication data before, during, and after dispensing to ensure appropriate medication decision making and positive patient outcomes. DURs are classified into three categories:

Prospective – evaluation of a patient's therapy before medication is dispensed

Concurrent – On going monitoring of drug therapy during the course of treatment.

Retrospective – review of therapy after the patient has received the medication.

DUR programs play a key role in helping managed health care systems understand, interpret, and improve the prescribing, administration, and use of medications. Employers and health plans find DUR programs valuable because the results are used to foster more efficient use of scarce health care resources. Pharmacists play a key role in this process because of their expertise in the area of pharmaceutical care. DURs help practicing pharmacists to identify trends in prescribing within groups of patients such as those with asthma, diabetes, or high blood pressure. Pharmacists can then recommend programs to improve drug therapy for both private and public set ups.

The Medicaid Drug Utilization Review (DUR) Program of USA promotes patient safety through state-administered utilization management tools and systems that interface with their Medicaid Management Information Systems (MMIS), Medicaid DUR is a two-phase process that is conducted by the Medicaid state agencies. In the first phase (prospective DUR) the state's Medicaid agency's electronic monitoring system screens prescription drug claims to identify problems such as therapeutic duplication, drug-disease contraindications, incorrect dosage or duration of treatment, drug allergy and clinical misuse or abuse. It also conducts retrospective DUR.

DUR will help to find out inappropriate use of medicines, both in private and public health care facilities and also help to find out the irrational prescription writing styles predominant in countries like India. In India DUR can be conducted on costly drugs, imported medicines, newer medicines and products like cardiac valves, stents for angioplasty so that the public will be benefitted very much.

Case Reports

It is an example of observational descriptive study in pharmacoepidemiology. It is a qualitative (descriptive) non-experimental method and is one of the simplest methods in pharmacoepidemiology. Quite often experts consider it as one of the weakest form of evidence for causation.

Case report is the presentation of the experience of a patient by his treating physician or other health care professional. The treating doctor could observe the emergence of an outcome for a particular drug exposure daily during his rounds in the hospital. Case report focuses an individual patient who is on drug use, but experience a particular outcome, generally adverse effect or event. Quick improvement of the condition of the patient is also of interest.

Case reports are hypothesis generating reports. They bring forth evidence that supports a hypothesis about drug effects to be tested with other more effective and rigorous study designs. A case report is not ordinarily used to make a report or statement on causation of an event. But it gives a signal that can make others alert to the possibility of causal association. In pharmacovigilance, case reports are important signal generating sources. The strength of case report rests on its ability to produce signals. But case reports are very weak in causation. It is to be noted that pharmacoepidemiology evolved with the publication of case reports in USA in the 1960s, mostly by hospital pharmacists and clinical pharmacists.

Illustration 1: Take the case of a patient who had taken four different drugs continuously for eight months developed aplastic anemia. The case report may suggest that one or more the four drugs used by the patient could have caused the aplastic anemia. This signal may help for further investigations or studies.

Illustration 2: The best classical example of a case report was that of Dr. William Mc Bride of Sydney, Australia, who published the first report indicating that thalidomide might be a human teratogen as a letter in the Lancet on 16th December 1961. (Mc Bride 1961). The signal generated later helped to confirm that thalidomide could produce fetal abnormalities. It was in fact responsible for the origin of teratology as a discipline.

Illustration 3: The case report of hyper-trichosis with the use of minoxidil for hypertension also helped for developing minoxidil as a topical preparation for baldness.

Case Reports help to promote research culture among health care professions and stimulate research into such areas where potential issues or problems were identified and reported. The case reports can straight away help the researcher to generate hypothesis for further research projects.

Case Series

Case series are also known as a Clinical series. It is a group or cluster of case reports generated by single/ group of clinicians or hospitals or pharmaceutical companies or regulatory agencies like Food and Drug Administration (FDA) or Drugs Controller.

It is a type of medical research study that tracks subjects with a known exposure, such as patients who have received same medicine, or examines their medical records for exposure and outcome.

Case series, like case reports are observational descriptive studies in pharmacoepidemiology. It is a qualitative (descriptive) non- experimental method and is considered stronger than Case Reports. A set of sequential case reports makes a case series. Case series are collections of patients all of whom have a single exposure and whose clinical outcomes are then evaluated and described. The patients can be identified for the case series either based on the exposure or on the outcome. The case series studies are useful in quantifying the incidence of an adverse reaction and are generally used for the study of newly licensed or marketed medicines. It is also useful to ascertain that the incidence rate of a particular adverse effects of concern does not occur in a population larger that the study population in the pre-license studies.

The greater the number of common experiences, the stronger will be the signal to support a conclusion. If six patients developed aplastic anemia after administration of the same medications, that can raise a strong suspicion compared to one person developing aplastic anemia. A classical example of Case Series occurred with Thalidomide induced phocomelia in the early 1960s when same type of malformations were reported in a cluster.

Case series does not have a formal trial protocol, but has many similarities with the open trial. They are very much useful to enlarge our knowledge about the medicines and their risks and help to confirm ADRs.

There are cases where an adverse event could be inferred from a case series study. The case of a rare event with a specific exposure combination is an example for this. Generally it is necessary to compare cases with a group of controls to identify risk factors. The lack of comparison groups is considered as a major disadvantage of the case series studies.

Surveys of Drugs

Surveys of medicines like case series and case reports are observational descriptive studies in pharmacoepidemiology. They are qualitative (descriptive) non- experimental method and are considered as effective tools in promoting health care and framing policy documents related to drug use. Surveys often take simple format and provide crude data. The health surveys have primarily had their origin in the charting of major diseases in the population and etiological research.

Pharmacoepidemiological research based on drug surveys has been scattered and taken place in different research groups at global levels in different settings. The extent has been very modest or poor, when considering that drugs comprise the most common treatment and one of the most rapidly increasing costs in health care. There may be several explanation for the low research out put. One of the reasons may be the poor access to information from issued prescriptions.

There are many areas in drug use where surveys can generate useful information and knowledge. University level surveys in the developed countries by pharmacy students helped to give an insight into drug use by breast feeding women versus non breast feeding women. Drug surveys will also help to compare the usages in various states or among various sections of society like educated and non-educated, working class and office staff, high income and low income groups, youths and adults etc.

In countries like US, UK, Canada etc. it is easy for the researchers to conduct surveys as they have a computerised databases for filling of prescriptions at hospital and community levels. However the Indian situation is totally different. We don't have a data base to analyse. Majority of Indian Community pharmacies are not computerised. Even the computerised pharmacies are not connected to net working and data banking. No agency exists in India to co-ordinate such activities. Same is the case with hospitals also. Medium and large hospitals are computerised, but keep the data as their private property and there is no agency to monitor and co-ordinate. Insurance in health care is yet to be popularised. Though the rough estimate of marketing data of drugs are available in the country that is having only very limited application in pharmacoepidemiology.

The potential for carrying out drug usage surveys in India is very high as it a country with over 1.3 crore population and annual production of drugs worth rupees one lakh crores. The Pharmacy students and working pharmacists can join together to conduct useful surveys at community levels or institutional levels. Drug Surveys are technically simple for students of pharmacy practice or PharmD programs.

Correlation Studies

A correlation is simply defined as a relationship between two variables. The whole purpose of using correlations in research is to figure out which variables are connected. Correlation research is looking for variables that seem to interact with each other, so that when you can see one changing, you have an idea of how the other will change. This often entails the researcher using variables that they can't control. For example, a researcher may be interested in studying the preference for a particular cosmetic item based on age of women.

Descriptive Cross Sectional Studies

A descriptive cross-sectional study is a study in which the disease or condition and potentially related factors are measured at a specific point of time for a defined population. Cross-sectional studies can be thought of as a "snapshot" of the frequency and characteristics of a condition in a population at a particular point in time.

This type of data can be used to assess the prevalence of conditions in a population. However, since exposure and disease status are measured at the same point in time, causal statements could not be made from this type of studies. It is usually not possible to distinguish whether the exposure proceeded or followed the condition.

(As Cross Sectional studies are used in both Descriptive and Analytic Studies in Pharmacoepidemiology, it is further discussed on page No 15 of Chapter 8).

Analytical Studies (Quantitative Models)

Analytical studies are non-experimental studies of pharmacoepidemiology. They are also known as explanatory studies. (Exploratory research is research conducted for a problem that has not been clearly defined. Exploratory research helps determine the best research design, data collection method and selection of subjects.)

Case Control and Cohort Studies are examples of analytical non-experimental studies. The analytic studies compare an exposed group with a control group and are usually designed as **hypothesis testing studies**. They help find the explanations and examine causal processes like why does the ADR occur in the population? Sometimes the study may cover both the descriptive and the analytical aspects of the non- experimental study.

The Case Control and the Cohort Study are widely two important major types of pharmacoepidemiological studies of analytical nature. The modified versions of Case Control and Cohort are also having applications in pharmacoepidemiology and hence briefly mentioned .

A sample of patients are taken for the studies. Their exposure status and outcome status are determined. Then the findings are compared with the results obtained from a group that represents the non exposed population or the control group. This comparison helps us to assess the relative benefits or hazards of the drug in question. This type of assessments help us to test the hypothesis about proposed relationships between exposures and outcomes of the drug in question.

Case Control

Case control is the simplest and most commonly used analytical strategy in epidemiology. It is designed primarily to establish the causes of a disease by investigating association between exposure to a risk factor and the occurrence of the disease. The design is simple. It is a **backward looking or retrospective** study based on exposure histories of cases and controls. The risk factor is something that happened or began in the past. Information about the exposure is obtained by taking a history and /or from records and registers. Sometimes the suspected factor or attribute is a permanent one like blood group or sex. Generally case control studies are conducted when the outcome of interest is rare.

It assembles a group of patients who have a common disease of interest. These are the 'cases'. If the researcher is interested in determining whether a particular drug can cause aplastic anaemia which is rare among the population, he would first identify patients with aplastic anaemia. The 'control' group would be people who are representative of the underlying population from which the cases came but are without the disease. The idea of case control study is to compare the prevalence of exposure between the cases and the control.

Like Cohort Study it utilizes comparison group. The exposure histories of the cases and the controls are determined to establish the extent of association between the exposures of interest and disease. Case control studies compare patients with a specific disease with a control group of similar people but not having the disease. Here attempts are made to identify risk factors for a disease by analyzing differences between cases and controls in the antecedent exposure variables like age, sex, disease severity and women of child bearing age.

Illustration 4: The issue of relationship between use of oral contraceptive and the occurrence of ovarian cysts in women of child bearing age can be conducted. Here prior use of oral contraceptive in the age group can be selected as the cases. The controls are those without the prior use of oral contraceptives. Matching is important in case control as it is not possible to randomise patients into groups as in the case of RCTs. Case control studies are used when outcomes are rare and exposure to the drug is also rare.

The case control studies are widely used to assess the safety of medicines. Some examples of case control studies that could establish the association between the drugs and the adverse events are

(i) diethylstilbestrol (DES) and vaginal cancer,

(ii) aspirin and Reye's syndrome,

(iii) NSAIDs and peptic ulcer and

(iv) oral contraceptives and venous thromboembolism. See Fig. 8.2.

Data from case control studies are used to calculate an odd ratio, which is the ratio of the odds of developing the disease for exposed patients to the odds of developing the disease for unexposed patients.

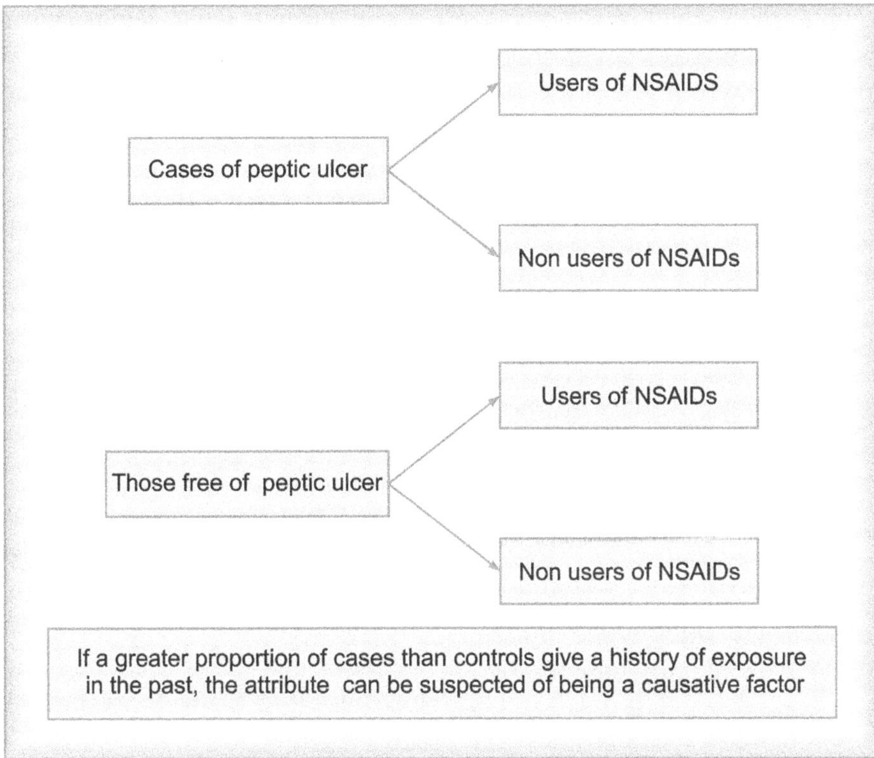

Figure 8.2 Example of case control study.

Nested case control study

A nested case control study is an efficient variation of a case control and a cohort study. In nested case control studies, all cases or a sample of all cases and only a random sample of all controls are chosen for study from the same defined population. The use of nested studies design was followed in studies to assess the role of potential confounding factors as in the case of study of inhaled corticosteroids and the risk of fatal and near-fatal asthma (Suissa.S. 2000).

Advantages and Disadvantages of Case Control studies

The main advantage of case control study for the drug outcome relationship is its efficacy for the study of rare or delayed outcomes. It measures strength or relationship, though causation is not certain. Compared to other methods like cohort study, it is relatively cheap. It is also quick and efficient. If results can be obtained from a database, then a study may be undertaken very quickly. It helps to assess not only rare outcomes, but also multiple exposures on a single outcome. It can be used to test hypothesis. Case control studies involve fewer participants in the study.

The disadvantage of the case control studies is their susceptibility towards certain types of bias including selection bias and information bias. Selection bias refers to systematic differences between those selected for study and those who are not.

Information bias is systematic differences in the quality of information gathered for study and comparison groups. It is inefficient for rare exposure. It is often difficult to establish temporal relationship between exposure and disease. Case control studies are inappropriate when outcome is not known.

Cohort Study

Methodologically cohort study is diametrically opposite of case control study. A cohort is a group. Hence a cohort study is a study of groups of patients having some common drug exposure of interest. Examples of Cohort include PharmD students of particular college of pharmacy, patients coming to a particular hospital, people with a particular genetic trait or adults admitted in a speciality hospital.

A cohort study assembles a group of persons without the disease of interest at the onset of the study. They are then followed over time and the experiences of the members of one cohort are compared with those in other cohorts in order to describe outcome among people whose exposure status is known. It helps to determine the development of disease in exposed and non exposed persons. Cohort studies involve the comparison of the incidence of one or more outcome events among those who received a drug with the incidence of events of the control group. To reduce the potential for bias, some researchers require that the study participants be members of the cohort for some time before the start of exposure. John Hopkins Hospital and the Boston Collaborative Drug Surveillance program developed the use of in-hospital monitors to perform cohort studies to explore the short- term effects of drug used in hospitals for the first time in the 1950s.

Cohort studies can be prospective or retrospective in nature.

Prospective Cohort Study

It is considered as the best type of cohort study as far as scientific evidence and control over the factors of interest are considered. It looks forward in time and allows the researcher maximum control over the study definition and its conduct. The potential confounding factors and variables that must be controlled in the study process can be defined and measured in prospective cohort studies. It is very expensive.

Retrospective Cohort Study

The retrospective cohort study looks back on existing data. Generally the data come from medical records and computer database. The major advantage of retrospective cohort study is its lower costs. The disadvantages include various forms of bias found in the study.

> **Illustration 5:** The risk of fatal cardiovascular diseases among oral contraceptive users has come from a study in which 23,000 oral contraceptive users were compared with 23,000 non- users chosen from the same British general practices. Records of death certificates were used to ascertain instances of fatal events during the follow up period (RCGP
>
> ***Contd...***

1974). It was a prospective study. Prospective cohort studies are one of the most valid types of observational study designs because exposure is measured and recorded prior to the development of the health outcomes of interest.

Hooten et al., studied the association between contraceptive methods and symptomatic urinary tract infection (UTI) in young women based on a prospective cohort study (Hooten TM, 1994). The study group recruited sexually active young women who were starting a new method of contraception and followed them for six months to determine the incidence of symptomatic UTI by contraceptive method.

Advantages and disadvantages of Cohort Studies

Cohort Studies are very useful for Hypothesis testing. It is one of the most powerful methods of pharmaco-epidemiology. Prospective cohort studies can provide strong evidence of association between drug and disease because the exposure is assessed before the outcome occurs. Some cohort studies may require large numbers of people for a long period of time and hence the study may become expensive, in some cases infeasible. Historical cohort study (retrospective cohort study) can overcome this limitation.

Very few non-experimental studies of drug interactions have been done. Since most patients are prescribed more than one drug at a time, the potential for drug interactions are ever present. Relevant studies can reduce potential interactions and their consequent effects. A cohort study can be a useful technique in this case.

Cohort studies utilize the natural history of diseases and determine multiple effect of single exposure. It helps to estimate incidence and risk of developing disease and can produce great deal of useful information.

The disadvantages of cohort study are many. The study requires large number of people as sample size. Even with large numbers there may not be sufficient patients to assess rare events. The studies are highly expensive and time consuming and may take years to complete. The study requires highly skilled management team. Validity of result depends on follow up and follow up is difficult in cohort studies.

Comparison of Case Control and Cohort Studies

Both Case Control and Cohort Studies are powerful analytical tools for testing Hypothesis in pharmacoepidemiology. The choice between them depends on the questions to be answered. Case Control studies are less expensive compared to Cohorts. In case control only the relative risk can be directly estimated with the help of odds ratio. In the case of Cohorts incidence rates can directly calculated and both relative and attributable risks can be determined. Cohort Studies often need large or huge number of patients while only a sample of the source population is needed in Case Control. Case control can give information on one or limited number of outcomes while Cohorts give information on a number of different outcomes.

Prospective and Retrospective Study Designs

A prospective study watches for outcomes, such as the development of an effect (beneficial or harmful) during the study period and relates this to other factors like suspected risk or protection factors. A retrospective study is a historic study where a search is made for a relationship between one phenomenon or condition and another that occurred in the past like exposure to a drug and the rate of occurrence of potential ADRs. We have seen that Case Control is often retrospective in nature while Cohort study can be prospective or retrospective or both.

It is to be noted that retrospective and prospective refer to the conduct of study rather than the actual design. A prospective Case Control study uses exposure date collected before the occurrence of outcome while a retrospective case control study uses exposure date collected after the development of the disease. Hence equating retrospective and prospective with Case Control and Cohort Study respectively is not correct. Hence if the study is appropriately designed and carried out, there is not much significance for whether it is retrospective or prospective in nature.

Other Methods Applied in Pharmacoepidemiology

Apart from the methods discussed in the earlier part, there are many other methods in pharmacoepidemiology which are used both in experimental and non-experimental studies. Some of them like Cross Sectional Study, Meta Analysis are having wide applications in all aspects of studies. Practicing health care professionals including pharmacists should need to know about the potential of Ecological studies in pharmacoepidemiology. We will discuss these methods in brief.

Cross-Sectional Study

Cross sectional studies may be of descriptive or analytical nature. Cross sectional studies are also known as "instantaneous studies", "simultaneous studies" or "prevalence studies". These are studies of the use of drugs at a specific point in time and are conducted through surveys, data base analysis or medication chart reviews.

Cross sectional studies help the collection of data on a cross section of population which may comprise the whole population or a proportion (sample) of it. This type of studies provides information about the situation that exists at a single time. A snap shot picture of the situation is obtained through a cross sectional study. This gives another name for the study - 'snapshot study'. This helps to provide an estimate of the prevalence of utilization and sometimes of the outcomes.

Many cross sectional studies do not aim at testing a hypothesis about an association, and are thus descriptive. They provide a prevalence at a particular point in time (point prevalence) or over a period of time (period prevalence).

In an analytical cross sectional study, the investigator measures exposure and disease simultaneously in a representative sample of the population. By taking a representative sample it is possible to generalize the results obtained in the sample for the population as a whole. Cross sectional studies measure the association between the exposure variable and the existing disease, that is the prevalence, in a defined population. (In cohort study the rate of developing the disease, that is the incidence is measured).

The cross sectional studies have been used to compare drug use between states or countries or regions. If the difference is very large, it suggests the reasons for those differences have to be studied to decide whether changes are to be made in the existing system. This type of studies can be used to analyze antibiotic use in a specific region or part. Such studies can identify problem areas and suggest where remedial actions are required.

Longitudinal study is also known as "time span study" and it provides data related to the study during a period of time. Studies, whether descriptive, analytical or both can be usefully categorized as *Cross sectional* or *Longitudinal* depending on the period of time covered by the observations.

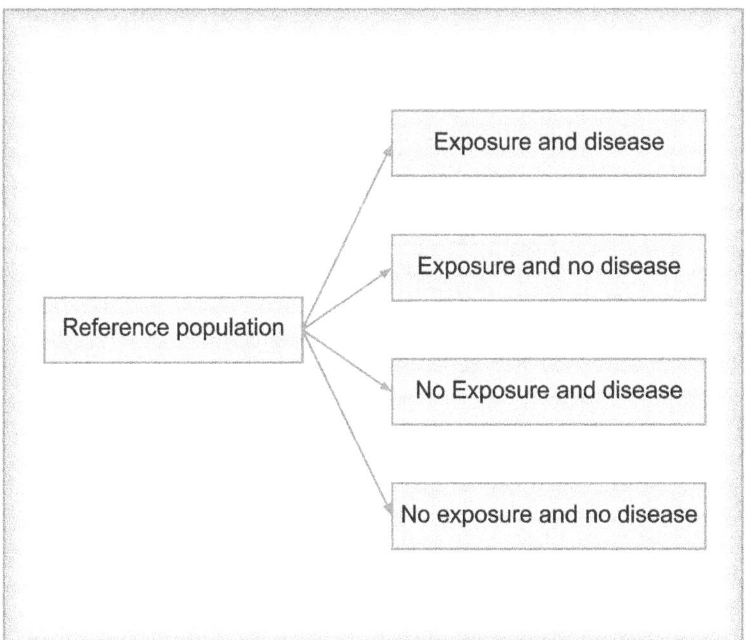

Figure 8.3 Example of design of cross sectional study.

Advantages and Disadvantages of Cross-Sectional Studies

Cross control studies have the advantage over case control studies of starting with a reference population from which the cases and controls are drawn. The studies can be of short term and therefore less expensive than prospective studies. The cross-sectional studies are the starting point in prospective cohort studies for screening out already existing conditions. They can provide a wealth of data that is of much use in health system research. Although not specific, cross sectional studies allow a risk statement.

The disadvantages include no direct estimate of risk and the scope for bias. Since exposure and disease are measured at the same point of time, it is not possible to establish temporality, that is, whether the exposure or presence of a characteristic preceded the development of the disease or condition.

Meta-Analysis

A meta-analysis (MA) is defined as systemic review that uses statistical techniques to integrate and summarise the results of included studies. Meta-analyses are often, but not always, important components of a systematic review procedure. A meta-analysis may be conducted on several clinical trials of a medical treatment, in an effort to obtain a better understanding of how well the treatment works.

Some people consider Meta-analysis as "conducting research about previous research." In Pharmacoepidemiology, it is the compilation of results from a group of studies to arrive at an overall summary estimate of the drug effect, namely benefit or risk. Meta analysis utilizes a variety of methods for aggregating results. The unit of analysis in a meta-analysis is the variable common to the studies being reviewed rather than the individual patient. It is a statistical analysis of a large collection of analytical results from, individual studies for the purpose of integrating the findings. It is a state of art review of literature employing statistical methods in conjunction with a thorough and systematic qualitative review. Meta analysis can be applied to RCT, Case Control or Cohort Studies. Meta-analysis combines the result of several studies that address a set of related research hypotheses.

Meta-analysis appears to be prone to the "garbage in, garbage out" phenomenon*. (**garbage in garbage out is used in computer or information technology to explain that the quality of output is determined by the quality of the input*) Combining a group of poorly done studies can produce a precise summary result made on a weak foundation. The method is not restricted to situations in which one or more variables is defined as "dependent." For example, a meta-analysis could be performed on a collection of studies each of which attempts to estimate the incidence of left-handedness in various groups of people.

Researchers should be aware that variations in sampling schemes can introduce heterogeneity to the result, which is the presence of more than one intercept in the solution. For instance, if some studies used 30 mg of a drug, and others used 50 mg, then we would plausibly expect two clusters to be present in the data, each varying around the mean of one dosage or the other. This can be modelled using a "random effects model."

Results from studies are combined using different approaches. One approach frequently used in meta-analysis in health care research is termed 'inverse variance method'. The average effect size across all studies is computed as a *weighted mean*, whereby the weights are equal to the inverse variance of each studies' effect estimator. Larger studies and studies with less random variation are given greater weight than smaller studies.

The first meta-analysis was performed by Karl Pearson in 1904. It was an attempt to overcome the problem of reduced statistical power in studies with small sample sizes. Analyzing the results from a group of studies can allow more accurate data analysis. Although meta-analysis is widely used in epidemiology and evidence-based medicine today, a meta-analysis of a medical treatment was not published until 1955. In the 1970s, more sophisticated analytical techniques were introduced in educational research.

Applications of Meta Analysis in Pharmacoepidemiology

Meta analysis can be used to solve the controversies when conflicting results are in existence in literature, by comparing the intensity and seriousness of differences with respect to their effects (both positive and negative). In one meta analysis relationship between cholesterol concentrations and occurrence of stroke was studied in 4,50,000 patients. In the case of non experimental studied (observational studies) the data will be more heterogeneous compared to experimental studies like RCT. Hence extreme care has to be taken while doing meta analysis on observational study data both for conducting the analysis and interpreting the results.

Strength and Weakness of a Meta-Analysis

The strength of the meta-analysis is that it includes all studies even though they are of differing quality. As a result of the meta-analysis, information from individual studies are lost. Another strength of meta-analysis is that it is not always reproducible by other analysts.

A weakness of the method is that sources of bias are not controlled by the method. A good meta-analysis of badly designed studies will still result in bad statistics. Robert Slavin has argued that only methodologically sound studies should be included in a meta-analysis, a practice he calls 'best evidence meta-analysis'. Other meta-analysts would include weaker studies, and add a study-level predictor variable that reflects the methodological quality of the studies to examine the effect of study quality on the effect size. Another weakness of the method is the heavy reliance on published studies, which may increase the effect as it is very hard to publish studies that show no significant results. This publication bias or "file-drawer effect" (where non-significant studies end up in the desk drawer instead of in the public domain) should be seriously considered when interpreting the outcomes of a meta-analysis.

Ecological Studies

In ecological studies, the unit of observation is an aggregate, a geographical administrative locality, a cluster of houses or hospitals, a town, a whole state or region or country. That is, a population is studied instead of a patient in ecological studies. There are situations when data are not obtained at the patient level, but there is interest in getting a preliminary understanding of the relationship between the use of the drug and an outcome. They help to relate the frequency with which some characteristic and some outcome is related in a geographic region. Ecological studies may take any of the forms of study like descriptive, case control, cross-sectional, cohort or experimental.

An example of the ecological study is the comparison of the number of prescriptions of â-adrenergic agonist inhalers dispensed in a country and the number of deaths from asthma. This type of relationship would be confounded by the increasing use of medication with increasing severity of illness. Sicker patients may use more â-adrenergic agonist inhalers. Another problem is that the investigator may not know whether the patients who died were even prescribed the medication. This dilemma of the investigator is known as "ecological fallacy".

Pharmacoepidemiology is the application of epidemiological methodologies for the study of drugs focusing on their use and effects in a large number of people. It is drug epidemiology.

CHAPTER 9

Systems to Study Drug Effects and Measurement of Outcomes in Pharmacoepidemiology

Chapter Mission

After learning this chapter you may be able to know:

- Systems to study drug effects at global levels.
- Facilities and system to study drug effects in India.
- Definition, need and classification of outcomes.
- Measurement of outcomes in pharmacoepidemiology.
- Common measures of outcomes in pharmacoepidemiology.

There are different systems to study the effects of drugs in populations. These systems are very much inter-related with Pharmacovigilance. Though they are often discussed along with Pharmacovigilance in detail, some of them are having important applications in pharmacoepidemiology and they are discussed in brief here.

Spontaneous Reporting

Spontaneous reports are so called because they take place instantaneously during the clinical investigation or normal diagnostic appraisal of a patient, or during a routine administration of medicines where a drug may be implicated in the causality of an adverse the event. The spontaneous reporting system is a widely used, effective, and relatively inexpensive method of collecting information on suspected ADRs. The spontaneous reporting system relies on vigilant physicians and other healthcare professionals who not only generate a suspicion of an ADR, but also report it. In many countries, the spontaneous reporting scheme has been extended to reporting from pharmacists, nurses, and even patients.

Spontaneous reporting is a cost effective system to follow the safety of all drugs during their entire lifecycle and also the most important source of information for regulatory actions such as taking a drug off the market or a label change due to safety problems. Spontaneous reporting of ADRs from health professionals is important for detection of signals indicating new ADRs. It is a basic method for post marketing surveillance. The spontaneous reporting in recent improved very much when new categories of healthcare providers like clinical pharmacists, hospital pharmacists and community pharmacists were included as reporters.

An adverse event is serious when it results in death, is life-threatening, requires inpatient hospitalization or prolongation of existing hospitalization, results in persistent or significant disability/incapacity, or is a congenital anomaly/birth defect . The World Health Organisation (WHO) in 1968 established the program for reporting adverse drug reactions. When a physician suspects a serious clinical event to be an ADR, they are encouraged to complete a questionnaire and notify the country's drug regulatory agency about the suspected ADR. The pharmaceutical industry and regulatory bodies collect and analyze these reports and utilize them in identifying previously unknown adverse reactions and where appropriate take action to minimize the risk due to the drug.

The spontaneous reporting questionnaire differs from country to country. However in general the information collected includes patient details like age, sex, weight etc., and details on the suspected drug like dose, duration of treatment, manufacturer, batch number etc. Details on the suspected reaction such as description of the event, seriousness, outcome, medical history of the patient, and other concomitant medication that the patient was taking are also registered for analysis. Withdrawals due to safety problems were often based on data from spontaneous reporting systems.

Limitations of Spontaneous Report System

The spontaneous reporting system has some shortcomings. Under-reporting is one. Another weakness of the system is that it only provides a numerator and the information on population exposed to the drug is lacking. Therefore, the risk associated with a drug is difficult to quantify accurately. The spontaneous reporting system is a passive surveillance method that solely relies on the healthcare professionals to detect and take the initiative to report an ADR. Reporting varies with the reporters' skill and experience to detect the ADR, their level of understanding of the spontaneous reporting system, and their workload. Furthermore, ADR reporting is also influenced by other factors such as the media, published literature, and age of the drug. Other weaknesses include variations in the quality of information provided and missing data. However, in spite of the limitations spontaneous reporting is the backbone of pharmacovigilance and provides valuable information on the safety of a drug throughout its life.

Effective Spontaneous Reporting Systems

The most effective spontaneous reporting systems include:

1. "Yellow card scheme" operated by the UK. Medicines and Healthcare Products Regulatory Agency (MHRA) and the Commission on Human Medicines,
2. Adverse Event Reporting System (AERS).
3. MedWatch operated by FDA of USA.

Yellow Card Scheme

The Scheme was established in 1964 after the thalidomide disaster. It was developed by Bill Inman. It is today run by the Medicines and Healthcare Products Regulatory Agency (MHRA) and the Commission on Human Medicines (CHM). Suspected ADRs are collected on all licensed medicines and vaccines, from those issued on prescription to medicines bought over the counter from a pharmacist or supermarket. The Scheme also includes all herbal preparations and unlicensed medicines. ADRs can be reported by anyone. Often the reporting is done by healthcare professionals like doctors, pharmacists and nurses. However patients and their care givers can also make reports under the scheme. Yellow card are available from all Pharmacies in UK.

ADRs that should be reported under Yellow Card System are:

ADRs that have caused death or a serious illness

Any ADR, however minor, if it is associated with a new medicine.

Any ADR however minor if associated with a medicine that is under continued monitoring (highlighted in the British National Formulary (BNF) with a ¼% black triangle.

Any ADR, however minor, if associated with a child (under 18 years of age) or in pregnancy.

The Adverse Event Reporting System (AERS) of USA

The Adverse Event Reporting System (AERS) is a computerized information database designed to support the post marketing safety surveillance program of U.S. Food and Drug Administration (FDA) for all approved drug and therapeutic biologic products. The FDA uses AERS to monitor for new adverse events and medication errors that might occur with their marketed products. AERS is a database of spon-taneous reports received by the US Food and Drug Administration (FDA) through the MedWatch form.

MedWatch of US FDA

MedWatch is the ADR reporting system of US Food and Drug Administration established in 1993 to collect data related to adverse events in health care including adverse event or sentinel event (an unexpected occurrence involving death or serious physical or psychological injury, or the risk thereof). The system includes publicly available databases and online analysis tools for professional.

The MedWatch system collects reports of adverse reactions and quality problems, primarily with drugs and medical devices. It also collects adverse effects for other FDA-regulated products like dietary supple-ments, medical food, infant items and cosmetics. Voluntary reporting by healthcare professionals, consumers, and patients is conducted on a single, one-page reporting form (Form FDA 3500).

Reporting can be done online, by phone 1-800-FDA-1088, or by submitting the MedWatch 3500 form by mail or fax 1-800-FDA-0178. In 2013, MedWatch introduced Form 3500B, which is designed to facilitate reporting by healthcare consumers. The MedWatch system is intended to detect safety hazard signals for medical products. If a signal is detected, the FDA can issue medical product safety alerts or order product recalls, withdrawals, or labelling changes to protect the public health.

Other Countries

Getting inspired from the impact of the UK and US systems of spontaneous report of ADRs of medicines and other items including dietary supplements and cosmetics, many other countries in the world introduced similar schemes in their countries including India, Japan and Australia.

In Canada, Health Canada is the regulatory body that approves drugs. Health Canada has a division called "Marketed Health Products Directorate" (MHPD) which coordinates Canadian post marketing surveillance. In European Union, the guidance document "MEDDEV 2.12-1 rev 8" offers a comprehensive guidance on best practice for 'medical device post-market surveillance' (materiovigilance). A manufacturer of medical devices is required to report incidents (serious adverse events) to the national competent authority of the member state the company resides in.

ARISg

ARISg is the Drug Safety Software used by Pharmaceutical Companies. ARISg is a leading pharmacovigilance and clinical safety system, with more than 300 major companies maintaining their critical drug safety data in ARISg worldwide. It provides all the functional requirements for managing adverse event reporting and adverse reaction requirements of different authorities around the world. ARISg enables companies to monitor their products and identify safety risks. Its activities extend from case entry to automatic generation of submission ready adverse event (AE) reports including CIOMS I, MedWatch 3500A and many more.

Spontaneous Reporting System in India

Inspired by the WHO initiative in 1968, pharmacovigilance programs were initiated in certain Indian hospitals like CMC Vellore in the late 1970s. Later it was extended to some other hospitals also and was in existence in India since 1980s in a planned and organised manner. However, the National Pharmacovigilance program was launched in 2005 by the Central Drugs Standard Control Organization (CDSCO) of the Government of India. CDSCO has initiated a nation-wide Pharmacovigilance Programme of India (PvPI) in collaboration with the Indian Pharmacopeia commission and established several pharmacovigilance centers in the country.

Prescription Event Monitoring

Prescription-event monitoring (PEM) is a non-interventional method for post-marketing drug safety monitoring of newly licensed medicines. PEM as a prescription-based monitoring system was introduced in UK in the 1980s at the Drug Safety Research Unit to study large cohorts of drug users. Utilizing the distinct structure of the UK National Health Service (NHS), PEM today enables the generation and testing of hypotheses regarding drug alerts or "signals" that may be of public health interest. PEM is a non-interventional, observational cohort form of pharmaco-vigilance. It is non-interventional in the sense that nothing happens to interfere with the doctor's decision regarding which drug to prescribe for each individual patient.

PEM is a hypothesis generating method like spontaneous ADR reporting. It is also used for testing hypothesis related to ADR in defined population of drug users. PEM and Spontaneous reporting constitute the backbone of the post marketing surveillance techniques developed to survey the use of newly marketed medicines.

Post Marketing Surveillance

Post marketing surveillance (PMS) is also known as post market surveillance. PMS is the practice of monitoring the safety of a drug or medical device after it has been released on the market and is an important aspect of pharmacovigilance. It evaluates drugs taken by individuals under a wide range of circumstances over an extended period of time. Such surveillance is much more likely to detect previously unrecognized positive or negative effects that may be associated with a drug.

Drugs are approved for marketing based on the basis of clinical studies/ trials which involve relatively small numbers of people who have been selected for this purpose. People involved in clinical trials normally do not have other medical conditions which may exist in the general population. PMS can further refine, or confirm or deny, the safety of a drug after it is used in the general population by large numbers of people who have a wide variety of medical conditions.

The majority of post marketing surveillance concern adverse drug reactions (ADRs) monitoring and evaluation. Other important post marketing surveillance components include unapproved or off-label drug use, problems with orphan drugs, and lack of paediatric formulations, as well as issues concerning international clinical trials in paediatric population.

Post marketing surveillance uses a number of approaches to monitor the safety of licensed drugs, including spontaneous reporting databases, prescription event monitoring, health records (both electronic and manual) patient register (both electronic and manual) and other administrative databases in health care. Such well-established PMS programs are available in countries like USA, UK, Canada and European Union. In USA the Food and Drug Administration oversees the program while the Medicines and Healthcare Products Regulatory Agency (MHRA) overlooks it in UK jointly with the Commission on Human Medicines. In Canada the drug regulatory body is Health Canada which has a division called 'Marketed Health Products Directorate' to supervise the PMS activities.

Why post marketing surveillance and ADR reporting needed?

The information collected during the pre-marketing phase of drug development is inevitably incomplete with regard to possible ADRs. This is mainly because:

- Tests in animals are insufficient to predict human safety.
- Patients used in clinical trials are selected and limited in number. The conditions of use differ from those in clinical practice and the duration of trials is limited.
- By the time of licensing exposure of less than 5000 human subjects to a drug allows only the more common ADR to be detected.
- At least 30,000 people need to be treated with a drug to be sure that you do not miss at least one patient with an ADR which has an incidence of 1 in 10,000 exposed individuals.
- Information about rare but serious adverse reactions, chronic toxicity, use in special groups (such as children, the elderly or pregnant women) or drug interactions is often incomplete or not available.

Thus, post-marketing surveillance is important to permit detection of less common, but sometimes very serious ADRs. Therefore health professionals worldwide should report on ADRs as it can save lives of their patients and others.

Record/ Data linkage Systems

In the past it was very difficult to maintain the registers and records in health care for long periods, say beyond 5 years. Though hospitals were maintaining the case sheets and registers in their record rooms or library, they were difficult to use after certain period of time due to damages or decomposition of papers and the writings. It was difficult to monitor the prescriptions and their dispensing in hospitals and community pharmacies. The analysis and compilation of data was very difficult and time consuming.

With the introduction of computers and the application of information technology in health care, record keeping and maintenance of registry became possible and easy. The data analysis and compilation became quick and perfect. However in India, the situation is not very much encouraging as the computerisation is yet to be introduced in many health care centers as well as in a large majority of Community Pharmacies. The net working is also very poor in the country in health care. The hospitals are keeping the data as their private documents due to the absence of agencies to govern such aspects.

We have already seen the Indian data system in par with those in other countries like USA, UK, Canada both in this chapter and other chapters of this book. In the case of using record linkage databases it is important to have validation process to get useful information and results.

Measurement of Outcome of Drug Use

Introduction

While discussing the systems of drug effects, we could see the inter-relationship between Pharmacoepidemiology and Pharmacovigilance. In the case of outcomes we can see the existence of a similar relationship between Pharmacoepidemiology and Pharmacoeconomics. Here in this chapter we are discussing the outcome of drugs from the view point of pharmacoepidemiology.

There is a wide range of important health outcomes. Historically, death and disease were the outcomes of interest to physicians. (Refer Box 9.1). However, disability, discomfort, and dissatisfaction now are also recognized as critically important outcomes. Disability, in particular, has received a great deal of attention as an important health outcome.

The World Health Organization International Classification of Function describes three separate levels of disablement-impairment, activity limitation, and participation restriction, all of which present separate measurement issues. Activity limitation is the focus of a wide range of outcome measures that differ greatly in terms of the specific activities included. These measures also employ a variety of measurement dimensions, including amount of assistance, degree of difficulty, frequency, time, and quality. In addition to disability measures, the broad concept of health-related quality of life (HRQOL) has become an outcome of interest.

Box 9.1 Outcomes of Disease - The 5 Ds

1. Death	:	A bad out come
2. Disease	:	A set of symptoms, physical signs, and laboratory abnormalities
3. Discomfort	:	Symptoms such as pain, nausea, and itching
4. Disability	:	Impaired ability to go about usual activities at home, work, or recreation
5. Dissatisfaction	:	Emotional reaction to disease and its care, such as sadness or anger

Definition of Outcome

Though an Outcome vocabulary has evolved in health care there is no consensus on the best approach to define and measure outcomes. Because of this situation, outcome means different to different people. The terminology uses by professionals involved health care outcome research is not standardized and hence definition used by one person or group of persons or an organization can vary significantly from that used by others.

In treatments and health care programs outcomes are the result of treatment or care and includes both positive and negative results. Outcomes are consequences or results of care or lack of care. Outcome assessment helps to evaluate the care delivery process. Patient's assessments of own health and evaluation of quality of care are also involved in the definition of outcome.

Outcomes in Studies

The outcome of a study is a broad term for any defined disease, state of health, or pharmacotherapy. In some studies, there may be multiple outcomes. The exposures and outcomes of interest are specific to study hypotheses and should always be clearly defined before the study starts. We measure health outcomes to help us make decisions about managing our patients.

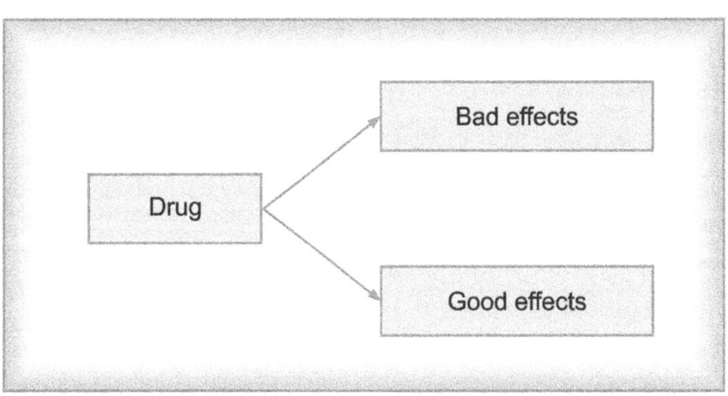

Outcome measures help us predict which patients will benefit most from a particular intervention and to document whether the patient improves after the intervention is provided. There is a wide range of important health outcomes, including disability and quality of life.

The term risk factor is often used to describe an exposure variable. The exposure of interest in one study may be the outcome in another. For example, smoking is clearly the exposure of interest in a study that examines whether smokers are more likely to develop lung cancer than non-smokers. It would be the outcome in a study examining the effectiveness of an anti-smoking intervention programme in reducing the frequency of smoking in a certain population.

Need for Outcome Studies

The health care costs are escalating continuously. It generates more and more interest in the area of cost containment programs without compromising quality of services. With the popularisation of health insurance in the developed countries, managed care organisations (MCOs) and large employer groups started using outcome measurement tools to identify, measure and evaluate the results of care. Even government agencies also examine their return on investments. These organisations measure and evaluate their return on investment to make effective business decisions for the future. Conduct of outcome studies help to empower the health care organisations to determine which treatment or therapy program gives better clinical, humanistic and cost effective outcomes for their members and also to validate the outcome of care. Clinical researchers, clinicians, epidemiologists, statisticians and economists are becoming more actively involved in outcome research and measurement.

Classification of Outcomes

Although outcome measures are continuously evolving, they give valid information to clinicians for choosing best therapeutic plan for specific conditions and situations. In the past clinical measures were focussed on mortality and morbidity. Today clinical effects go beyond the traditional markers of morbidity (disease) and mortality (death) and include a number of other aspects like economic and humanistic aspects. It also address the effects of treatment on the patients quality of life and ability to function.

It can be seen that often outcomes are classified according to the perspective of the users of the data. Managed Care Organisations including Insurance firms choose outcomes that focus on cost effective service in the set ups, balancing cost and quality of care by improving the care delivery activities. Physicians are interested in the clinical results. Clinical measures are also known as physical measures. Patients are interested on aspects like functional status (performance level) and Patient satisfaction. Functional status is also known as performance level and take into consideration factors like ability to work, need of supervision or support by care givers or others.

Patient satisfaction is measured based on a number factors of like impact on their health, quality of life and hazards or inconveniences caused or effects of daily activities. Clinical or therapeutic outcomes can be grouped into Improvement (success) or deterioration/ worsening or no change in the condition. See Box 9.2.

Box 9.2 Classification of Outcomes

Clinical results	Improvement in the condition, deterioration/worsening of condition or no change in the condition.
Functional Status	Factors like ability to work, level of functioning, whether supervision needed or not.
Patient satisfaction	Various aspects of care like delivery care, effect on daily activities or life satisfaction.
Economic measures	Here the factors like cost of financial burden and the benefits obtained are noted.
Humanistic measures	Various aspects of quality of life (QOL) are included here.

Measurement of Outcome and the Tools Used

Measurement is an abstraction. It involves developing a set of rules to assign numbers to represent a concept. The rules must provide a precise system for assigning numerical values to different levels of the concept. To understand something, we must be able to measure it. Without measurement we may be able to say that someone is fat or thin. However, without some way of assigning numbers to represent body mass, it would be very difficult to accurately determine whether someone is fatter than someone else or whether someone's body mass has increased or decreased. It would certainly be impossible to determine how body mass relates to other things, such as fitness, health, or risk of disease. We measure health outcomes to help us make decisions about providing care for our patients. Outcome measures help us predict which patients will benefit most from a particular intervention and to document whether the patient improves after the intervention is provided.

Definition of outcome measurement

Outcome measurement is defined as the systematic quantitative analysis of the outcome indicators at a point of time. These measures are used to find out whether the goals of patients were identified and achieved. The outcome indicators measure performance of *functions, process* and *outcomes* over a period of time.

Research groups are continuously designing outcome tools that will help to measure the results of various interventions in health care. They are searching for effective and efficient treatments and programs that can produce positive outcomes when implemented in day-to-day clinical practice and pharmacotherapy programs.

Common Measures of Pharmaco-epidemiological Outcomes

Pharmacoepidemiological outcomes are generally measured by statistical methods like prevalence, incidence, cumulative incidence and incidence rate. Drug use measures like number of prescriptions, units of drugs dispensed, monetary units, defined daily doses (DDDs) and prescribed daily doses (PDD) are widely used in pharmaco-epidemiological research throughout the world. Apart from such methods surveys of therapy and diagnosis are also used to measure the outcomes in pharmaco-epidemiology.

Prevalence

Prevalence in pharmacoepidemiology is the proportion of people affected with the exposure of a particular drug in a population at a specified time. It is a measure of the 'status quo' of people affected or exposed to a drug in a population at a fixed point of time or during a specified period. Prevalence is the proportion of people affected by or exposed to a drug at the specified point or period of time.

Prevalence is typically obtained from cross sectional studies like surveys and occasionally based on registers of people exposed or affected. It can vary between 0 and 1 and is often expressed as cases per 1000 exposures or population. The prevalence at any given time is called the "point prevalence" and for a year is called "annual prevalence". If there are 1000 patients with epilepsy in a district of 10,00000 population, the prevalence of epilepsy in that district will be 1000 / 10,00000 or 1/1000 or 0.01 per cent. Prevalence (P) depends on previous incidence (I) and the duration of the disease (D). When both the incidence and the duration are relatively stable, P = (I x D). Hence prevalence can change over time depending on changes in incidence, changes in disease duration or intervention programs.

Incidence

Incidence measures the occurrence of new cases of disease or outcome. It is a measure of the frequency with which new disease events occur, and the rate at which people free from disease develop the disease during a specified period of observation. Generally a period of one year is used for the measure of incidence. The important aspects of incidence are

(i) the need to define the population of interest which is often known as 'inception cohort',

(ii) all the persons in the inception cohort should be free of disease,

(iii) a period of observation should be specified,

(iv) all persons should be followed for the specified period,

(v) in the case of incomplete follow up (as in the case of follow up for less than the specified period) the estimates of incidence should be appropriately adjusted.

In the case of descriptive studies two measures of incidence are commonly used – cumulative incidence and incidence density or incidence rate.

Cumulative Incidence

When all the people in the population of interest have been followed up for the specified period, the number of new cases of disease / out come divided by the size of the population gives the cumulative incidence. It is a proportion and is a measure of risk of acquiring the disease or outcome in that population over the specified period. It is a longitudinal measure, that is time dependent. It is normally measured with an inception cohort. That is, a large group of population is observed over a period and the number of cases or outcome is measured. The cumulative incidence is expressed either as a percentage or proportion per unit time. If there are 100 new cases of epilepsy in a district of 10,00000 population, the incidence of epilepsy in that district will be 100 / 10,00000 or 1/10000.

Incidence Density or Incidence Rate

It is the number of new cases that appear over the amount of person- time at risk. It is generally expressed as cases/ person – year exposures. For example in a study of ADR of Ampicillin, 100 patients were followed for six months, and 100 patients were followed for one year. A total of 40 persons developed GI discomfort. The total observations is 1800 person- months or 150 person-years. Here the incidence density or incidence rate will be 40/150 person-years of exposure to ampicillin.

Drug Use Measures

Pharmacoepidemiological outcome measures like prevalence, incidence, cumulative incidence and incidence rate data regarding drug use in population is needed. Various sources can be used for such situations and some of them are mentioned here.

Number of Prescriptions

Prescriptions are widely used in pharmaco-ecomic studies as they are easy to obtain. The prescriptions need to be produced in community pharmacies and hospital pharmacies for obtaining medicines. However there may be variations with respect to dose, dosage form and duration of use in individual prescriptions. The quantities dispensed from the pharmacies may vary with the prescribed quantity for various reasons. Normally prescription number analysis is used to get rough estimates like percentage of analgesic drugs, oral contraceptives or antibiotics used by the population. It helps to give a comparatively good estimate of number of people exposed to certain drugs or number of episodes of treatment programs in our health care. This type of studies also help to find whether there is increase in the number of prescription during certain periods.

Units of Drugs Dispensed

Units of drugs represent measures like number of capsules or tablets or doses of vaccines. Compared to number of prescriptions, it is easy to find the number of drug dispensed. This type of studies help to analyze the drug use trends in various countries or various states or territories of a country. It too has limitations like units of drugs dispensed need not always reflect the actual number of drugs used by population. People may not use certain dispensed medicines for various reasons. However studies on units of drugs dispensed helps to compare the hypotheses generated related to drug use like over use or under use.

Monetary Units

The most common and generally used practice in estimation of drug use is to quantify the value of medicines in monetary units like rupees, dollar, pounds, euros or other similar units. This will help to find the percentage of financial burden for individuals, family, society, organizations or governments for drug use. It will help for comparisons at various levels from persons to global. A paracetamol tablet may cost one rupee in India can have a cost of five rupees in the middle east countries and 15 rupees in USA. In such a situation the measurement of drug use in monetary units may net help to give a clear picture when countries are compared. However it is useful in comparing within a similar set up. Similarly a drug may have different dosage forms and strengths in market and the price may vary for them. Unless corrective measures are taken there can be errors while estimating the monetary value of drug use.

Defined Daily Doses (DDDs)

The defined daily dose (DDD) is a statistical measure of drug consumption, defined by the World Health Organization (WHO). It is used to standardize the comparison of drug usage between different drugs or between different health care environments. The DDD is not to be confused with the therapeutic dose or with the dose actually prescribed by a physician for an individual patient.

According to WHO "The DDD is the assumed average maintenance dose per day for a drug used for its main indication in adults." If the DDD for a certain drug is given, the number of DDDs used by an individual patient or (more commonly) by a collective of patients is as follows.

$$\text{Drug usage (DDDs)} = \frac{\text{Items issued} \times \text{Amount of drug per item}}{\text{DDD}}$$

For example take the case of Paracetamol (Acetaminophen) as a pain killer (analgesic). If it is having a DDD or 3 g, it means that an average patient who uses Paracetamol as a pain killer (main indication) uses 3 grams in a day or within a period of 24 hours. This is equivalent to six standard tablets of 500 mg each. If a patient consumes 24 such tablets (12 g of paracetamol in total) over a certain span of time, this equals a consumption of four DDDs.

$$\text{Drug usage (DDDs)} = \frac{24 \times 500\,\text{mg}}{3\,\text{g}} = 4$$

Doses for individual patients and patient groups will often differ from the DDD and will necessarily have to be based on individual characteristics (e.g., age and weight) and pharmacokinetic considerations. For the optimal use of drugs, it is important to recognize that genetic polymorphism due to ethnic differences can result in variations in pharmaco-kinetics of drugs. The DDD should reflect the global dosage irrespective of genetic variations of drug metabolism.

Drug consumption data presented in DDDs only give a rough estimate of consumption and not an exact picture of actual use. The DDD provide a fixed unit of measurement independent of price and dosage form. It helps the researcher to assess trends in drug consumption and to perform comparisons between population groups.

Drug utilization expressed in DDDs is generally reported by controlling for population size differences (e.g., per 1000 persons), providing a measure of drug exposure or "therapeutic intensity" in a defined population. This allows for the comparison of results across various time periods and populations groups. The following measures are commonly used

DDD per 1000 inhabitants per day

This measure is generally employed for medication used in the treatment of chronic conditions. A result of 10 DDD per 1000 inhabitants per year is interpreted as follows: in a representative group of 1000 inhabitants, 10 DDDs of the drug are utilized, on average, on any given day of the year studies.

DDD per inhabitant per year

This measure is normally employed for drugs generally used in acute treatment. A result of 10 DDD per inhabitant per year is equivalent to an average of 10 days of treatment with a certain medication per inhabitant per year.

DDD per 100 bed days

This measure is applied in analyses of in-hospital drug use. A result of 10 DDD per 100 bed days is the equivalent of 10% of the in-patients receiving the medication, on average, daily.

Advantages and Disadvantages of DDDs

The DDDs was developed as a standard measure of drug utilization that solves the problems of number of prescriptions, units of drugs dispensed and the monetary units of drug use. However it has certain limitations. The DDD is a technical unit of comparison and many drugs are not yet assigned the DDDs. Pediatric uses are often not considered in the calculations. Problems can also arise when doses vary widely as in the case of Aspirin which in low doses are used in cardiology while high doses are used for inflammatory conditions.

Prescribed Daily Doses

The prescribed daily dose (PDD) is defined as the average dose prescribed as calculated from a representative sample of prescriptions. The PDD gives the average amount of a drug that is actually prescribed. The PDD can be determined from studies of prescriptions or medical or pharmacy records. It is important to relate the PDD to the diagnosis on which the dosage is based.

The PDD is useful for validating the DDD. In the case of drug drugs where the recommended dosage differs from one indication to another (e.g., the anti-psychotics), it is important to link the diagnosis to the PDD. Pharmaco-epidemiological information (e.g., on sex, age, number of drugs in use) is also important in order to interpret a PDD.

The PDD can vary according to both the illness treated and national therapeutic traditions. In the case of anti-infectives, PDDs can vary according to the severity of the infection treated. The PDDs also vary substantially between different countries and this should always be considered while making international comparisons.

It should be noted that the PDD does not necessarily reflect actual drug utilization. Some prescribed medications are not dispensed, and the patient does not always take all the medications that are dispensed. Specially designed studies including patient interviews are required to measure actual drug intake at the patient level, that is, . the *consumed daily dose* .

Survey of Therapy and Diagnosis

Survey data related to prescriptions of clinicians and the rates of diseases encountered in practice are also useful in pharmacoepidemiological studies to measure the outcomes. In many countries established organizations and agencies are collecting such information and make it available in their databases. In India researchers have to depend on local data collected by themselves as no computer system is in existence to survey the prescriptions or registering the details for the use of studies and research.

Pharmacoepidemiology is the application of epidemiological methodologies for the study of drugs focusing on their use and effects in a large number of people. It is drug epidemiology.

CHAPTER 10

Areas in Pharmacoepidemiology Research

Chapter Mission

After learning this chapter you may be able to know:

- Problems of pharmacoepidemiology in India.
- Areas of research in pharmacoepidemiology.
- Pharmacoepidemiological publications in India.
- Need for research in pharmacoepidemiology in India.
- Role of pharmacists in pharmacoepidemiology.
- Design of research projects in pharmacoepidemiology.

Pharmacoepidemiology is an emerging bridge between the fields of Clinical Pharmacology and Clinical Epidemiology. Pharmacy Practice can provide valuable contributions to Pharmacoepidemiology which can help to frame policies based on principles of 'evidence based medicine'. There is tremendous scope for pharmaco-epidemiological research in India where the drug consumption is so large.

Problems in Pharmacoepidemiology in India

The field of pharmacoepidemiology faces problems in certain key areas. These problems include methodological as well as logistical. In the case of methodological problems there is difficulty in studies of rare effects of infrequently used medicines as the sample to be attained is huge. There is also difficulty in studying drug effects. Available databases have not been in existence for long enough to make this type of study reliable and efficient. Data collection is also very poor and ad hoc in nature. There is also difficulty in identifying reliable screening methods for adverse drug effects and Case reports have led to many false positive findings in the past .

Among the logistical problems faced by Indian Pharmacoepidemiology, manpower requirement for the studies constitute one of the lead problems. With the increase in interest and funding of drug related projects and the introduction of programs like PharmD in 2008 in India, it may be solved in the very near future. Another related problem is training of the interested individuals in this field. Many Universities in the world including Indian institutions offer courses on Pharmacoepidemiology at PG (both degree and diploma) and / PhD levels. Today pharmacoepidemiology has emerged as a bridge between the fields of Pharmacy Practice and Clinical Epidemiology. There is tremendous scope for research in the area Pharmacoepidemiology in India as the production and consumption of medicines are very high in terms of quantity.

Pharmacoepidemiological Studies in Medical Field

Factors like lack of financial support for research from the administration of medical and other health institutions, the difficulty in procuring and maintaining laboratory animals, control and monitoring on recruiting patients or healthy volunteers, problems faced in conducting experiments etc., compelled many medical researchers to opt pharmacoepidemiology as their area of research during the past few decades. During the 1990s and 2000 AD, the number of papers presented in the regional and national conferences in this discipline has been on the rise, but not seem to add anything new to the existing knowledge of drug use in our country. Pharmaco-epidemiology has found a niche among pharmacologists who are happy to embrace it as "pencil and paper" research, more for reasons of convenience rather than that of genuine interest (Geetanjali B 2003).

According to the editorial appeared on Indian Journal of Pharmacology in 2003, the problems associated with Pharmaco-epidemiological studies in India included issues like serious methodological flaws, improper or non-existent sampling techniques, lack of calculation of sample size, absence of statistical analysis and very superficial treatment of the subject matter. Though Pharmacoepidemiology, by its very definition, lends itself to large variety of study designs, for reasons not well known, Indian researchers seem to be interested in conducting only quantitative drug utilization studies leaving qualitative and experimental aspects in total. While these studies are necessary for hypothesis generation, why researchers are found not much interested in testing a hypothesis or conducting interventional studies? (Geetanjali B 2003).

Till 2010, most of the Indian study papers in the area of Pharmacoepidemiology consisted of analysing a specific number of prescriptions and looking at the different classes of drugs prescribed, the number of drugs per prescription, the number of fixed dose drug formulations, injectables and so on. However, in recent times, studies from pharmacy practice took the studies to further steps of assessing whether the prescriptions are rational or not wherever standard treatment guidelines are available. Quantifying the drug use with the support of internationally accepted measures such as 'Defined Daily Dose' and 'Unit Dose Dispensing' are also conducted by certain practicing pharmacists and students of pharmacy practice in their local situations.

Pharmacoepidemiological Studies by Pharmacists

Clinical Pharmacists and Pharmacologists planning to carry out research in pharmaco-epidemiology should take care to learn and understand the essential concepts of epidemiological research and ensure that the basic principles are reasonably addressed during planning and design of the study. It is to be noticed that till 1990s, studies which compared the drug utilization patterns of various departments in health care facilities by looking at "n" prescriptions were "publishable" material in standard Journals in India.

Any study describing factors which affect drug use in the community, be it compliance to therapy or genetic factors of patients, must use the appropriate sampling techniques and methods to draw valid conclusions. Citing the example of earlier studies which lacked these requisites is no more justifiable in India. As in any other field, research should be conducted using methods appropriate and commensurate with the achievements in the field.

The prudent use of antibiotics can be analysed from the following aspects:

(a) Rational use

(b) Extent of adherence to local therapeutic guidelines and antibiotic policies and

(c) Reversal of resistance trends.

(d) Compliance/ Adherence

(e) Serious Adverse Drug Reactions

However often it is found that only the first component is studied, that too in a cursory manner. Not taking their research further and deeper, most researchers prefer to study another class of drugs using the very same setting, design, questionnaire so that they can have another study without efforts. Why are Indian researchers restrict themselves to observational studies and are seemingly wary of conducting interventional studies and RCTs? We have to examine and analyse seriously.

Areas of Research in Pharmacoepidemiology

The areas of research in the discipline of Pharmacoepidemiology is vast. In the past most research in Pharmacoepidemiology were focussed on the study of selected areas of drug use like usage and adverse effects. Even with adverse effects, the information collected was only partial. There are many areas for carrying out research in Pharmacoepidemiology and some of them are noted below:

Drug Usage Studies

Drug usage studies at periodic intervals in a general population covering urban and rural areas are vital in pharmacoepidemiological studies. If carried out once it can serve as a barometer for the future health model and help to predict changes in the usage of prescription and non-prescription medicines. In this era of computers, large pharmacoepidemiology databases can be created with the help of internet for drug utilization studies with the individual user as the statistical unit. Various measures of drug utilization are currently known and can be applied in studies.

Drafting of Policies Related to Drug Usage

Policy makers in health care and the health care professionals always aim to improve medication use and ensure medicine safety. They require information as to how to integrate strategies and interventions that have been shown to be effective. Study report on overall system of events that are implemented to improve medication use are highly useful. Once done, policy makers can be provided with information on how to coordinate and orchestrate the activities that support quality use of medicines. Pharmacoepidemiological studies help to draft policies by providing evidence in 'evidence -based medicine'

Studies on Pharmacogenomics

Patient response variations due to genetic variation. It is an area which needs due consideration. The Pharmacogenomics look after such aspects in medicine use. The genetic response to drug metabolism and pharmacokinetics needs to be studied under the discipline of either pharmacogenomics or genetic epidemiology. Population characteristics are studied by invoking principles in population genetics, molecular biology, biostatistics and pharmacoepidemiology. The ultimate focus of the area will be the optimal usage of drugs based on the genetic classifications. In India there is lot of scope and need for such studies.

Drug and Therapeutic Committees

Drug and Therapeutic Committees (also known as Pharmacy and Therapeutic Committees) play an important role in the determination of drug utilization by patients in hospitals. It is important to study the structure, activities and drug selection processes followed by these Committees. Studies are also needed with respect to the responsibilities, and the guidelines of these Committees. Studies in other countries found that these Committees quite often work without guidelines and transparency . They often pass the responsibilities to the hospital pharmacists or clinicians. In India it is essential to study the formation and functioning of such Committees in order to ensure optimal drug utilization.

Hospital Formularies

Hospital Formularies can influence the prescribing behaviour of clinicians very much. The prescribing quality may be changed by the way the formulary is laid out, information highlighted and updated. It is imperative that the Formularies available at different hospital set-ups in the country are evaluated and the deficiencies corrected. Hospital Formularies will also help to promote generic prescription both in public and private set ups, if they have a practice oriented approach.

Clinical Pharmacies in Hospitals

The presence of modern Clinical Pharmacy services in Indian hospitals, especially after the introduction and popularization of Doctor of Pharmacy programs (Pharm.D) is considered as a watershed area for pharmacoepidemiological studies in the hospital scenario. The clinical pharmacies in hospitals can bridge the gap between clinicians and biostatisticians in terms of most of the medicine related studies.

Pharmacovigilance

Monitoring of ADRs are essential factors in any pharmacoepidemiological study. The monitoring of adverse drug reactions will also receive a boost through such pharmacoepidemiological studies. ADR programs that highlight the incidence of ADR and define the risk/ benefit ratio taking account of the pathophysiological variations of patients will be of immense benefit in the long-term usage of drugs.

A new approach is on preventing adverse effects resulting from inappropriate, excessive, or therapeutically incompatible drug use. This information can reduce costs by preventing adverse effects and their treatment.

Drug Interactions

Profile of drug interactions is another area wherein the Clinical Pharmacy Unit can supplement the clinician's therapeutic prowess. Compared to all other health care professionals, pharmacist are the most competent people to associate with or take up the projects on such areas. Very few non-experimental studies of drug interactions have been done. Since most patients are prescribed more than one drug at a time, the potential for drug interactions are in existence. Relevant studies like cohort study can reduce potential interactions and their consequent effects.

Drug Surveillance at Local, Regional and National Levels

Primary Drug Surveillance includes keeping a check on the use of medicaments dispensed through pharmacies at community and hospital levels. Since in India, primary health centres form an important facet of the health set up, long-term descriptive observational studies can be done in these centres. The number of visits to the pharmacy, number of medicaments dispensed, adverse effects to medicaments etc., can be surveyed. Comparison between age groups and men and women need to be made.

Prescription data available from hospital pharmacies and community pharmacies (rural and urban) can be used as an instrument in improving prescribing behaviour. For this to be useful in an epidemiological context, pharmaco-therapeutic audits are very helpful. Aspects like quality of drugs, volume, cost, refill of prescriptions etc., can be discussed for making recommendations.

Considering the possible problems and pitfalls when new drugs are introduced into the market and the monitoring of existing drugs, a national system of drug surveillance is needed. How it can be set up? What are the various methods through which the drug surveillance needs to be done? This aspect is discussed separately as a case study in **Chapter 11** of Pharmacoepidemiology.

Studies on New Drugs

When a new drug is introduced into the market, it is having only limited safety study information with it. Less than five thousand humans may have been exposed to the drug. Serious adverse reactions occurring less frequently, may be difficult to detect. Post marketing safety mainly relies on spontaneous reporting of adverse reactions. Such reporting is often incomplete. Observational epidemiological studies can be used to investigate drug risk hypotheses, but they are expensive, time consuming and dangerous if the hypothesis is correct.

Marketing and dispensing of new (or restricted use) drugs is increasing in India every year as in other developing countries. Since very little safety-monitoring infrastructure exists in such countries, the onus is on the sponsors to monitor for adverse reactions. This can be done by maintaining patient records and using simple methods to promote and facilitate reporting of unusual clinical events to an expert committee or body. Such agencies shall include pharmacoepidemiologists who can play an active role in collaboration with the government and other agencies. The Pharmacovigilance program currently available in India needs to be strengthened.

Age based Medicine use and its Analysis

Life expectancy is increasing and the entire world is aging. Age based consumption studies of medicines and analysis of its regression models is a dire need. Causal age based dependence of drug consumption level needs to be found in an analytical form. The optimum regression model for this dependence needs to be sought by methods of regression and correction analysis. Epidemiological studies of the aged tend to avoid estimations of medication prevalence and adverse effects. This may be due to the difficulty of capturing medication data. Now a number of versatile coding systems for medication data entry are available which will make the studies more easy.

Some other areas for research in Pharmacoepidemiology are:

1. Identifying and quantifying less common adverse effects and delayed adverse effects.
2. Evaluation of efficiency and toxicity of drugs in specific patient groups like children, elderly, pregnant and lactating women.
3. Studies on unanticipated adverse effects of drugs. (Using cohort study and case control designs, these adverse effects can be studied).
4. Studies on anticipated adverse effects of drugs. (Here experimental study, cohort study or even case series can be applied).
5. Studies on un identified beneficial effects of drugs. (Here the research methodology used can be cohort study that focuses on the drug in question. Case control studies and voluntary case reports are also possible).
6. Studies on expected beneficial outcomes of drugs. There are certain questions that need to be addressed here including :
   (a) Efficacy of drug vs. change in drug regimen – dose per unit time, distribution of dose over time, duration.
   (b) Variations in characteristics of patients – age, sex, genetics, diet, compliance, other diseases, concurrent drug usage.
   (c) Efficacy of drug for other secondary indications and drug comparisons.

   (Studies of drug efficacy in general require randomised clinical trials).
7. Reviews of drug utilization can be carried out on overuse of drugs or use of costly drugs.
8. Reliable information (Data bases) on the usage and variation in drug therapies is essential for health care delivery. Areas that can be reviewed include:
   (i) Characteristics of the routine practice according to circumstance, patient population and physician characteristics.
   (ii) Validity issues dealing with data sources and their potential for outcomes research.
   (iii) Data sources divided into primary and secondary types based on their features, advantages and limitations.
   (iv) Procedures for analysing secondary data.

The future of pharmacoepidemiology in India will be determined by the actions taken by experts in the field of Pharmacy Practice, Pharmacoepidemiology, Clinical Epidemiology and Clinical Pharmacology as well as those interested in the combined subject. A great deal of work needs to be done in the areas of drug toxicity, drug interactions, indigenous drugs, and pharmaco-genetics among others. The subsidiary area of pharmacoeconomics is also extremely relevant to the Indian situation. The gulf between the rich and the poor is ever widening and many drugs will soon be out of reach for the poor. Studies need to be done to find out cost effective alternatives. Many other areas of interest in pharmacoepidemiology are existing in the health care and pharmacotherapy.

Information from the studies could contribute to population based care and regulatory decisions on drugs. The integration of medical and epidemiological knowledge helps for good choice of medication at the, institutional as well as individual levels. Pharmacoepidemiological database could provide vital information regarding safety, drug use and evidence based pharmacotherapy.

Pharmacoepidemiology is the application of epidemiological methodologies for the study of drugs focusing on their use and effects in a large number of people. It is drug epidemiology.

CHAPTER 11

Evidence based Medicine and Concepts of Risks in Pharmacoepidemiology

Chapter Mission

After learning this chapter you may be able to know:

- Definition and genesis of evidence based medicine.
- Role of pharmacoepidemiology in evidence based medicine.
- Concepts of risks and their classification.
- Calculation of risks.

Evidence based Medicine

Medical decision making has gone through a fundamental change in the last 50 years more. The foundation for decision making has shifted away from subjective judgments and reliance on authorities toward a formal analysis of evidence. In the past, treatments were recommended if physicians believed patients would benefit. Now, before recommending a treatment, physicians ask - What's the evidence?

What caused this change?

Evidence based medicine (EBM) as we know it today is the confluence of several related but initially separate lines of research, and everyone who participated in the movement has his or her own story. But Dr David M Eddy and Dr David Sackett are the pioneers, the former in USA and the latter in Canada, in making and popularising the concept of EBM at the global levels.

"Evidence based medicine (EBM) is an approach to medical practice intended to optimize decision taking by emphasizing the use of evidence from well designed and conducted research studies". Although all medicine based on science has certain extent of empirical support, EBM goes further. It classifies evidence by its epistemological (the study of the nature and grounds of knowledge) strength and requiring that only the strongest types (coming from meta- analysis, systemic reviews and RCT) can yield strong recommendations. Weaker studies like Case Control can yield only weak recommendations.

Evidence based medicine (EBM) is the process of systematically reviewing, appraising and using clinical research findings to aid the delivery of optimum clinical care to patients. See Fig. 11.1.

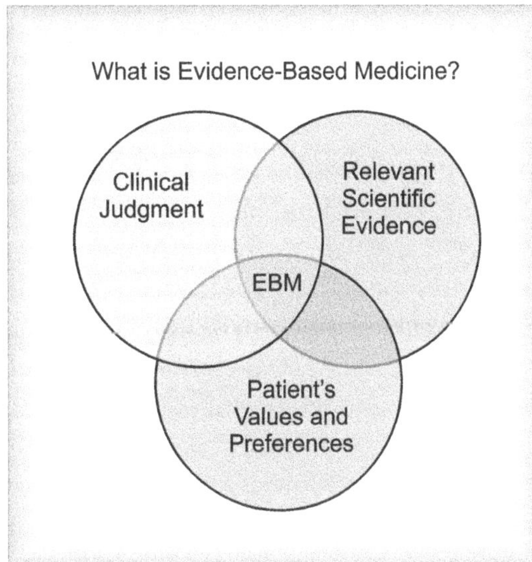

Figure 11.1 Position of EBM in patient care.

The most common definition of Evidence Based Practice (EBP) is from Dr. David Sackett. Evidence Based Practice is defined as "the conscientious, explicit and judicious use of current best evidence in making decisions about the care of the individual patient. It means integrating individual clinical expertise with the best available external clinical evidence from systematic research."

EBP is the integration of clinical expertise, patient values, and the best research evidence into the decision making process for patient care. Clinical expertise refers to the clinician's cumulated experience, education and clinical skills. The patient brings to the encounter his or her own personal preferences and unique concerns, expectations, and values. The best research evidence is usually found in clinically relevant research that has been conducted using sound methodology.

Evolution of EBM Concepts

The term was originally used to describe an approach to teaching the practice of medicine and improving decisions by individual physicians about individual patients. Use of the term rapidly expanded to include a previously described approach that emphasized the use of evidence in the design of guidelines and policies that apply to groups of patients and populations ("evidence based practice policies"). It has subsequently spread to describe an approach to decision making that is used at all levels of health care and related programs as evidence based practice. It believes that to the extent possible, decisions and policies should be based on evidence, not just the beliefs of practitioners, experts, or administrators. It can be applied to medical education, decisions about individuals, guidelines and policies or administration of health services. In its broadest form, evidence-based medicine is the application of the scientific method into healthcare decision-making. Medicine has a long tradition of both basic and clinical research.

The term "evidence based" was first used by David M. Eddy in the course of his work on population-level policies such as clinical practice guidelines and insurance coverage of new technologies. He first began to use the term "evidence based" in 1987 in workshops and a manual commissioned by the Council of Medical Specialty Societies to teach formal methods for designing clinical practice guidelines. The manual was widely available in unpublished form in the late 1980s and eventually published by the American College of Medicine

Eddy first published the term "evidence based" in March, 1990 in an article in the 'Journal of the American Medical Association' that laid out the principles of evidence based guidelines and population-level policies, which Eddy described as "explicitly describing the available evidence that pertains to a policy and tying the policy to evidence. The policy must be consistent with and supported by evidence. The pertinent evidence must be identified, described, and analysed. The policymakers must determine whether the policy is justified by the evidence. A rationale must be written. He discussed "evidence-based" policies in several other papers published in *JAMA* in 1990s.

The term evidence based got a big push when David Sackett and his colleagues used it in the title of a paper they published in *JAMA* 2 years later (Sackett 1996). Later both of them together developed the term "Evidence Based Medicine" (EBM) and "Evidence Based Practice" in their own way (Eddy 2005). Evidence based medicine now has a life of its own, with scores of books, courses, programs, and even departments in medical schools dedicated to it. Current students and younger physicians now take for granted the requirement for evidence and explicit formal analysis, barely knowing that this was not the case just a few decades ago.

By 2000, "evidence-based medicine" had become an umbrella term for the emphasis on evidence in both population-level and individual-level decisions. In subsequent years, use of the term "evidence based" had extended to other levels of the health care system. An example is "evidence based health services", which seek to increase the competence of health service decision makers and the practice of evidence-based medicinc at the organi-zational or institutional level.

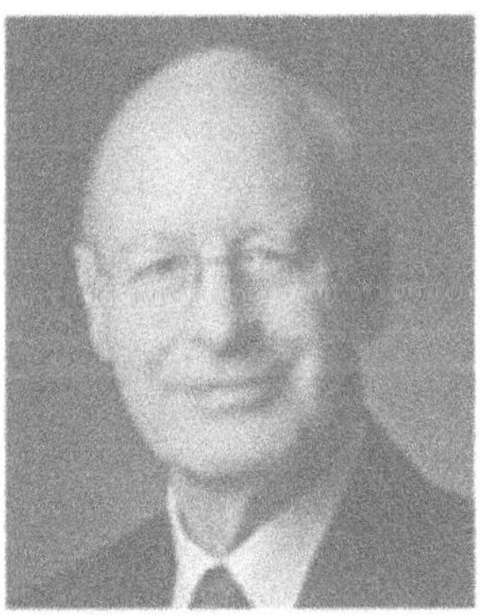

David M Eddy USA

David M. Eddy, MD, PhD is a physician, mathematician, and healthcare analyst who has done seminal work in mathematical modelling of diseases, clinical practice guidelines, and evidence based medicine. Four highlights of his career have been summarized by the Institute of Medicine of the National Academy of Sciences: "more than 25 years ago, Eddy wrote the seminal paper on the role of guidelines in medical decision-making, the first Markov model applied to clinical problems, and the original criteria for coverage decisions. David M Eddy was the first to use and publish the term 'evidence-based'.

Eddy was Chief of the Bioengineering Branch of the US Army Medical Research and Development Command from 1971 to 1973. After obtaining his PhD, he was an assistant professor (1978) and then professor (1980) of Engineering Economic Systems at Stanford. In 1981, he went to Duke University, where he was Professor of Health Policy and Management. He was the Director of the WHO Collaborating Center for Research in Cancer Policy from 1984 to 1996. He is responsible for the policy framed under Medicare and other insurance schemes in USA.

Dr David Sackett started his career in 1967 as the Head of Clinical Epidemiology and Biostatistics at McMaster Canada. Eddy was Chief of the Bioengineering Branch of the US Army Medical Research and later got associated with the insurance and other health policies of USA and also the WHO. Their research and epidemiological backgrounds empowered them to the establishment and popularisation of the EBM and EBP. In the first chapter we have seen that Pharmacoepidemiology has a strong chemical bonding with clinical epidemiology.

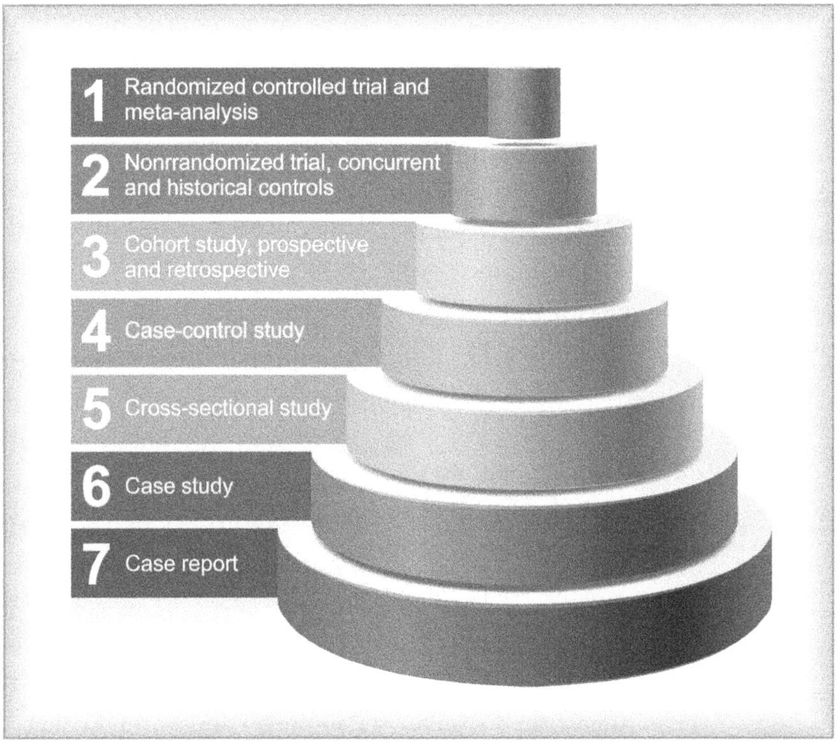
1 Randomized controlled trial and meta-analysis
2 Nonrrandomized trial, concurrent and historical controls
3 Cohort study, prospective and retrospective
4 Case-control study
5 Cross-sectional study
6 Case study
7 Case report

Figure 11.2 Relationship between pharmacoepidemiological research methods and the 'E" in EBM.

Role of Pharmacoepidemiology in Evidence based Medicine

The term "evidence based medicine", as it is currently used, has two main tributaries. Chronologically, the first is the insistence on explicit evaluation of evidence of effectiveness when issuing clinical practice guidelines and other population-level policies. The second is the introduction of epidemiological methods into medical education and individual patient-level decision-making.

Pharmacoepidemiology is a study of unintended effects of treatments. Pharmacoepidemiological studies are used for post-clinical trial evaluation of effectiveness and safety of treatments and procedures in real-life clinical settings. Thus, pharmacoepidemiological research is a key contributor to evidence based medical practice.

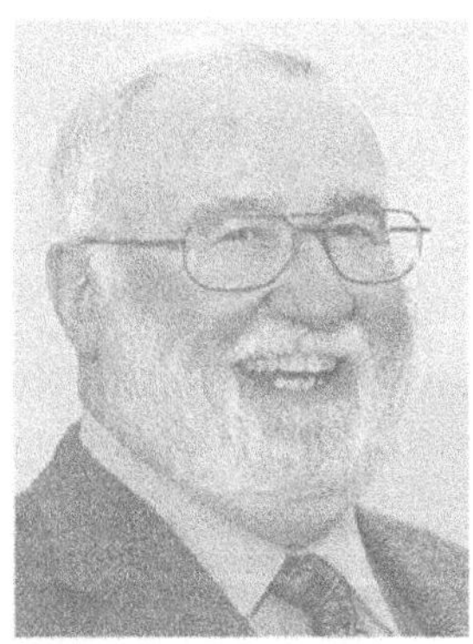

Dr David Sackett Father of EBM

David Sackett, MD
(17 Nov 1934-13 May 2015)

The reputed father of evidence based medicine (EBM) David Sackett was born in Chicago in November 1934 and after taking degrees in internal medicine, nephrology and epidemiology, he started his career as the founding Chair of Clinical Epidemiology & Biostatistics at McMaster, Ontario Canada. In 1967, he then started to design, execute, interpret, monitor, write and teach about randomized clinical trials, an activity that continued till his death. He worked as the physician in chief and head of the division of Internal Medicine at McMaster Hospitals.

During his stay at McMaster for 26 years he pioneered for the development of Clinical Epidemiology, Randomised Clinical Trials (RCT) and Evidence Based Medicine. In 1968 he established the first department for Clinical Epidemiology and Biostatics in Canada. In the early 1980s he demonstrated the beneficial effects of Aspirin for patients with angina which established the rationale for the use of Aspirin in the prevention of cardiovascular diseases (Cairns JA 1985). Today Aspirin remains a foundational component of the treatment of angina and preventing heart attacks and strokes.

In 1994, he joined University of Oxford in England as Director of the NHS R&D Centre for Evidence-Based Medicine (CEBM). In 1996 he defined Evidence Based Medicine (EBM) as the "conscientious explicit and judicious use of current best evidence in making decisions about the care of individual patients." He sought to combine individual clinical expertise with the best available external clinical evidence for systematic research.

Retired from clinical practice at age 65, he returned to Canada and established the Trout Research & Education Centre. He taught about RCT and research there till his end. He lived long enough to see physicians using smartphones to look up practice guidelines at a patient's bedside, an inevitable outcome of the movement he spawned.

Concepts of Risk

The concept of risk has a commonplace in discussions on health and its aspects of research studies. A risk approach is used when thinking about the causes of health and illness issues or positive and negative outcomes. In spite of this widespread focus on the concept of risk, there is no clear consensus on definitions. The Oxford dictionary defines risk as *a chance or possibility of danger, loss, injury or other adverse consequences.* Risk is *the likelihood or the probability of experiencing some type of harm, or losing something that one values.* The specific interpretation of the definitions of risk vary widely.

Risk was originally proposed to refer to causal factors that were neither necessary nor sufficient. Risk factors are variables or characteristics (biological, environmental or psychosocial) associated with an individual that make it more likely that he or she, as opposed to another person randomly selected from the population, will develop a problem.

Risk factors:

- exist before a disorder or problem;

- may be time-limited or may continue over time;
- can derive from the individual, the family, the community, institutions or the general environment; and
- can play a causal role or be a marker for a problem.

Characteristics of Risks

Risk is not certain. Risk is based on probability. Therefore, not everyone who is exposed to a risk condition or factor will have an adverse outcome. Risk factors are *"linked to"* and *"associated with"* negative outcomes. Therefore, in most cases, especially those relating to mental health and psychosocial outcomes, it would be inaccurate to assume a direct cause and effect relationship between a given risk factor and a specific outcome. There are, however, some specific biological outcomes which have cause and effect relationships. Two examples are certain teratogenic drugs, such as thalidomide, and environmental toxins such as lead.

Risk is a relative concept— Risk factors range from those that are only markers to minimally harmful situations to those that are markers to life-threatening situations. According to the Canadian Association on Gerontology, the personal risk exists on a continuum, from those that individuals vigorously pursue as opportunities, to those over which they have little choice. This is explained in the Fig. 11.3.

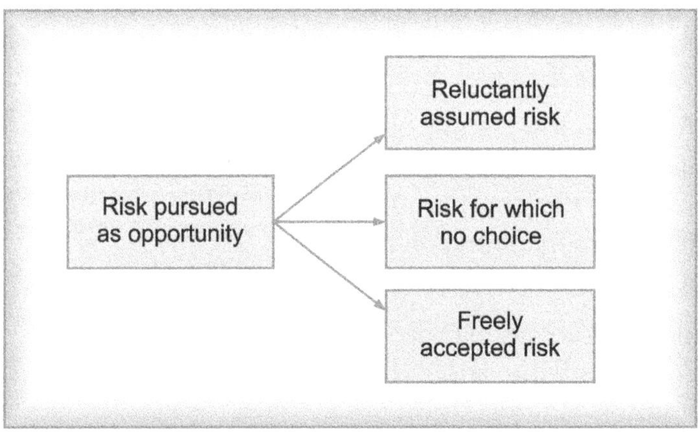

Figure 11.3 Personal risk continuum.

There is also a social continuum of risk, ranging from risks which society views as inevitable or are willing to accept, to risks which are considered unacceptable or unreasonable. While the personal risk continuum is based on choice, the social risk continuum is based on societal notions of acceptable and unacceptable outcomes. Therefore, *risk is not a neutral concept,* it involves determining what are acceptable or unacceptable consequences.

Risk factors work together over time to influence the likelihood of a negative outcome. The longer the exposure to risk factors, the greater the likelihood the health problem will occur. Risk identification exists in a social context. Since other people define risk for individuals and groups, usually health and other service providers and community agencies, the identification of risk will be partially based upon their values, biases, experience and knowledge.

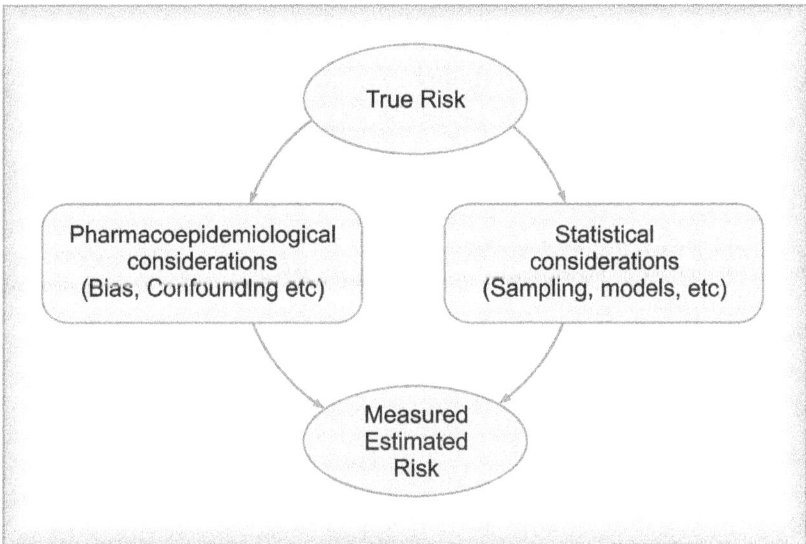

Figure 11.4 Flow of risk in pharmacoepidemiology.

Fig. 11.4 indicates the flow is from a true, but unknown, risk to a final estimate of the risk. Similarly risk can flow from initial hypothesis, through the design of the experiment, the analysis of the data, and the final estimate of the true risk.

Risk in Pharmacoepidemiology

Health research involves the estimation of risk. In the case of drug related research, it is important to understand the concept of risk. It is the probability of developing an outcome when exposed to a drug. A drug is approved for human use only after measuring the risks and benefits associated with it. The health care professionals including pharmacists who give advice and education to patients should know the magnitude and frequency of the risk involved in the drug in use. Each drug outcome has its own risk. It is a probability and depends on a variety of factors like age, sex, physical conditions, food habits, other diseases, other medicines, kinetics of drugs etc. The risk may harm the patient. A harm is a hurt of damage or injury suffered by the patient due to the adverse effect of the drug. Measures of the risk vary according to the type of the variable and the study design.

Risk is essentially a measure of probability. Almost all aspects of statistical analysis of epidemiological data can be viewed in terms of the concepts of probability.

Measurement of Risk

To accurately and precisely measure risk, one needs a tool that is accurate and precise enough for the measurement being made. We know that a meter stick is inadequate for measuring length to a precision of 0.1 mm.

When measuring risk in epidemiology, precision and accuracy depend on many factors including the degree to which the experimental data and analysis are free of the errors associated with experimental design flaws (i.e., confounding, bias, reliability, measurement error and misclassification, potential alternate risk factors), and statistical analysis errors (i.e., sampling error, violations of model assumptions, model shopping, multiple subgroup analyses, reliance on significance levels or *p*-values).

Attributable Risk

In pharmacoepidemiology and epidemiology, *attributable risk* is the difference in rate of a condition between an exposed population and an unexposed population. Attributable risk is mostly calculated in Cohort Studies, where individuals are assembled on exposure status and followed over a period of time. Investigators count the occurrence of the diseases. The cohort is then subdivided by the level of exposure and the frequency of disease is compared between subgroups. One is considered exposed and another unexposed.

$$AR = R_{exposed} - R_{non\text{-}exposed}$$

where R is the rate of the outcome of the interest or the Incidence.

Attributable Risk =

Incidence in exposed – incidence in unexposed.

Per cent of AR can be calculated as

$$\%\,AR = 100 \times \frac{R_{exposed} - R_{non\text{-}exposed}}{R_{exposed}}$$

Illustration of Attributable Risk in Pharmacoepidemiology

The risk of a drug has to be assessed within the environment or atmosphere where it is used. We cannot attribute all incidence of GI discomfort in people taking ampicillin capsules to the drug since some may have it for other reasons than the drug use. If the risks due to other reasons than the drug are reduced from the overall risks, we will get the attributable risks. It is simple to calculate and easy to understand. Mathematically it is expressed as

$$AR = R_{exposed} - R_{non\text{-}exposed}$$

where R is the rate of the outcome of the interest.

Attributable risk is also known as *risk difference* or *rate difference*. In clinical outcomes the rate difference simply quantifies one rate in comparison with another. If amoxicillin is 90 percent successful in treating a specific type of infection and ampicillin is 65 percent successful in treating the same infection, the rate difference 90 percent – 65 percent = 25 percent.

Relative Risk (RR)

Both in statistics and pharmacoepidemiology, *relative risk* or *risk ratio* (RR) is the ratio of the probability of an event occurring (for example, developing an ADR to a drug) in an exposed group to the probability of the event occurring in a comparison, non-exposed group.

Relative risk includes two important features:

(i) a comparison of risk between two "exposures" puts risks in context, and

(ii) "exposure" is ensured by having proper denominators for each group representing the exposure

$$RR = \frac{\text{Prevent when exposed}}{\text{Prevent when non} - \text{exposed}}$$

It is a ratio of two risks, the risk of the outcome/event in the treated group compared with the outcome in those not exposed (control group).

RR = Proportion of events in experimental group/ proportion of events in control group

A relative risk above 1 means that the treatment /exposure is associated with the outcome and the value below 1 means that the treatment is negatively associated with the outcome. Relative risk is also known as risk ratio. When the rate in the exposed group is equal to the rate in the comparison group RR will be equal to 1 or unity. An RR of 2 means that the rate in the exposed group is twice that in the non exposed group. An RR of 0.5 means that the rate in the exposed persons is half that of non exposed persons.

Illustration of RR

Consider an example where the probability of developing allergy among users of perfume was 20% and among those not using perfume 1%.

Table 11.1 Relative risk

Risk	Allergy status	
	Present	**Absent**
Perfume users	a	b
Perfume Non-users	c	d

This situation is expressed in the 2 × 2 table (Table 11.1)

Here, $a = 20$,
$b = 80$,
$c = 1$,
and $d = 99$.

Then the relative risk of allergy associated with users of perfume would be

$$RR = \frac{a/(a+b)}{c/(c+d)} = \frac{20/100}{1/100} = 20$$

Perfume users would be twenty times as likely as perfume non- users to develop allergy.

Different types of RR

The RR is derived from study designs where the study population is selected on the basis of exposure (e.g., cohort study), or disease (e.g., case-control design) and may have different names depending on the context:

- In a cohort mortality study the RR is called a standardized mortality ratio (SMR).
- In a cohort incidence study the RR is called a standardized incidence ratio (SIR).
- In a morbidity cohort or cross-sectional study the RR may be called a prevalence ratio.
- In a case-control study the RR is called an odds ratio (OR).

Odds Ratio (OR)

Odds ratio in statistics and epidemiology is commonly abbreviated as 'OR'. It is a measure of association between an exposure and an outcome like Risk Ratio (RR). In clinical studies and many other settings, the first parameter of greatest interest is the RR and next one is OR. We saw that Risk Ratio is determined probabilities. In OR instead of probabilities odds are used.

> **Illustration: How to find odds?**
>
> There are two sample groups, one consisting of 100 men and other 100 women were identified from city residential area. In a dinner party out of 100 men, 90 drank beer, while out of 100 women only 20 drank beer.
>
> The odds of a man drinking wine are 90 to 10, or 9:1, while the odds of a woman drinking wine are 20 to 80, or 1:4 = 0.25:1.

Computation of OR

The OR represents the odds that an outcome will occur given a particular exposure, compared to the odds of the outcome occurring in the absence of that exposure. For example OR helps to quantify how strongly the presence or absence of property 'X' is associated with the presence or absence of property 'Y' in a given population.

If each individual in a population either does or does not have a property "X", (e.g., increased blood sugar level), and also either does or does not have a property "Y" (e.g., use of statins) where both properties are appropriately defined, then a ratio can be formed which quantitatively describes the association between the presence/ absence of "X" (increased blood sugar level) and the presence/absence of "Y" (use of statins) for individuals in the population. This ratio is the odds ratio (OR) and can be computed by following these steps:

1. For a given individual that has "Y" compute the odds that the same individual has "X"
2. For a given individual that does not have "Y" compute the odds that the same individual has "X"
3. Divide the odds from step 1 by the odds from step 2 to obtain the odds ratio (OR).

The term "individual" in this usage does not have to refer to a human being, as a statistical population can measure any set of entities, whether living or inanimate.

If the OR is greater than 1, then having "X" is considered to be "associated" with having "Y" in the sense that the having of "Y" raises (relative to not-having "Y") the odds of having "X". Note that this is not enough to establish that 'Y' is a contributing cause of "X": it could be that the association is due to a third property, " Z", which is a contributing cause of both "X" and "Y" (Confounding).

Illustrations of OR computation

Illustration 1: Take the same illustration given for finding odds above. Now we can find the OR as shown below

The odds ratio (OR) is 9/0.25, or 36. It shows that men are much more likely to drink wine than women.

The detailed calculation is:

$$\frac{0.3/0.1}{0.2/0.8}=\frac{0.9\times0.8}{0.1\times0.2}=\frac{0.72}{0.02}=36$$

This example also shows how odds ratios are sometimes sensitive in stating relative positions. In this illustration men are 90/20 = 4.5 times as likely to have drunk beer than women, but have 36 times the odds.

Illustration 2:

Table 11.2 Odds ratio contingency

	Cases	Control	Total
Exposed	a	b	a + b
Un exposed	c	d	c + d
Total	a + c	b + d	(a + b) + (c +d)

$$OR=\frac{a/c}{b/d}=\frac{a\times d}{b\times c}$$

Imagine a group of 20 friends went out to the pub – the next day a 7 were ill. They suspect that it may have been something they ate, maybe the fish casserole. Here are the numbers:

	Cases (Illness)	Control (No Illness)	Total
Exposed (ate fish)	5	3	8
Un exposed (didn't eat fish)	2	10	12
Total	7	13	20

- Odds of exposure in cases = a/c = 5/2 = 2.5
- Odds of exposure in controls = b/d = 3/10 = 0.3
- Odds Ratio = (a/c) / (b/d) = 2.5/0.3 = 8.33

Interpretation: What does this mean?

OR of 1 would suggests that there is no difference between the groups; i.e., there would be no association between the suggested exposure (fish) and the outcome (being ill).

OR of > 1 suggests that the odds of exposure are positively associated with the adverse outcome compared to the odds of not being exposed.

OR of < 1 suggests that the odds of exposure are negatively associated with the adverse outcomes compared to the odds of not being exposed.

In the example above, we can conclude that those who ate the fish casserole (exposure) were 8.3 times more likely (OR = 8.3) to be ill (outcome), compared to those who did not eat the fish casserole.

Advantages

- Appropriate to analyse associations between groups from case-control and prevalent (or cross-sectional) data.
- For rare diseases (or diseases with long latency periods) the OR can be an approximate measure to the RR (relative risk)
- Doesn't require denominator (i.e., total number in population) unlike measuring risk
- Good method to estimate the strength of an association between exposures and outcomes

Disadvantages

- Association does not infer causation.

Time Risk Relationship

Is the outcome of an exposure to a drug is related to the time? The answer is always yes. Some drugs act quickly while others may take time to get the effects. If injection morphine is giving pain relief immediately, certain vaccines will give protection after a period of time only. It is also true with risks associated with medicines. There is always a time related association of risk in pharmacoepidemiology. Certain events like anaphylactic reactions happen immediately after taking an injection while certain other risk events occur after days or months or even years. Prazosin (Minipress) is a blood pressure medicine known as an alpha-blocker. Its main effect is dilation of veins and arteries which leads to a reduction in blood pressure. Prazosin is also sometimes used for a condition called benign prostatic hyperplasia (BPH), which is commonly known as an "enlarged prostate. To minimize the impact of the first dose effect, prazosin is normally taken at bedtime. Other drugs of the same family, doxazosin and terazosin, can also cause this phenomenon, though less frequently.

Delayed reactions to medications commonly begin more than six hours after exposure but sometimes occur days after exposure. For example, delayed adverse drug reactions to amoxicillin classically start between 7 to 10 days of exposure and may even begin 1 to 3 days after the patient has stopped taking the medicine. Medications that cause delayed reactions include heparin, quinine, sulphonamides, vancomycin, gold compounds, beta lactam antibiotics and non-steroidal anti-inflammatory drugs. Lomustine is an anti-cancer drug used in different types of cancer. It has adverse effect of producing leucopoenia, which can occur up to six weeks after a dose of lomustine.

The above mentioned aspects of medicines demonstrate that the exposure time must always be considered and the risk should be expressed as a function of time wherever possible in pharmaco-epidemiology. The risk can be estimated for different time slots. The duration of exposure is significant in the case of certain medications. The risk of breast cancer development was found to be more with women who had taken oral contraceptives for a long period. In the case of statins both the duration of exposure is found to be associated with the risk of producing type 2 diabetes.

Confidence Intervals (CI)

Confidence intervals are a range of values within which the true population value probably lies. When the risk estimators like RR or OR are calculated they are presented with a confidence interval (CI). Generally a 95 percent confidence interval (CI_{95}) is calculated. It means that we are 95 percent confident that the true value lies between these limits.

Absolute Risk

The risk of having a disease at any point in time is known as absolute risk. It is the incidence. If the incidence of epilepsy is 1 in 10,0000 then the absolute risk is 0.001 percent.

Experimental Event Rate (EER)

It is the proportion of patients in the treated group in whom an event is observed. If out of 100 treated patients (a+b), the event is observed in 27 (a), the EER = 0.27, that is

$$EER = [a/(a+b)]$$

Control Event Rate (CER)

It is the proportion of patients in the control group in whom an event is observed.

$$CER = c/(c+d).$$

CHAPTER 12

Sample Size and Causation in Pharmacoepidemiology

Chapter Mission

After learning this chapter you may be able to know:

- What is sample size?
- Need to calculate sample size.
- Application of sample size in pharmacopidemiology.
- Softwares used in pharmacoepidemiology.

Sample Size

'How many is sufficient?' is a question that pharmacoepidemiologists, clinical epidemiologists, epidemiologists and researchers in health care and medicine ask themselves when they plan to conduct a new study. Researchers want to enrol a large number of people so that statistical errors are minimized, but the cost, time and labour to be acceptable. Sample size calculations remind us of complex and complicated formula. In this book no formula is given, but only discuss certain aspects that will help us to carry out the studies.

Illustration of Need to Calculate Sample Size

When we would like to know an attribute of a population like a mean cholesterol of the people of India, it may not be feasible or possible to study the entire 130 crores of people due to cost or time issues. Apart from the cost or time issues, it is not ethical to study the entire population, if accurate enough results can be obtained by studying a sub group of the population. For such reasons we need to study a sample size of the population.

The results may vary from sample to sample and they be somewhat different from the true mean of the Indian population. For example one sample of 500 Indians may have a mean cholesterol of 180 mg/dl and another sample may have a mean of 184 mg/dl. However as the sample size increases, the probability of obtaining a result close to the true mean for the population increases. The basic question is how large the sample size should be to make the difference narrow from the true mean. There are certain principles which apply to all sample size calculations some them are noted below.

Variation in the Variable of Interest

The more the variation in the variables of interest, the larger is the required sample size. If there is no variation, even a sample size of n = 1 is sufficient.

Illustration 1: There are 100 community pharmacists in a chain pharmacy set up. If all the 100 pharmacists get exactly the same salary INR 20000 per month, knowing the salary of only one is sufficient to know the mean.

Illustration 2: There is a disease which is universally fatal. There is no variation in its outcome in terms of death and life. If a new drug cures only one case of this disease, that single case is enough to accept that the drug works provided the diagnosis is correct. (This was the situation when Penicillin was used for septicaemia during the World War II period).

Magnitude of Error that we Accept

The less the magnitude of error that we accept , the larger should be the sample size. Larger sample size is the price we are paying for less error.

Illustration 3: A researcher wants to estimate the mean weight of a population. Any sample would be most likely estimate the mean weight with some error. If the real mean weight is 58.00 kg, a sample may estimate it as 56.00 kg. It means 2 kg error. If we want to be relatively certain that our sample mean has no more than 1 Kg error, the sample required size is much larger than the earlier one.

Probability of making a Certain Magnitude of Error

The smaller the probability of error, the larger the sample size should be. In the Illustration 3 above, we are not sure that the error is going to be less than 2 kg if we increase the size. In a large population there are many heavy weight people. It could turn out that a random sample, having a mean weight of 3 kg more than the entire population.

We can only increase the sample size to the extent that with a large probability say 95 % or 99%, the sample size mean be within 1 kg from the true population mean. If we want 99% certainty , we need a larger sample size than we accept 95 % certainty. This is again saying that larger sample size is the price we pay for more certainty.

The following are examples of other factors affecting the sample size:

(i) Main objective of the study. It is primary factor in selecting the formula for calculating the sample size.

(ii) Design of the study. Cross over trials often need smaller sample size.

(iii) Proportion of participants distributed in each study arm.

Non-statistical Considerations

Non-statistical considerations. like funding, ethical issues, fixed number of population available to researcher, novelty of study and conduct of similar studies in other places can also influence the sample size.

If the researcher has funding to study only 20 subjects, he may not be able to take a study requiring 100 participants. In the case of RCT, with new drugs, it is unethical to increase the study population than the actual required. Sometimes the sample size is almost fixed. For example a researcher may have been able to find the data regarding occurrence of Stevens–Johnson syndrome with a sulpha drug. Over his 30 years of service he might have identified 20 cases. If the sample has to be increased, he has wait for years (without guarantee) or collaborate with other centers in the world which again may not be feasible. In such situations sample size formula can be used, but not to determine the sample size, but to learn about the power to detect certain difference.

Novelty of the study is also significant. When the first report on AIDS was published in 1981, only five cases of the disease among homosexuals were collected. Today a report of far larger number of such cases may not be interesting enough to publish in reputed journals.

Application of Sample Size in Pharmacoepidemiology

From the earlier discussion we have seen that the sample size for pharmaco-epidemiological studies must be large enough to have sufficient statistical power to detect the differences deemed important. One of the problems often encountered in epidemiological investigations is figuring out how large a sample we need to answer a specific question. Our sample size must be big enough for the study to have appropriate statistical power – the ability to demonstrate an association if one exists. We base sample size calculations on a number of study design factors like:

- prevalence
- acceptable error
- the detectable difference.

Box 12.1 Criteria of sample size calculation

The following information is needed before the calculation is made:

- Required level of statistical significance of the ability to detect a difference.
- Acceptable error, or chance of missing a real effect.
- Magnitude of the effect under investigation.
- Amount of disease in the population.
- Relative sizes of the groups being compared.

There are numerous formulae and computer programs that simplify the task considerably

Sample size calculations can be done with standard formulae or with the support of biostatisticians. A practical guide for determining sample size in health studies was published by WHO (Lwanga SK, Lemeshow S). Sample size determination in health studies. Geneva, World Health Organization, 1991) in 1991 to have a uniform concept and solution to the issue of sample sizes in health care studies.

Application of Software to Calculate Sample Size

Sample size can be calculated using almost all commercial statistical software like STATA and SAS. *Sampsi* command of STATA and PROC POWER of SAS can do the work for a variety of research designs. Other freely available and easy to use software designed for sample size calculation are in wide use. *PS Power and Sample Size Calculation Program* written by Dupont and Plummer at Vanderbilt University provides a step- by- step guide to calculate sample size. Another example is the *Power* program written by Lubin and Garcia Closas at US National Cancer Institute. Another highly useful free software for statistical analysis and power calculation is *Epi Info* developed by US Centre for Disease Control and Prevention. (Farin Kamangar, 2013). Also see the section Soft wares in Pharmacoepidemiology.

In reality, sample size is often determined by logistic and financial considerations, and a compromise always has to be made between sample size and costs. The precision of the study can be improved by ensuring that the study groups are of appropriate sizes. In the Case-Control studies where a decision is required on the number of controls to be chosen for each case, it will become an issue of concern. It is not possible to be definitive about the ideal ratio of controls to cases, since this depends on the relative costs of accumulating cases and controls. If cases are scarce and controls plentiful, it is appropriate to increase the ratio of controls to cases.

> **Illustration 4:** Between 1959 and 1960 hundreds of monsters (without limbs) were born in Federal Republic of Germany when the pregnant women took Thalidomide tablets to cure their 'morning sickness' during the early period of pregnancy. A case control study was conducted in 1961 comparing 46 affected children with 300 normal children. The Case group consisted of 46 mothers who gave birth to limbless children. Out of them 41 were found to have taken thalidomide during the 4th and 9th weeks of pregnancy. The Control group consisted of 300 mothers whose children were normal.

In general, however, there may be little point in having more than four controls for each case. However it is important to ensure that there is sufficient similarity between cases and controls when the data are to be analysed by, for example, age group or social class. If there are large number of cases and only a few controls were in the older age groups, the study would not be able to account for the confounding factor of age.

Softwares in Pharmacoepidemiology

Quality assurance of all bio-statistical data, including pharmacoepidemiological analysis is becoming mandatory. Statistical soft wares may be classified into four categories: easy-to-use general public soft wares with limited functions, such as EPI INFO; simple reference soft wares with satisfactory user-friendliness and performing most of the statistical analyses, such as PCMS, STATISTICA or STATA; complex reference soft wares intended for statisticians (EPILOG PLUS, SAS); specific cases such as EGRET performing only multivariate analysis or SUPERANOVA performing only analysis of variance.

'EPI INFO' is a public domain statistical soft ware for epidemiology developed by Centers for Disease Control and Prevention (CDC) in Atlanta, Georgia (USA). Epi Info has been in existence for over 20 years and is currently available for Microsoft Windows.

'PCMS' - Property & Casualty Management Systems, Inc. is an American company founded in 1999 best known for providing insurance related software and services. PCMS is a privately held company based in Dallas, Texas and is a Microsoft Certified Partner.

'STATISTICA' is an advanced analytics software package originally developed by Stat Soft which was acquired by Dell in March, 2014. Statistica provides data analysis, data management, statistics data mining machine learning, text analytics and data visualization procedures.

'STATA' is a general-purpose statistical software package created in 1985 by Stata Corp. Most of its users work in research, especially in the fields of economics, sociology, political science, biomedicine and epidemiology. Stata's capabilities include data management, statistical analysis, graphics, simulations, regression, and custom programming.

'EPILOG PLUS' is Statistics package for epidemiology and clinical trial

'SAS' (Statistical Analysis System) is a software suite developed by SAS Institute for advanced analytics, multivariate analysis data management, predictive analytics and business intelligence. SAS was originally developed at North Carolina State University in 1966.

'EGRET' software is a statistical package that provides specialized modeling and graphics capabilities to investigators conducting epidemiological and biomedical studies.

ActivEpi Web, is an electronic textbook for teaching epidemiology, available free on-line. This unique instructional tool can be accessed using the link: http://activepi.herokuapp.com.

Cytel is a multinational statistical software developer and Contract Research Organization (CRO) with, headquarter at Cambridge, Massachusetts, USA. Cytel provides clinical trail design and implementation services and specialized statistical products primarily for the biotech and pharmaceutical development markets. Cytel specializes in adaptive trials – a new type of RCT that allows modifications of on going trials while aiming to preserve the statistical validity and integrity of the study. Top pharmaceutical firms and FDA utilise their services.

Some examples of web links that provide epidemiological soft wares are shown in **Table No 12.1.**

Table 12.1 Examples of epidemiology Soft ware Links (both free and paid)

ActivEpi	A collection of tools for learning epidemiology.
CDC Wonder	Public health information system. Free.
Cytel	Epidemiological computing software.
Disease Surveillance On-Line	Disease statistics in Canada.
DoEpi	Teach epidemiology and Epi Info. Free.
EpiCalc 2000	Statistical calculator for pre-tabulated data. Free.
EpiData	Data entry and data documentation. Free.
Epigram	Vitalnet software for analyzing mortality data.
Epi Info	Make questionnaire; enter data; analyze data. Free.
EpiMeta	Performs meta-analysis. Free.
Epitools	R package for epidemiologic computing and graphics.
EpiWorld	Discussion Group listserv.
Georgia OASIS	Accesses Georgia health data.
iEpidemiology	iPhone app for analysis of epidemiologic study data. Free.
Life Table Analysis System	Occupational cohort mortality studies.
MedTrend	Vitalnet software for analyzing hospital discharge data.
MIX	Meta-analysis learning; teaching; and exploration.
NetEpi	Open source tools for epidemiology and public health.
Ohio DW	Ohio DOH Data Warehouse.
OpenClinica	Open source clinical trials software.
OpenEpi	An online epidemiologic and statistical calculator.
PEPI	Computer Programs For Epidemiologic Analysis.
PopTrend	Vitalnet software for analyzing population data.
PregData	Vitalnet software for analyzing pregnancy data.
Public Health Associate	Builds differential diagnosis lists of infectious diseases.

Table 12.1 *Contd...*

Real-Statistics.com	Real Statistics Using Excel
SampleLQ	Sampling plan calculator for lot quality assurance sampling surveys.
SampleRate	Sample size calculator.
SampleXS	Sample size calculator for cross-sectional surveys.
Sampsize	A utility to compute sample size for surveys.
SaTScan	A free software that analyzes spatial temporal and space-time data.
SigmaD	Assists in standardising epidemiological measurements.
SDA	Survey documentation and analysis - UC Berkeley.
StatPages.org	Web Pages that Perform Statistical Calculations.
Utah Hospital Discharge Query System - 1	Descriptive statistics section.
Vitalnet	Software and services for analyzing health-related data sets.
WEAT	Web Enabled Analysis Tool - BRFSS.

Causation in Pharmacoepidemiology

Causal inference is the term used for the process of determining whether observed associations are likely to be causal. The process of judging causation is very difficult and contentious. It has been argued that causal inference should be restricted to the measurement of an effect, rather than as a criterion-guided process for deciding whether an effect is present or not. Causation is an essential concept in epidemiology, yet there is no single, clearly articulated definition for the term in epidemiology discipline.

Before an association is assessed for the possibility that it is causal, other explanations, such as chance, bias and confounding, have to be excluded. The steps in assessing the nature of the relationship between a possible cause and an outcome are shown in **Figure 12.1.**

Scientific research has a goal - to observe, describe and finally relate the observations to some cause or causes. It is difficult to tease out different threads of causation. There is no definite list or set of methods that help us to determine whether an association is causal or not. One set of often used causality criteria consists of

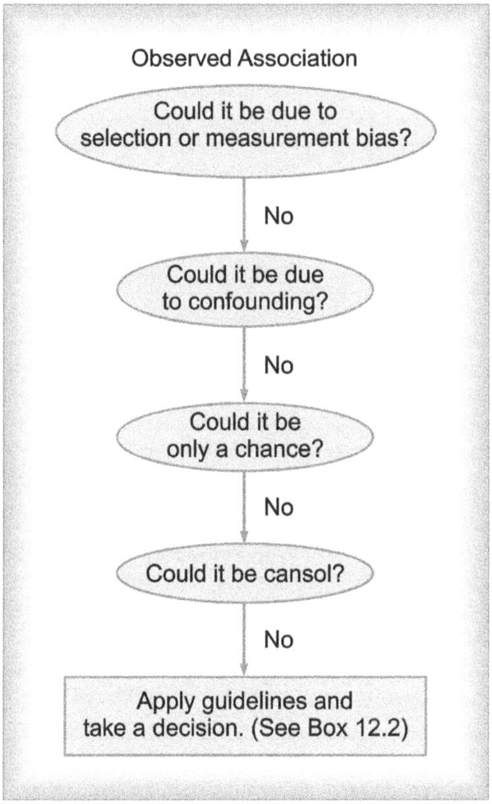

Figure 12.1 Relationship between cause and outcomes.

Box 12.1 Causality criteria

Strength	Between cause and Effect (Relative Risk)
Consistency	Have similar results in other studies?
Specificity	One particular effect only?
Temporality	Does the cause precede the effect?
Biologic gradient	Dose response. Increased exposure with increased Effect ?
Plausibility	Is the association consistent with other knowledge?
Coherence	Pathophysiology support the disease ?
Experimental Evidence	It is the reversibility. Does the removal of cause help to reduce the risk?
Analogy.	Judging the evidence with other theories?
Study Design	Is the evidence based on a strong study design?

Illustration 5: A systematic approach to determining the nature of an association was used by the United States Surgeon General to establish that cigarette smoking caused lung cancer. This approach was further elaborated by researchers.

The risk of lung cancer in smokers is about 10 times more than in non-smokers. In general the idea of strength is used to convey a sense of risk.

If the risk of disease in people exposed to a factor or event is not much higher than it is in the unexposed people, the factor is a 'weak' cause. The second criterion Consistency applies when the same general association is observed for different groups of people in different situations. For a cause to be specific it must least to one particular effect only which is a difficult requirement to fulfil. Temporality requires that the exposure come before the disease or the risk. In this case in order to develop a smoking related cancer the person must have smoked first.

A biologic gradient is present when there is a positive dose- response relationship. When the dose increases, the chance of developing disease also increases. Here in our case, it is the exposure to smoking. A plausible hypothesis is one that makes a sense or reason. This is often subjective and depends on other factors. If the mechanism of action of the drug is not known, it is difficult to establish plausibility. Coherence is similar to plausibility, and requires that the explanation suggested must not conflict with what is known about the pathophysiology of the disease. In this case it is the indicators of damage to bronchial tissue due to cigarette smoking.

The criterion of experimental evidence refer to the fact that if the risk factor is removed, that will help to improve the situation. Here it means that if the smoking is absent, that will reduce the incidence of disease considerably. Analogy refers to the ability to conceive of more complicated theories of the relationship between the suggested cause and risk under study.

Critical Analysis of the Criteria

The strength of a cause is often relative, that is it depends on whether other causes are known. Smoking is a strong cause of lung cancer compared to radon gas (Radon is a naturally occurring radioactive gas and comes from the natural breakdown (radioactive decay) of uranium. It is usually found in igneous rock and soil, but in some cases, well water may also be a source of radon) as more cases of lung cancer are ascribed to smoking. If smoking is totally eliminated, other causes may appear to be stronger causes of lung cancer. Consistency is relatively poor indicator between exposure and outcome because causality is a function of exposure and the genetic features of the person and the environment have important role in the genesis of the risk.

The relation between the cause and effect are often inconsistent because a cause can have many effects, many exposure and many results. Regarding the temporal relationship, it is often difficult to establish a time line as records are often incomplete or human memory is fallible. The situation become more complicated when the exposure occurs long time before the outcome or when the exposure is intermittent. Plausibility requires the observer to make a subjective decision or judgement which may or may not match with his own point of view. Coherence and analogy are inherently not clear. Experimental evidence may or may not be available and hence cannot be generalised in application. Because of this type of limitations some experts are of view that causation has to be approached from the approach of refutation, that is, considering opposing viewpoints and refuting conflicting views.

Applications of Causation in Pharmacoepidemiology

Epidemiology has provided society with many benefits by providing clues to the causes of adverse effects of medicines and identifying factors that contribute to the bad effects of medicines and therapy programs. Causal knowledge allows quick and effective preventive measures to lessen or halt the risks without a full understanding of the underlying mechanism.

Pharmacoepidemiology is the application of epidemiological methodologies for the study of drugs focusing on their use and effects in a large number of people. It is drug epidemiology.

CHAPTER 13

Case Studies in Pharmacoepidemiology

Chapter Mission

After learning this chapter you may be able to know:

- Background and implications of selected studies.
- Understand the theory and practice of selected designs.

Case 13.1: Pharmacoepidemiology and Drug Safety

Case: "Wide use of medicine after being introduced for marketing will help to identify many additional risks and sometimes some additional benefits". Citing examples from epidemiological studies, illustrate the statement.

Answer: Pharmacoepidemiological studies during the post marketing period help to get important information to assist in optimizing therapeutic responses to drugs. Such studies help us to find the relationship between the drugs and adverse and beneficial effects. More information emerges only at the post marketing stage of the drugs. There are many examples of serious adverse effects discovered after the drugs were put in wide use.

In 1937 over 100 children died in the US due to renal failure as a result of the use of sulfanilamide syrup marketed by Massengill Company. The firm manufactured the syrup by using di-ethylene glycol (DEG) as the solvent. In response to this incident, the Food, Drug and Cosmetics Act 1938 was passed in the US. Through the Act, pre-clinical toxicity testing was made mandatory for drugs for the first time. The manufacturers were also required to gather clinical data about drug safety and submit the same to Food and Drug Administration (FDA) before marketing drugs. Little attention was paid to the adverse reactions of drugs until the early 1950s, when it was found that Chloramphenicol could cause serious adverse effects like aplastic anemia (Wallerstein RO 1969).

In 1956, Dr.Muckter and his colleagues of the German company, Chemie Grunenthal, synthesized thalidomide which showed considerable promise as a sleeping pill. The manufacturer started selling *thalidomide* in Germany in October 1957 under the name "Countergan" and in England the Distillers Company started to sell it under license as "Distaval". In the early 1960s thousands of deformed babies known as "thalidomide babies" were born throughout the world. On 16 December 1961 Lancet published the first report in the British Medical Press indicating that *thalidomide* might be a human teratogen. It was a letter by Dr. William McBride of Sydney, Australia, that was published by Lancet. Epidemiologic studies established its cause to be *in utero* exposure to *thalidomide*. Later a number cases of adverse effects were reported of newly marketed drugs through the post marketing surveillance studies.

(German Apothecary and scientist at Bayer company), Felix Hoffmann discovered Aspirin in 1897 as a less-irritating replacement for standard common salicylate medicines. Aspirin's popularity grew over the first half of the twentieth century, spurred by its effectiveness in the wake of Spanish flu pandemic of 1918. Aspirin's profitability led to fierce competition and the proliferation of Aspirin brands and products. Aspirin's popularity declined after the development of Paracetamol (Acetaminophen) in 1956 and Ibuprofen in 1962. In the 1960s and 1970s, John Vane and others discovered the basic mechanism of aspirin's effects.

In the 1980s Dr David Sackett, father of 'Evidence Based Medicine" and then Professor of Clinical Epidemiology and Biostatistics at McMaster, Ontario, Canada through RCTs established Aspirin's efficacy as an anti-clotting agent that reduces the risk of clotting diseases. Aspirin sales revived considerably in the last decades of the twentieth century, and remain strong in the twenty-first with widespread use as a preventive treatment for heart attacks and strokes. Today Aspirin remains a foundational component of the treatment of angina and preventing heart attacks and strokes.

The adverse effects on human fetus can be estimated only through observational methods, not through experimental methods. Such cases help us to remind about the inherent limitations of the drug development process and the need to study populations receiving medications through routine prescriptions of doctors.

Case 13.2: National Drug Surveillance

Case: Considering the possible problems and pitfalls when new drugs are introduced into the market and the monitoring of existing drugs, an effective national system of drug surveillance is needed for India. How to establish a surveillance set up? What are the various methods through which the drug surveillance needs to be done?

Answer: In this context, it is useful to know how the surveillance system works in France. The French system of drug surveillance is a well-established . There is a network of more than thirty regional drug surveillance centres. A causality assessment method is used to assess the causal relationship between an adverse effect and one or more drugs. If needed, additional evaluation is done using various pharmacoepidemiology methods.

A Technical Committee and a National Commission of Drug Surveillance have been set up. These bodies collect and assess all the data in order to provide a consensual advice to the relevant authorities on necessary measures in order to prevent or reduce a drug related adverse effects. If there is an inquiry, the drug surveillance department of the pharmaceutical company and the network of regional drug surveillance centres pool their data with the aim to exchange information and ideas.

We have seen the Indian situation along with the Yellow card system of UK and the MedWatch of USA (Chapter 9). When we see the situations in other countries, it is easy to understand the limitations of our existing system. In India we need a Drug Surveillance unit in each state, with pharmacoepidemiologists playing a primary role in surveillance. These state units have to linked to a national central unit at Delhi or nearby place.

Case 13.3: Quasi Experiment

Case: The "XYZ" is a health insurance company for years. One of schemes "Health Plan One" was in existence in the country since 2005. For the treatment of peptic ulcer other than antacids two H2 receptor antagonists / H2 Blockers namely Cimetidine and Famotidine two Proton Pump Inhibitors (PPI) Omeprazole and Rabeprazole were originally included. In 2015 the policy got changed and instead Rabeprazole and Lansoprazole was included. Is there an increase in the use of Omeprazole after the policy change?

Answer: The research question "Is there an increase in the use of Omeprazole after the policy change in 2015?" can be studied with the help of an observational study by recording the number of Rabeprazole used per 1000 population over the 10 years period of policy (2005 to 2015) and then compare the pattern with the period after the change in policy. The data system of the insurance firm "XYZ" will help to make the study easy for the researcher. However with the change of policy in 2015, there is an intervention affecting the society. It is true that the intervention was not made by the researcher or the experimenter. This is an example of a Quasi- experimental study.

Case 13.4: Prospective DUR/Patient Ounselling

Case: Mr " B" is patient being treated with warfarin to prevent blood clots for some time. Recently he was prescribe Diclofenac tablet for pain by another physician. The patient is in the Community Pharmacy with the prescription of Diclofenac.

Answer: If this patient takes Diclofenac tablets along with his regular drug Warfarin, that will adversely affect INR and could experience internal bleeding. Upon reviewing the patient's prescriptions, the pharmacist can contact the prescriber and alert him / her to the problem or take other appropriate steps in this case

A Prospective DUR involves evaluating a patient's planned drug therapy before a medication is dispensed. This process allows the pharmacist to identify and resolve issues before the patient actually receives the medication. Pharmacists routinely perform prospective reviews in their daily practice by assessing a prescription medication's dosage and directions and reviewing patient information for possible drug interactions or duplicate therapy

In the DUR process the following issues are commonly addressed by the pharmacist.

1. Drug Disease Contraindications
2. Evaluation of Prescription for correctness of drugs
3. Drug allergy issues

> In countries like USA and Europe pharmacists discuss issues related to therapeutic interchange, generic substitution and drug safety issues with the patients focussing on the pharmacoeconomic issues. This will empower the patients to make
>
> ***Contd...***

decisions. According to the Pharmacy Practice Regulations of 2015, pharmacists in Indian community and hospital pharmacies are responsible for patient counselling and prescription checking and scrutiny.

Case 13.5: Ad hoc Cohort Study

Case: A pharmaceutical firm in USA in the 1970s conducted a Phase IV post marketing surveillance (PMS) study of Prazosin. The purpose of the study was to find the incidence of first dose syncope of the drug in the American population. The investigators collected data from over 20,000 newly exposed subjects recruited through the sales force of the manufacturers. The study expense was over one million US $ excluding the cost of the time of sales executives. Why it is considered as an Ad hoc Cohort study?

Answer: The usual method of recruiting patients for pharmacoepidemiology cohort study is using the medical representatives or sales executives of pharmaceutical manufacturers. These representatives will approach the physicians for enrolling the patients for whom they prescribe the drug in study. In India this can be done only at the hospital level as the physicians are not keeping a registry for their prescriptions in their practice centers. The physicians then provide follow up information on the results of the treatment. This type of practice is still followed in India also.

Prazosin, (trade name Minipress, Vasoflex, Lentopres) is a sympatholytic drug used to treat high blood pressure. It is an alpha-adrenergic blocker that is specific for the alpha-1 receptor. It was first approved by US FDA in 1976 and is still used for treatment of hypertension. These days prazosin is usually used in combination with other anti-hypertensive drugs.

First dose syncope (Sudden and severe fall in blood pressure that can occur when changing from a lying to a standing position when drug is used for the first time. It can result in a syncope or fainting and was considered as 'threat' by the manufacturers when the drug was approved and marketed.

Why this is considered as an Ad hoc Study?

It suffers from certain aspects of a standard study like

1. It was highly expensive.
2. There was no control group.
3. The physician recruited patients are not the representatives of all physicians.
4. There is no way to monitor whether the physician select patients are true representatives of all their patients.

Here a control group was not necessary for the investigators to get answers to the research questions designed. They just wanted to quantify the frequency of events in those exposed to the drug, rather than to test hypothesis about whether the drug caused particular outcome. Without a control group one cannot determine whether the observed frequency of the event is larger or smaller than expected. This type of studies are still continued in the case of medicines and is mainly for marketing than for the scientific information it will generate.

Case 13.6: Both Case Control and Cohort Designs

Case: On the night of 2–3 December 1984 methyl isocyanate (MIC) gas leaked from the factory plant of M/s Union Carbide India Limited (UCIL) pesticide plant in Bhopal, Madhya Pradesh. Over 500,000 (half a million) people were exposed to methyl isocyanate (MIC) gas and other chemicals. The toxic substance made its way into and around the area located near the plant. About 20,000 people died and 1,20,000 people still suffered health hazards with the gas exposure beyond 2010 AD. What type of pharmacoepidemiological studies are possible?

Answer: The acute effects of the exposure were studied with Cross-Sectional design. More subtle chronic effects and those developing only after long latency period are still being studies using Cohort Study design.

Cohort Studies are called prospective studies with respect to the timing of data collection process only. Cohort studies can be both prospective and retrospective in relation to the exposure and outcome studies.

Case 13.7: Alternate Names and Applications of Selected Designs

Case: What are the applications and degree of suitability of common Pharmacoepidemiological studies. Why some studies are known by different names in different books?

Answer: Pharmacoepidemiology evolved from the concepts of Epidemiology and Clinical Epidemiology. Early researchers of pharmacoepidemiology used such terms and names as they were used in Epidemiology and Clinical epidemiology while writing reports. The Table 13.1 shows the names of common types of pharmacoepidemiological studies having alternate names. The units of study are also noted.

Table 13.1 Alternate names and applications of designs

Name of design	Alternate name	Unit of study	Applications and degree of fritability
Experimental Studies	*Intervention Studies*		
Randomized Controlled Trials	Clinical Trials (CT)	Individuals	To study of effects of interventions A^{++}
Community Trials	Community Interventions	Healthy People Communities	To study outcomes influenced by social conditions and prevention efforts target group behavior A^{++}
Non-Experimental	*Observational Studies*		
Case control	Case reference	Individuals	1. Study of multiple exposure A^{+} 2. Investigation of rare diseases A^{++} 3. Investigation of long latent periods A^{+}
Cross Sectional	Prevalence	Individuals	Testing multiple effects of cause B^{+} Study of multiple exposure B^{+}
Cohort	Follow up (Prospective)	Individuals	Investigation of rare cause A^{++} Testing multiple effects of cause A^{++} Measurement of time relationship A^{++} Direct measurement of incidence A^{++} Study of multiple exposure A
Ecological	Correlational	Populations	Investigation of rare disease A^{+} Investigation of rare cause B^{+}

PHARMACOEPIDEMIOLOGY AND PHARMACOECONOMICS

CONCEPTS AND PRACTICE

Pharmacoepidemiology is the application of epidemiological methodologies for the study of drugs focusing on their use and effects in a large number of people. It is drug epidemiology.

CHAPTER 14

Practical Pharmacoepidemiology - Review for Researchers

Chapter Mission

After learning this chapter you may be able to know:

- How to conduct a pharmacoepidemiological study?
- How to write a protocol for pharmacoepidemiological study?
- General considerations for a pharmacoepidemiological study.
- How to read a study paper on pharmacoepidemiology?

How to Conduct a Pharmacoepidemiology Study?

Doing a pharmacoepidemiological research necessitates a number of aspects including understanding of the concepts of epidemiological studies, choice of research question, good protocols, ethical approval, funding sources, and other factors including applications of the results and publication of the study. The researcher and his team should complement their pharmacoepidemiological knowledge with what is known about clinical epidemiology, pharmacotherapy, pharmacovigilance, pharmacoeconomics and the regulatory aspects in practice. Though individual drugs can be selected for the study, it is better to focus on specific risk factors in pharmacoepidemiology.

A basic understanding of a specific risk epidemiology requires knowledge of the aspects like natural history of the individual, etiology, risk development in different groups, preventive and curative aspects of the risk and impact on society and policies.

Keeping informed, even in a narrow field, is difficult because of the huge quantity of material that is published. Finding, sorting through, and understanding relevant and valid information is a crucial skill that can only be acquired through practice and experience. The effort spent for reading and learning references is benefitted when it comes to designing research.

Planning a Research Project

The steps involved in planning a research project include:

- Choosing the project
- Writing the protocol
- Getting approval
- Doing the research
- Analysing the data
- Disseminating the results.

Choosing a Project

Ideally, the project should be of significance and of relevance to some health care activities related to use of medicines. Projects may focus on a wide range of subjects like drug safety, drug use evaluation, medication adherence in cases like diabetes, hypertension etc., drug interaction among specific groups like antihypertensive, NSAIDs etc., adverse effects of a particular drug or groups of drugs like statins, PPIs etc.

General Considerations for Pharmacoepidemiology Studies

The choice of study design and methods is a crucial part in every pharmacoepidemiological study and starts with the formulation of a relevant research question. A working example is 'whether non-steroidal anti-inflammatory drugs [NSAIDs] increase the risk of gastro-intestinal bleeding?' The study design and methods should follow the research question and are naturally interrelated.

Pharmacoepidemiological studies involving multiple objectives are not so uncommon. One approach for a given study might be to consider the study population as a cohort in which to implement the most appropriate design for each objective, thus ensuring alignment of each objective to the best possible design and analysis. Indeed, for studies involving primary collection of data, it may be particularly useful to adopt an approach that also incorporates strategies for appropriate minimisation of the possible sources of bias and confounding problems identified by the design.

In a descriptive study, the research question is to describe a population with respect to pre-defined parameters. In analytical studies, the research question drives three key sequentially structured phases in the design and conduct of an epidemiological study:

(i) Relation of a parameter of incidence to a determinant or a set of determinants (e.g., the incidence rate ratio of gastro-intestinal bleeds among users and non-users of NSAIDs),

(ii) Collection of data to empirically document this relation (e.g. collection from a database of exposure [use of NSAIDs] and outcomes data [gastro-intestinal bleeding] in a cohort of patients that are/have been NSAIDs users), and

(iii) Analysis of data (from raw data to quantification of associations).

These three phases are not independent. A hypothesised relation may lead to an array of designs for data collection based. In the given example, on different data sources available on use of NSAIDs (exposure) and occurrence of gastro-intestinal bleeds in patients (outcomes). Each design for data collection will be followed by only a few appropriate designs of data analysis. If applicable, the selection of appropriate electronic health data sources will be an important aspect of the design of data collection, but depending on the research question, other sources of data may be needed (e.g., some claims databases may not have a 'reason for stopping' a NSAID whereas another may have).

The choice of epidemiological methods to answer a research question is based on principles rather than on rules. These principles may provide opportunities for creativeness and new innovative methods, when appropriate and needed. However, there are certain 'dos and don'ts' and certain standards in order to assure validity and robustness of the study results.

Many research organisations (including those owning or hosting databases) have scientific review boards ensuring scientific standards are met. Some national competent authorities also have their own review board for registering/approving studies. In addition, it is good practice to invite experts to review the protocol and study report, and any publications and/or communications thereof. The role of scientific committees in governance is of particular importance in any study.

General aspects of study designs, their relevance to types of research question and issues relating to internal and external validity, including biases and confounding, are covered by many textbooks on epidemiology and pharmacoepidemiology.

> List of textbooks recommended for consultation on pharmacoepidemiology .
>
> 1. Pharmacoepidemiology 5th Edition (B. Strom, S.E. Kimmel, S. Hennessy. Wiley, 2012).
>
>   It provides a complete review of epidemiological methods applied to the study of drugs.
>
> 2. Pharmacoepidemiology and Therapeutic Risk Management 1st Edition (A.G. Hartzema, H.H. Tilson and K.A. Chan, Editors. Harvey Whitney Books Company, 2008).
>
>   In addition to a general review of drug specific methodologies, this textbook illustrates practical issues with a large number of real life examples.
>
> 3. Dictionary of Pharmacoepidemiology (Bernard Bégaud. Wiley, 2000) illustrates definitions with practical examples.
>
>   It is very useful for pharmacovigilance aspects of pharmacoepidemiology.
>
>   Researchers may find other textbooks more appropriate to their specific needs.

Research Question

The research question and the associated objectives describe the knowledge or information to be gained from the study. It is important that current knowledge gaps are properly identified. Existing guidance on this aspect includes the Guidelines for Good Pharmacoepidemiology Practices (GPP) of International Society for Pharmacoepidemiology (ISPE) and the European Network of Centres for Pharmacoepidemiology and Pharmacovigilance (ENCePP) Checklist for Study Protocols. These guidance documents emphasise that it should be clearly explained why the study is to be conducted (e.g., to answer an important public health concern, to confirm or further characterise a risk identified in a Risk Management Plan, to assess a new or emerging safety issue or to determine health outcomes or the benefit /risk profile).

It also should be clear whether the results that will be reported represent pre-formed hypotheses or research questions, or are data driven. If there is no pre-formed hypothesis, this should be clearly stated. The European Network of Centres for Pharmacoepidemiology and Pharmacovigilance (ENCePP) Checklist for Study Protocols also suggests that the research objective should briefly state the target population, primary endpoints, questions of dose dependency and the main outcome measures.

A critical and thorough review of the literature usually forms the basis for the background description and theoretical framework of the research question and should be included in a protocol. Such review aims at evaluating the pertinent information and at identifying gaps in knowledge.

According to the GPP of ISPE the review should include findings of relevant animal and human experiments, clinical studies, vital statistics and previous epidemiological studies. The findings of similar studies should be mentioned and gaps in knowledge that the study is intended to fill should be described. In addition, previous findings are useful for the methodological planning of the current study. They may be used to discuss how the findings of the previous research may support the background, significance, research question, hypotheses, and/or design of the proposed study. They may also serve to determine the expected magnitude of the event(s) under study and, if available, in the target population, to characterise the various risk factors for the event and to identify the outcomes and measures that have been used in previous studies.

The review assists in providing an assessment of the feasibility of the proposed study. In addition to seeking information, the review should be a critical appraisal of the evidence in order to assess, analyse and synthesis previous research, and place it in its current context.

General Aspects of Study Protocol

The Study Protocol/ Research Protocol is the core document of a study. A protocol should be drafted as part of the initial steps in any research project. It can be amended and updated as needed throughout its course. Amendments should be justified. It must precisely describe everything that will be done in the study, so that the study can be reproduced. It is usually and profitably based on standard protocol outlines, which could be prepared for different types of studies (e.g. cohort or case-control studies based on field data or database studies that include different information according to study type). Research protocols are subject to intense scrutiny, and are the basis on which you are going to seek funding and ethics approval for your study. Some journals may solicit protocols for peer review also.

Chapter II of the Guidelines for Good Pharmacoepidemiology Practices (GPP); International Society for Pharmacoepidemiology June 2015 provides guidance on what is expected of a pharmacoepidemiology study protocol. The guideline states that the protocol should include a description of the data quality and integrity, including, for example, abstraction of original documents, extent of source data verification, and validation of endpoints. As appropriate, certification and/or qualifications of any supporting laboratory or research groups should be included, as well as validation steps taken or considered to standardise laboratory methods proposed.

The guidelines recommend description of data management, statistical software programs and hardware to be used in the study, description of data preparation and analytical procedures, as well as the methods for data retrieval and collection. It should be borne in mind that, as stated in the GPP, adherence to guidelines will not guarantee valid research. The European Network of Centres for Pharmacoepidemiology and Pharmacovigilance (ENCePP) Checklist for Study Protocols also seeks to stimulate researchers to consider important epidemiological principles when designing a pharmacoepidemiological study and writing a study protocol.

The protocol should cover at least the following aspects:

1. The research question the study is designed to answer, which might be purely descriptive, exploratory or explanatory (hypothesis driven). The protocol should include a background description that expounds the origin (scientific, regulatory, etc.) and the state of present knowledge of the research question. It will also explain the context of the research question, including what data are currently available and how this data can or cannot contribute to answering the question. The context will also be defined in terms of what information sources can be used to generate appropriate data, and how the proposed study methodology will be shaped around these.
2. The main study objective and possible secondary objectives, which are operational definitions of the research question. In defining secondary objectives, consideration could be given to time and cost, which may impose constraints and choices, for example in terms of sample size, duration of follow-up or data collection
3. The source and study populations to be used to answer the research question. The protocol should describe whether this population is already available (such as, in a database) or whether it needs to be recruited *de novo.* The limits of the desired population will be defined, including inclusion/exclusion criteria, timelines (such as index dates for inclusion in the study) and any exposure criteria and events defining cases and exposed study groups.
4. Exposures of interest that need to be pre-specified and defined, including duration of exposure or follow-up, visits or time-dependent appraisals and details of which data are collected when, using what methods.
5. Outcomes of interest that need to be pre-specified and defined, including data sources, operational definitions and methods of ascertainment such as data elements in field studies or appropriate codes in database studies.
6. The covariates and potential confounders that need to be pre-specified and defined, including how they will be measured.
7. The statistical analysis of the resulting data, including statistical methods and software, adjustment strategies, and how the results are going to be presented.
8. The identification of possible bias.
9. Major assumptions, critical uncertainties and challenges in the design, conduct and interpretation of the results of the study given the research question and the data used.

10. Ethical considerations, as described in the section on governance of the current document.
11. The various data collection forms including the Case Report Form (CRF) or descriptions of the data elements may be appended to the protocol, allowing having an exact representation of the data collection. The study protocols could include a section specifying ways in which the CRF will be piloted, tested and finalised. Amendments of final CRFs should be justified. For field studies, physician or patient forms would be included depending on data collection methodology. Other forms may be included as needed, such as patient information, patient-oriented summaries, etc.

Doing the Research

Once you have written the protocol, it needs to be circulated for comments and revised as necessary. With major epidemiological studies there is often a long delay between preparing the protocol and starting the project, caused by the processing of a grant application. Small projects including students' projects should be designed in such a manner that they can be done quickly, as the time available is often very limited. Students' projects should not require major resources, and the supervisor should be responsible for acquiring any resources that are necessary. The supervisor should also be charged with submitting the project for ethical approval in good time.

Group projects require a reasonable division of labour and it is often helpful if one member of the group communicates with the supervisor. You need to review your progress together regularly, and allow time to pre-test questionnaires and do a pilot study of the sampling and data collection process.

Analysing the Data

There is a wide choice of software for statistics and epidemiology, ranging from spreadsheets which can do limited analyses, through software made for specific analyses, to "all-purpose" software which can do almost all the statistical analyses required for epidemiological research. A catalogue of epidemiological resources which are available free or at minimal cost has been produced by Epidemiology Monitor (http://www.epimonitor.net). Rothman's Episheet program can be downloaded from http://77www.oup-usa.org/epi/rothman.

Public domain programs, such as "OpenEpi" or the CDC's 'EpiInfo'TM are also distributed free; commercial programs can cost as much as several thousand US dollars. In choosing software, you may wish to evaluate how the program handles data entry and missing variables, what the program's capacity is for updating and merging data sets, the types of analysis that it can do, and the presence of any report-writing features or graphics and mapping options.

Getting Published

You should think about where you are going to submit your work for publication throughout the planning stages. The best way to resolve disputes over authorship is to avoid them in the first place, which means deciding early who in your research group is going to be the authors and what order? How much of the writing each of you will do.

How to Read and Evaluate a Study Paper for Empowering to do Research?

When reading a pharmacoepidemiology paper we may consider various aspects of the risk or outcomes of exposures like source of risk, factors influencing and the driving forces . Take a step wise approach to read and learn the paper.

Step 1: What is the research question?

The first step is to determine the objectives of the study – the question that the researchers wish to address or the hypothesis that they wish to test.

Step 2: If the research question is valid, are the results relevant to my work?

If yes, keep reading.

If no, start again with another paper.

Step 3: What kind of study is this?

Cross-sectional studies address questions about the prevalence of a risk factor or outcome. Cohort studies address questions about natural history or prognosis and causation. Case-control or cohort studies identify possible causal factors. Randomized controlled trials (RCT) are usually the most appropriate design for answering questions about the efficacy of treatment or other interventions. (See Chapters 7, 8 and case studies and illustrations)

Step 4. What is the study population?

Who is included and who is excluded?

Are the subjects a sample of the target population?

If not, why not?

How have the samples been selected?

Is there evidence of random selection, as opposed to systematic, or selfselection?

What possible sources of bias are there in the selection strategy?

Is the sample large enough to answer the question being addressed?

Step 5 A: For experimental studies, are the methods well described?

How were the subjects assigned to treatment or intervention: randomly or by some other method?

What control groups were included (placebo, untreated controls, both or neither?

How were the treatments compared?

Were measurements supported by quality assurance procedures?

Is the hypothesis clearly stated in statistical terms?

Is the statistical analysis appropriate, and is it presented in sufficient detail?

If this is a randomized controlled trial, was the study done with an "intention to-treat" analysis - e.g., are all the people who entered the study accounted for?

Were the outcome or effects measured objectively?

Step 5 B: For observational studies, are the methods well described?

Was the data collection process adequate (including questionnaire design and pre-testing)?

What techniques were used to handle non-response and/or incomplete data?

If a cohort study, was the follow-up rate sufficiently high?

If a case-control study, are the controls appropriate, and adequately matched?

Step 6: How are the data presented?

Are there sufficient graphs and/or tables?

Are the numbers consistent? Is the entire sample accounted for?

Are standard deviations presented with means, confidence intervals, or other statistics, as well as the raw data?

Step 7: Evaluating and interpreting the results

If you are satisfied with the Steps up to 6, and found that the study is valid and relevant. Proceed . If you are not good enough to deal with the statistics and related issues, it is advisable to seek the opinion or advice of a bio- statistician.

If it is an experimental study,

Do the researchers find a difference between the treatment and control groups? If there is no difference, and you can rule out the possibility of a Type II error, then this is a negative study – which does not mean that the results are of no consequence. If the authors have found a difference, are you confident that it is not due to chance or bias?If there is a statistically significant difference, is it enough of a difference to be clinically significant?

If it is an observational study

Were the findings in the control group consistent with what you would expect – are the averages similar to the general population? Do the researchers find a difference between exposed and control groups or cases and controls? Can Type I or Type II errors be ruled out?Is there a statistically significant difference between groups? Could the results be of public health significance, even though the difference is not statistically significant? (This may highlight the need for a larger study.)

Final evaluation

In weighing the evidence, you should ask the following questions

Was the research question worth asking in the first place, and what could be the consequences of the various possible answers?

Did the research provide suggestions for action?

Has the researcher made an adequate attempt to answer the question?

Could the study design have been improved?

Does missing information prevent you from fully evaluating the study?

Did the researcher account for results of previous studies?

If you are again satisfied with the information obtained so far and confident that the study of published papers give the information and strength, proceed with the planning, protocol and other related works of your new project.

Pharmacoepidemiology is the application of epidemiological methodologies for the study of drugs focusing on their use and effects in a large number of people. It is drug epidemiology.

CHAPTER 15

References used in the Pharmacoepidemiology Chapters

Chapter Mission

After learning this chapter you may be able to know:

- Important references used in various Chapters of this book.
- References for further reading.

References for Further Reading

Abenhaim L, Moride Y, Brenot F, et al. Appetite suppressant drugs and the risk of primary pulmonary hypertension. N Engl J Med 1996; 335: 609-616.

Biomedical evidence for determining causality. In: US Public Health Service: The health consequences of smoking- cancer. A report of the Surgeon General. Washington. 1982; 13.

Cairns JA, Gent M, Singer J et al, Aspirin, sulfinpyrazone or both in unstable angina- results of a Canadian multicenter trial. New England Journal of Medicine 1985; 313: 1359-1375.

Connolly HM, Crary JL, Mc Goon MD, et al. Valvular heart disease associated with fenfluramine-phentermine. N Engl J Med 1997; 337: 581-588.

Collett JP, Boissal JP. Pharmaco-epidemiology: Epidemiologic approach to the study of drugs. Post marketing surveillance 1991. 5: 3-14.

DeTricornot, B., Saddier, P., Bons, B. et al. Proposal of guidelines for the set up of pharmacoepidemiological studies in drug surveillance. Therapie. Nov – Dec; 1997; 52 (6): 579-585.

Dictionary of Pharmacoepidemiology; Bernard Bégaud Wiley, 2000.

Eddy DM. Probabilistic reasoning in clinical medicine: problems and opportunities. In: Kahneman D, Slovic P, Tversky A, eds. *Judgment under Uncertainty: Heuristics and Biases*. New York: Cambridge University Press; 1982: 249-267.

Eddy DM. Evidence-based medicine: a unified approach. *Health Aff (Millwood)*. 2005; 24(1): 9-17.

Experimental carcinogenesis with tobacco smoke. In: US Public Health Service: The health consequences of smoking- cancer. A report of the Surgeon General. Washington. 1982; 181.

Faich GA, Stadel BV. The future of automated record linkage for post marketing surveillance of drug safety. A response to Shapiro. Clin Pharmacol Ther 1989; 46: 387-389.

Farin Kamangar, Farhad Islami; Sample size calculation for epidemiologic studies: Principles and methods. Archieves of Iranian Medicine 2013;16 (5) 295-300.

Fayers PM. Generalisation from phase III clinical trials: Survival, quality of life and health economics. Lancet 1997; 350: 1025-1027.

Fletcher RH, Fletcher SW, Wagner EH. Clinical Epidemiology, The Essentials. 3rd ed. Baltimore, Williams & Wilkins, 1996.

Geetanjali B, Editorial. Indian Journal of Pharmacology 2003; 35:137-38.

Geiling EMK, Cannon PR, Pathogenic effect of elixir of sulfanilamide (diethylene glycol) poisoning. JAMA 1938; 111: 919-926.

Guidelines for Good Pharmaco-epidemiology Practices (GPP); International society for Pharmacoepidemiology. June 2015.

Hill AB. The environment and disease: association or causation? Proc R Soc Med 1965; 58: 295-300.

Hooten TM, Scholes D, Hughs JP, et al. A prospective study of risk factors for symptomatic urinary tract infection in young women. N Engl J Med 1996; 335: 468-474.

Lwanga SK, Lemeshow S. Sample size determination in health studies. Geneva, World Health Organization, 1991.

Mc Bride WG. Thalidomide and congenital abnormalities. Lancet; (Letter) 1358, 1961.

Mc Bride WG. Cited in Mann RD. Modern Drug Use- A enquiry on historical principles. Lancaster: MTP Press- Kluwer, 1984; 606.

Moore RD, Smith CR, Lietman PS. Increased risk of renal dysfunction due to interaction of liver disease and amino-glycosides. Am J Med 1986; 80: 1093-7.

Pharmacoepidemiology 5th Edition (B. Strom, S.E. Kimmel, S. Hennessy. Wiley, 2012).

Pharmacoepidemiology and Therapeutic Risk Management 1st Edition (A.G. Hartzema, H.H. Tilson and K.A. Chan, Editors. Harvey Whitney Books Company, 2008).

RCGP- Royal College of General Practitioners. Oral contraceptives and health. London, Pitman, 1974.

R Bonita R Beaglehole, T Kjellstrom Basic Epidemiology 2nd Edn. World Health Organization Geneva, Switzerland.

Revikumar K G, Miglani BD, Pharmacoepidemiology; A Text Book of Pharmacy Practice. Career Publication Nashik, India. 2009.

Revikumar K G, Veena R; Doctor of Pharmacy Education in India - Its Genesis and Prospects: A Critical Study based on the Global Vs. Indian Scenario. Int. J. Pharm. Sci. 24(2), Jan – Feb 2014; 46, 280-287.

Sackett DL, Rosenberg VM, Gray JA, Haynes RB, Richardson WS. Evidence-based medicine: what it is and what it isn't. *BMJ.* 1996;312(7023):71.

Shapiro S. The role of automated records linkage in the post marketing surveillance of drug safety. A critique. Clin Pharmacol Ther 1989; 46: 371-386.

Storm BL, Carson JL, Use of automated database for pharmacoepidemiology research. Epidemiol Rev 1990; 12: 87-107.

Storm BL ed. Pharmacoepidemiology Third Edn. John Wiley & Sons New York 2000.

Suissa.S. Ernst P, Benayoun S, et al. Low dose inhaled corticosteroids and the prevention of death from asthma. N Engl J Med 2000; 343: 332- 336.

The European Network of Centres for Pharmacoepidemiology and Pharmacovigilance (ENCePP). Guide on Methodological Standards in Pharmacoepidemiology (Revision 2). EMA/95098/2010. Available at http://www.encepp.eu/standards_and_guidances.

Wallerstein RO, Condit PK, Kasper CK. Statewide study of chloramphenicol therapy and fatal aplastic anemia. JAMA 1969; 208: 2045-2050.

PART II

PHARMACOECONOMICS

PHARMACOEPIDEMIOLOGY AND PHARMACOECONOMICS

CONCEPTS AND PRACTICE

Pharmacoeconomics is the description and analysis of cost of drug therapy to health care systems and society. It is a health care discipline of placing a value on drug therapy.

CHAPTER 16

Introduction to Pharmacoeconomics

Chapter Mission

After learning this chapter you may be able to know:

- Genesis and development of health economics and pharmacoeconomics.
- What is Pharmacoeconomics and how it can be defined?
- Evolvement of Pharmacoeconomics as a research method in health care.
- The objectives of Pharmacoeconomics.
- Why is Pharmacoeconomics important in pharmacotherapy?

Introduction

Resources like materials, products and other consumables are scarce or finite. Their possible uses are infinite and ever increasing. It may be impossible for one to obtain or achieve all the good things that he or she desires. Some hard choices have to be made to tackle the situation. One has to learn the technique and skill to manage the situations with available logistics and other resources. It is very much true in the case of health care where the demand for items including medicines are increasing day by day and year by year. The important role of economics rests on finding an acceptable solution to the unlimited demands of the members of the society with respect to the limited production or availability of goods and services in the society. Economics help to teach the society what to be produced, how to be produced and for whom to be produced. It also enlighten them the need for allocating scarce resources in a proper and justifiable manner.

Economic analysis is a systemic and scientific method of determining the optimum use of scarce resources and involves comparison of two or more alternatives in achieving targeted objectives under specific conditions of assumptions and constraints. According to Samuelson, "economics is the study of how men and society end up choosing, with or without the use of money, to employ scarce productive resources that could have alternative uses, produce various commodities and distribute them for consumption, now or in future, among various people and groups in society. Economics analyses the costs and benefits of improving patterns of resource allocation"(Samuelson P.A., 1976).

The Samuelson definition of economics makes clear that:

(i) Resources are limited everywhere. It is true both in rich and poor societies.

(ii) There are unlimited competing demands on these limited, scarce productive resources.

(iii) Individuals and the society have choices about how the resources are to be used. They can be used for manufacture, distribution, services or for other purposes.

(iv) With each choice comes an associated cost for that choice.

(v) Economics defines the most efficient use of the available limited resources recognizing the costs associated with that choice.

Health Economics

Health care is becoming more and more product oriented demand in increasing number of items and services for treatment and care. It is also becoming expensive and cost sensitive. The increasing cost of health care is causing concern in the society. This concern of cost of items and services is taken up, analyzed and evaluated by the science and arts of economics. Appraisal of goods and services in health care goes beyond evaluation of safety and efficacy and consider the economic impact of these goods and services on the cost of health care. It is a challenge for all health care professionals to provide quality patient care with minimum cost. In economics, efficiency and cost are the key concepts. It is very applicable in health care and related treatment programs where one has to use drugs and services. Application of the principles of economics in health care helps to design strategies for buying the greatest amount of benefit for a given resource use.

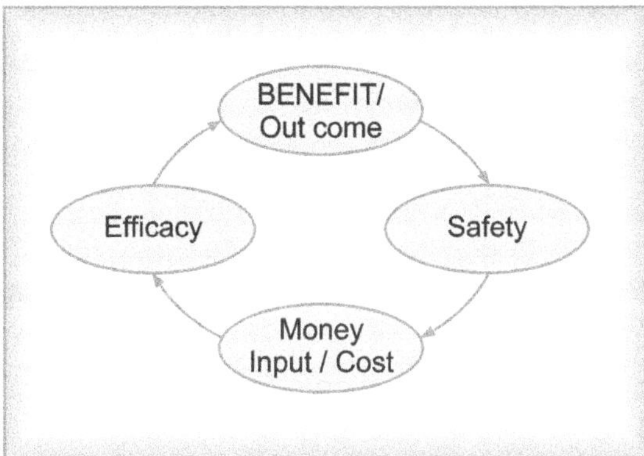

Figure 16.1 Health care concepts.

Application of economic principles in health care constitute the area of health economics. Health economics studies the supply and demand of health care resources and the effect of health services on the society or its members. Health economics can be defined as that branch of economics concerned with matters related to efficiency, effectiveness, values, styles and behaviour and their consequences in the production and consumption of health and health care. Health economists study the functioning of health care systems and life styles like use of alcohol, smoking, non-vegetarian food etc.

The concept of health economics originated in the 1960s as a way of analyzing and evaluating problems and issues related with health care. Health economics considers health care as a commodity, It accepts the fact that health care as a commodity has many characteristics different from other traditional or conventional commodities. Today health economics helps to evaluate the behaviour of individuals, firms and markets in health care. It generally focuses on cost and benefits (consequences) of health care interventions like the use of drugs, health care products, procedures, services and programs. Cost is the input and consequences are the outcomes.

Clinicians, pharmacists, economists, epidemiologists, operation researchers and other health scientists have contributed to the development of health economics as a discipline and emergence of specialized areas like 'clinical economics' and 'pharmacoeconomics' in it. Clinical economics is founded on the principle that choices must be made among alternative uses of the scarce resources. It also teaches that decision making in health care should consider cost and health benefits. Clinical economic analysis are performed mainly to assess the health outcomes achieved with respect to alternative health care interventions in relation to their costs. The purpose of clinical economics is to maximize health benefits for people with respect to the limited resources and their constraints. Today one cannot find much difference between the terms clinical economics and pharmacoeconomics.

In the beginning there were resistances and hesitance in introducing economic principles in health care as some clinicians considered it as an intrusion or invasion into their territory. It is true that there were both philosophical and methodological differences between health care and economics as disciplines. However both health care and economics gained much from the experience and have mutually enriched their research methodologies. The traffic and exchange of ideas and concepts started in both directions - from economics to health care and health care to economics and the researchers got benefited. By 1980s some understandings were developed which later lead for mutual acceptance and integration. Debates, deliberations and discussions were conducted before taking decisions. The results of such collaboration and exchange helped very much to popularize pharmacoeconomics throughout the world in the subsequent decades. The scientific community has benefited very much out of the integration and association.

Genesis of Pharmacoeconomics

The concept of pharmacoeconomics as it is understood today, originated in the 1970s in USA. The evolvement of pharmacy as a clinically oriented discipline and the incorporation of clinical pharmacy in the pharmacy curriculum contributed positively for the genesis and development of pharmacoeconomics as a super specialty in Health Economics. The Pharm D program started in the 1950s in some Universities in USA helped very much to popularize pharmacoeconomics as a subject in academic programs first in USA and then other parts of the world.

Pharmacoeconomics evolved as a subdivision of health economics. The first book on health economics was published in 1973 (Cooper MH 1973). In 1976 McGhan, Rowland and Bootman introduced some course materials related to pharmacoeconomics into the undergraduate and graduate pharmacy curricula at the University of Minnesota, USA. In 1978, McGhan introduced the concept of cost-effectiveness and cost-benefit analysis in pharmaceutical literature (McGhan, 1978). In 1979 Bootman et al., published a research article in which cost benefit analysis was used to evaluate the outcome of individualizing aminoglycoside dosage in seriously burned patients with gram negative septicemia using sophisticated pharmacokinetic protocols (Bootman JL 1979). However the term pharmacoeconomics was not used till 1982.

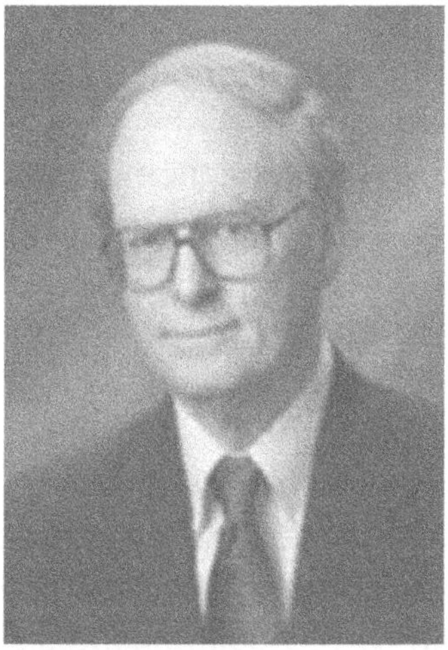

William F. McGhan, PharmD, PhD

Dr. McGhan is a known Professor of Pharmacy and Health Policy in USA . He is the head of Department of Pharmacy Practice and Pharmacy Administration, at the Philadelphia College of Pharmacy, University of the Sciences in Philadelphia.

He is founding director of the USP Graduate Program in Pharmacy Administration and also one of the founders of the USP graduate programs emphasizing health policy and pharmaceutical business.

He obtained his Doctor of Pharmacy and Clinical Residency Training from the University of California, San Francisco. He was a recipient of the American Foundation for Pharmaceutical Education (AFPE) fellowship for his Ph.D. training in economics and administration at the University of Minnesota.

Dr. McGhan has generated substantial amounts of outside funding as principal investigator on numerous grants and contracts. He has also worked at other prestigious Universities like University of Southern California, University of Arizona as director of evaluation for the innovative program of drug prescribing by pharmacists and as a founder of Center for Pharmacoeconomics. He is a past President of the Academy of Pharmaceutical Research and Science and has served on the board of directors of the American Association of Pharmaceutical Scientists and the American Association of Colleges of Pharmacy.

He was the recipient of the American Society of Consultant Pharmacists' highest honor, the Archambault Award, for outstanding professional contributions. He was the founding President of the International Society for Pharmacoeconomics and Outcomes Research (ISPOR). He is a speaker and consultant for numerous companies and organizations around the world. His research focuses on decision analysis, outcomes research, and clinical economics.

The term pharmacoeconomics was introduced in literature in 1982 by Townsend (Townsend RJ, 1986), though it was coined by some others in early 1980s. In 1983, Ohio State University College of Pharmacy initiated a specialized pharmacy academic program with the objective of providing an overview of the application of cost benefit and cost effective analysis in health care with emphasis on their application to the delivery of pharmaceutical care. In 1992, a journal was started for pharmacoeconomics with the name 'Pharmacoeconomics'. By 1990s pharmacoeconomics became an integral component of MS/ M.Pharm programs and Pharm D. When pharmacy practitioners started to apply the result of pharmacoeconomic research to therapeutic decision making, the patients started getting increased positive outcomes. By 2014 pharmacoeconomics became a critical and vital component of pharmacy curriculum at global levels.

Definition of Pharmacoeconomics

The term pharmacoeconomics is the outcome of the union of two words 'pharmacon' (means drugs) and 'economics'. Hence the literal meaning of pharmacoeconomics is economics of drugs. Pharmacoeconomics is the economics of drugs and health care based on the use of drugs. In the beginning pharmacoeconomics was defined as the "analysis of the costs of drug therapy to health care systems and society" (Townsend RJ 1986). This definition was concerned with costs alone. It did not consider the results from the use of drugs. These days such a definition is not treated as true pharmacoeconomics and is more appropriately known by the term cost analysis.

In 1990s the concept of pharmacoeconomic research was specified as "assessing the implications of projected outcomes and costs of pharmaceutical products for the decision whether to continue or stop development of a drug and for global pricing policy" (Clemens K 1993). This expanded, broader definition helped to integrate pharmacoeconomic research with the process of drug development covering pre Phase 1 (inception) to Phase IV (post marketing surveillance).

Pharmacoeconomics is the health care discipline of placing a value on drug therapy. It helps to measure the cost and consequences of various therapeutic decision making process in health care. It also helps the decision makers as a guide for earmarking resources for health care and planning process specifying priorities. Pharmacoeconomics helps the pharmacists and other health care professionals to answer questions like - "what is the value of pharmaceutical products and services provided to the patient?" or "which drug therapy or treatment program is economical to the patient"?

> *Pharmacoeconomics can be defined as the study of how individuals and groups choose to allocate scarce pharmaceutical and health resources among competing alternative uses and opt to distribute the products and services among members of the society.*

It is the description and analysis of the cost of drug therapy to health care systems and society. It gives importance to the concepts of various perspectives (like individual / patient or his family, institutional / employers, social or societal, governmental or third parties/ insurance firms) from which the health care programs are approached and evaluated. The International Society for Pharmacoeconomics and Outcomes Research (ISPOR) defines Pharmacoeconomics as 'the field of study that evaluates the behaviour of individuals, firms and markets relevant to the use of pharmaceutical products, services, and programs, and which frequently focuses on the costs (inputs) and consequences (outcomes) of that use' (Pashos C., 1998).

Prescription Costs and Factors Influencing the Demand for Pharmaceutical Products

Cost of medicine has a significant role to play in health care economics. It is well realized that the cost of medicines is not limited to their purchase price alone, but includes many accompanying costs. In order to contain costs, there should not be any compromise on quality of patient care.

Access to medicines is governed by health care service activities. In the case of other commodities, the consumer or the actual user is the deciding factor whether to buy or use the particular items. In health care the patient approaches the physician and he or she advises which medicines the patient has to use through a direction known as prescription. The demand for medicines is often a 'directed demand' and the patient has no choice but to take the medicine. This directed demand is also supplemented by a 'derived demand' - the demand based on its benefit or utility. The patient's demand for medicines are often price inelastic, that is, price increase will not lead people out of the market or decrease in price may not attract more people.

Medicines are used for specific disease conditions. The demand for a particular drug or a particular group of drugs depends on the total need of medicines for that particular disease condition they can cure. If there is no scheme to issue medicines free of cost or to subsidize, the effective demand for a sufficiently available drug at a given price may be lower to the total physical needs of patients. However in the case of scarce medicine, the situation may be different. If the physicians prescribe medicines to patients who don't require medicines or in excess of what is actually required, the effective demand can exceed total physical needs. It is also true in the case of non- prescription or over the counter (OTC) drugs.

Generic Prescribing Vs Brand Name Prescribing

Medicines once approved by the licensing authority will generally have three names - chemical name, generic name and the trade name or brand name. Chemical name is usually complicated and tongue twisting and an ordinary man may find it difficult to read or pronounce. It is usually reserved for the scientific community. The generic names are for common people and are universal in nature. The brand names are names given by the manufacturers to their products and are specifically for the trade or marketing purposes and will vary from manufacturer to manufacturer. In countries like India, there are hundreds or even thousands of brand names for a single generic product. Even educated people may find it difficult to co-relate the generic names with the various brand names of certain medicines.

Internationally branded products are very much costlier compared to their generic products. Brands are 60 percent to 300 percent or more costlier than their generics. A brand name medicine and its generic version will have same active ingredient, dosage, safety, usage directions, quality, performance and intended use. Generic drugs are as safe and strong as branded items. When a firm or manufacturer develops a new drug and applies for approval or license, they get a 20 year patent for the product which prevents other firms from selling the drug during the life of patent. Only after the patent period others can market its generic versions. Once generics are allowed competition keeps the price down.

In India the brand name prescriptions are predominant both in government and private sectors for products outside the patent periods. It is interesting to note that the students of medical sciences including medicine, pharmacy and nursing are taught the various subjects related to medicines based on their generic names during the academic courses in the country. However the medical practitioners start writing brand names of medicines right from the day one of their practice because of their mentors and preceptors. Because of this practice, the out of pocket expenses of medicines and the treatment are increased exorbitantly. Such situations necessitate the active role to be played by the practicing pharmacists through patient education, pharmaceutical care and counselling.

Why are prescribing costs increasing? There are many reasons. Some of them are the following:

(i) As a result of identification of newer health screening programs and improved diagnostic techniques previously non-identified diseases are now identified. Such identifications necessitates newer items and services for their treatment.

(ii) New medicines are introduced regularly in to the market. Many of them are more effective and less toxic compared to the existing agents. Newer medicines are generally more costly.

(iii) Medicines are increasingly used in preference to invasive treatments.

(iv) The use of existing medicines become more and more widespread as a result of their additional therapeutic uses.

(v) Increase in the life span of the people necessitates more medicines. Long life of aging population has increased the need for pharmaceutical products and services.

Applied Pharmacoeconomics

Applied pharmacoeconomics is the application of pharmacoeconomic principles, methods and theories in practice with the objective of quantifying the value of pharmaceutical products and pharmaceutical care as used in the normal and real environment.

Over the years, pharmacoeconomics has been used mainly by professionals working in pharmaceutical industry and academic settings. In industry pharmacoeconomics is used during various phases of clinical research or trials and drug development and also in post marketing studies to justify the value of medicines and other health care supplies. In academia the focus was on definition of various principles and theories and developing various methodologies for research. Unfortunately proper attention was not paid to the practice set ups like hospital pharmacy and community pharmacies. Pharmacoeconomics is a powerful, effective and persuasive tool to justify the value of the products and services provided by community pharmacists, hospital pharmacists and clinical pharmacists in any country. In a large number of countries pharmacoeconomics has been successfully applied in pharmacy practice from micro level, that is, individual patient to macro level like health care system. We will discuss it in detail in formulary system later.

Applied pharmacoeconomics will provide powerful benefits to practicing pharmacists in hospital and community pharmacies in India. Some of these benefits are shown in **Box 16.1.** How, when and where we apply these principles and methods to maximize the benefits of pharmacy services is a challenge and task to the Indian pharmacists.

Box 16.1 Benefits of applied pharmacoeconomics for pharmacists in pharmacy practice aea

- Pharmacoeconomics will provide data empowering to make better and more informed medication use decisions.
- Pharmacoeconomics will help the pharmacists to inform their administrators the evidence to choose better treatment from the alternatives currently available in the country.
- Pharmacoeconomics will help the pharmacists in justifying the need and necessity to implement the Pharmacy Practice Regulations 2015 in India.
- Pharmacoeconomic analysis will help the pharmacists to highlight the importance of generic prescription writing in India.
- Pharmacoeconomic studies related to medication errors will help to promote prescription writing as per the format specified by the Medical Council of India (MCI) and the filing of prescriptions as per the Pharmacy Practice Regulations 2015.
- Pharmacoeconomics will help the practicing pharmacists to justify the need for implementation of various pharmaceutical care services in India.
- Pharmacoeconomics can empower the pharmacists to do exercises balancing cost with patient outcome in various pharmacotherapy decisions.

Pharmaceutical care has been defined as the responsible provision of drug therapy for the purpose of achieving definite outcome (Hepler CD, 1990). There is a strong and clear relationship between pharmacoeconomics, outcome research, and pharmaceutical care. Through the concept of pharmaceutical care, the pharmacy practice accepts responsibility of managing drug therapy so that positive outcomes are produced.

Pharmacoeconomic studies are designed to provide the different information needs of health care purchasers and regulatory authorities. Economic data from Phase III studies are used to endorse the initial pricing of new therapies and are used in professional and educational activities by pharmaceutical firms. Post-marketing economic studies are used for comparing new therapies with existing therapies. They are also used to confirm the initial phase III economic assessments of the item. In the early phases, pharmacoeconomics helps to identify commercially viable options and find a market niche that could be commercially exploited. In the later phases, it permits informed decision making with regard to appropriate use of drugs that have been developed.

Pharmacoeconomics can assess the value of a product or service from single or multiple perspectives. Since the results of pharmacoeconomic valuation depend heavily on the perspective taken (e.g., patient perspective, doctors perspective, government perspective etc.), it is always essential to clarify the perspective in the pharmacoeconomic studies. For example, we can make a comparison of insulin injection with insulin pumps or pens from the perspective of the patient. Here personal factors like nature, position, occupation, etc., of the patient have to be taken into consideration for relating outcome with cost. Pharmacoeconomic studies of drugs like alteplase (tPA) and streptokinase, heparin and low molecular heparin (fragmin heparin), etc., are other examples that necessitate the relevance of perspective clarification. Once the perspective is made clear, then the evaluation of the cost can be initiated.

Applications of Pharmacoeconomics in Drug Therapy and Related Areas

Pharmacoeconomics is having applications in various aspects of health care where drugs and other services / programs are used for the positive benefit of the members of the society. Pharmaceutical industry, health scientists, academicians, pharmacy practitioners, medical professionals, economists and other health care professionals are the important users of pharmacoeconomic concepts. Practicing pharmacists have to stay abreast with the latest pharmacoeconomic studies on products and services in health care. Their knowledge should be used to analyze the economic and other claims made by the pharmaceutical manufacturers and the prescribers.

The application of the principles and concepts of pharmacoeconomics in health care aspects depends on the following factors:

(i) Availability of competent and effective professionals capable of conducting the pharmacoeconomic studies from the perspective of the people of state/ nation.

(ii) Availability of people having the capacity to learn and understand the implications of pharmacoeconomic studies and their findings in the policy makers team of the state or nation.

(iii) Availability of defined methodologies and guidelines for the conduct of pharmacoeconomic studies and their evaluation in medical interventions.

In India the health insurance system usually cover only the inpatient care which necessitates hospital stay for insurance claims. This results in increased cost. It is necessary to have some modified form of mechanism which helps to expand insurance services. Introduction of pharmacoeconomic principle in the hospital administration and treatment protocols will help both the patients and the insurance industry.

Pharmaceutical Industry and Pharmacoeconomics

Indian pharmaceutical industry is not very old as it was started only by 1900. At the time of independence the country was producing medicines worth only Rs. 10.00 crores which increased to about Rs 1,20,000.00 crores by 2015. By 2014 India became one of the world leaders in pharmaceuticals and has attained 3rd or 4th position in the quantity of production of drugs. Indian medicines are of world class quality and the lowest priced in the world. However there are certain issues adversely affecting the industry and its services in the country. The industry has a responsibility to improve and modernize the pharmacy practice services in the country by strengthening the activities like pharmaceutical care, pharmacovigilance and pharmacoeconomic studies. The industry has to play a pro-active role in ensuring rational, safe and prudent use of medicines. Serious steps have to be taken to address the issue of availability of spurious, fake and misbranded medicines in market.

The industry is expected to actively involve in the research and development of newer safe and cost effective medicines needed for the Indian population and to address the health care needs of the society. The industry has to promote access to medicines (ATM) by supporting the governments and the other non-governmental agencies (NGOs) in the country and promote manufacturing and distribution set ups accordingly .

Pharmacoeconomics in the Selection of Medicines

Medicines account for about 20 per cent of the expenditure in hospital budgets and drug therapy plays an important role in health care. In India health insurance covers about 21 per cent of the population as on 2015 AD. Government health care programs and schemes help to cover the requirements of about 40 per cent of the society who utilize the services of public health care settings extending from primary level to tertiary care level. A sizable amount of drug cost is paid by the patients out of their pocket and this expense is increasing year by year.

Pharmaceutical products are conventionally evaluated for parameters like efficacy, effectiveness, purity and safety for which well developed methodologies were established and carried out. Drug regulatory rules require that studies of safety and efficacy be performed prior to marketing of new drugs. In recent times, with the applications of principles of pharmacoeconomics, health care researchers from various disciplines managed to develop new techniques for the evaluation of the economic effects of clinical care including drug therapy. Even though the various stakeholders like physicians, decision makers, payers and patients have their own interest in a product, pharmacoeconomics helps them to take a wise decision best suited for the situation.

Pharmacoeconomics in the Discovery and Marketing of Medicines

Pharmacoeconomic research helps to evaluate the study of drug development right from the identification of a new molecule to post marketing surveillance. In order to obtain market access and retain the market manufacturers should be capable of demonstrating clinical and economic evidence to decision makers, providers, payers and users. It is true that the role of pharmacoeconomics varies with different phases of drug development. In the beginning pharmacoeconomics helps to take a decision whether we should proceed with the new drug discovery or not to proceed. Similarly after the approval of the drug and its marketing, the pharmacoeconomic importance will be given to other aspects like safe and effective prescriptions by doctors, dispensing by pharmacists and prudent use by the patients. The principal objective of pharmacoeconomics remains to ensure efficient and cost effective use of the limited resources in all situations and circumstances.

Pharmacoeconomics in the Selection of Treatment Programs

Pharmacoeconomics is increasingly being used to help determine the effect of new classes of therapy programs on patients before they are brought to the market. It also helps to determine appropriate clinical and economic outcomes for the clinical development program. Pharmacoeconomics research involves the process of identifying, measuring and comparing the costs, risks and benefits of programs, services, or therapies and determining which alternatives produce the best health outcome for the resources invested (Drummond M., 1988). It helps to measure the added advantage of a new product or service with respect to its added cost. Pharmacoeconomics helps for optimal healthcare allocation of resources in a scientific, transparent and convincing manner (Pooja Desai, 2013).

Pharmacoeconomics in Pharmacy Practice

Pharmacoeconomic studies in pharmacy practice has both academic and practice significances. The pharmacy practice curriculum must have required components and contents of pharmacoeconomics, pharmaceutical care, pharmacovigilance and pharmacokinetics required to polish their skills to provide patient care and to conduct outcome research studies. The clinical pharmacists can provide many important services in patient care areas.

Knowledge about pharmacoeconomics will help the pharmacists to quantify the products and services in terms of money value. The valuation of products and services can help to balance the costs and outcomes of various treatments and programs. This will help to identify which option gives best outcome per rupee or dollar spent. Economic, Clinical and Humanistic outcomes (ECHO) are assessed in taking decisions on pharmacotherapy programs.

With the support of knowledge in matters related to pharmacoeconomics and outcome research, pharmacists can effectively communicate with various stakeholders, program implementing agencies and patients and convince that even though certain medications are expensive, they can be beneficial in long term from the angle of both expenditure and health care outcomes. Pharmacists can enlighten the doctors by discussing the relationship between cost of pharmaceuticals and their estimated outcomes to the patients. This will help them in making most appropriate individual therapy decisions. Prudent and appropriate use of drugs and other materials in health care will reduce the overall cost and help to avoid or reduce expensive services like hospitalization and emergency department visits.

Through pharmacoeconomics, practicing pharmacists can become the key players in ensuring that drug therapy and related pharmaceutical services are safe, effective and provide real value in economic, clinical and humanistic terms. In community and hospital settings they can weigh the cost of providing pharmaceutical products or services against the outcomes (consequences) of the use of the product or service. They can also determine which alternative yields the optimal outcome per rupee spent. This will help the clinicians to choose the most cost effective treatment options.

Pharmacoeconomics in the Choice of Policies and Decisions

Pharmacoeconomics has an important role to play in the process of finalizing certain policies and decisions in health care like health policy, drug policy, and user policies or guidelines like standard treatment guidelines (STG) and preparation of essential drug list (EDL). It is vital tool in the inclusion of drugs in the Formulary of the establishment, organization or region and Government health insurance programs. Cost minimization analysis, cost utility analysis and cost benefit analysis will help the insurance schemes and agencies to select and identify the medicines for various treatment programs as is done by Medicare and Medicaid programs in USA. Cost effectiveness analysis data will help to take decision on matters related to addition and deletion of medicines from the Hospital Formulary/State Formulary. Pharmacoeconomics studies can be used to determine the values of existing services in health care including pharmacy services. It is a useful tool to estimate the money value of new services proposed to be implemented in health care. Pharmacoeconomics is the scientific method to value the various cognitive and clinical interventions in health care. When various health care programs and services compete each other for resources and approval from the authorities and organizations, pharmacoeconomic studies are important as they can provide necessary data showing the service that maximize resource allocation in the existing set up.

Pharmacoeconomics will particularly help to optimize access, cost and quality of care of the society in developing countries. Pharmacoeconomics directly and indirectly influences aspects like dosage regimens and prescription practices, national pricing policies, subsidization policies, prescribing advices and dispensing practices of medicines. It can influence policies and programs for populations of a particular region or national disease prevention programs including immunization.

Pharmacoeconomics in Formulary System

Limited or finite health care resources necessitates effective Formulary management system in health care. Formularies help to promote rational and prudent use of medicines in the society. Formularies have grown from simple drug lists to comprehensive systems of medication use policies intended to ensure safe, appropriate, and cost effective use of pharmaceuticals in patient care.

A formulary includes, but is not limited to, a list of medications and medication-associated products or devices, medication-use policies, important ancillary drug information, decision-support tools, and organizational guidelines. It represents the clinical judgment of physicians and the wisdom of pharmacists, and other experts in the Pharmacy and Therapeutic Committee (P&TC) in the treatment of disease. A formulary system is the on-going process through which a health care organization establishes policies regarding the use of drugs, therapies, and drug-related products.Today, formulary systems are considered an essential tool for health care organizations.

Traditionally, most formulary decisions were made on the basis of relative clinical efficacy, safety, drug interactions, pharmacokinetics, pharmacology, and drug acquisition costs with little consideration for the overall health-systems costs. Pharmacoeconomic evaluations help to make cost effective use of medicines. Economic evaluations have to be conducted in some cases when reviewing new medications.

The pharmacoeconomic valuations explicitly state the perspective of the analysis (e.g., patient, health care provider, payer) and include consideration of all costs and consequences relevant to that perspective. When new medications being considered are found to be therapeutically equivalent to existing alternatives (having equivalent efficacy and safety), then the cost-minimization approach is used. Cost-effectiveness analysis and Cost-benefit analysis are also useful in formulary systems on certain situations.

Strategy for Application of Pharmacoeconomics in Indian Situations

We should have an idea regarding the strategies for applying pharmacoeconomic principles in Indian Pharmacy practice settings. The implementation of pharmacoeconomic principles in the hospital, community and clinical pharmacy services is really a challenge as our pharmacies were traditionally managed by non-professionals and traders. However with the popularization of pharmacy practice education at post graduate level (M.Pharm) during the post 1990s period and the introduction of PharmD in 2008, the Indian scenario of pharmacy practice is getting serious changes both in physical facilities and service contents. Highly qualified pharmacists are opting community pharmacies and hospital pharmacies. A large number of Indian hospitals have introduced clinical pharmacy settings either as part of their hospital pharmacies or independently during the post 2010 periods. The situation is matured enough to introduce innovations in pharmacy practice in India. It is almost similar to the situation in USA in the 1960s when innovations were introduced in their community and hospital pharmacies. The existence of PharmD programs in a large number of pharmacy schools and colleges, the introduction of Pharmacy Practice Regulations of 2015 and the recent judgments of various Indian high courts regarding promotion of generic prescriptions, legible prescription writings by physicians and the need to avoid medication errors make the Indian situation more convenient for introduction of newer concepts in pharmacy practice.

The various strategies that can be considered for applying pharmacoeconomics are listed below. Which strategy is more appropriate depends on the local situations and the set up. Before selecting a strategy the pharmacists should try to find answers for the following questions

1. What is possible impact of the strategy on quality of care delivered?
2. What is the potential impact of the strategy on cost of care provided?

Strategy 1. Evaluate and use the study publications

A number of pharmacoeconomic and outcomes evaluations have been published in various medical, pharmacy and health economic journals during the last two or three decades. Select quality publications and evaluate them. Try to introduce the suggestions in the local situations with necessary modifications wherever needed.

Strategy 2. Use economic modeling techniques

During the post 2000 AD period, there is tremendous increase in the use and popularity of economic modeling as an application strategy for introduction of pharmacoeconomics in health care. Modeling can be performed with the help of popular techniques like decision analysis, Markov modeling and MAUT models.

Strategy 3. Conduct local pharmacoeconomic study

Studies can be conducted at institutions or on specific plans. Compared to the earlier two strategies, this may need more costs, time and labour. But is often more effective and proved to have significant impact. Because the studies are conducted locally, the result generated will have high significance as they are specific to the settings.

Strategy 4. Transfer results from other countries

Data from other countries can be used to educate local decision makers. Care should be taken to see whether the studies are technically correct and applicable for local decision making process. Can the study be generalized with respect to cost and practice patterns?

Strategy 5. Application of Sensitivity analysis to findings of other studies.

When trying to apply the results of a published study to a specific decision, sensitivity analysis will help to tailor the results to local situations (Bootman JL et al., 2005).

Strategy 6. Conductance of Meta-Analysis

It is very much useful for pharmacy practice areas. It is important to become familiar with the methodology of meta-analysis prior to conducting a full meta- analysis of the literature.

Strategy 7. Replicate the study on a smaller scale or as pilot project

A well conducted pharmacoeconomic study in another country or place or institution can help the Indian pharmacists to apply the results (with necessary changes) in decision making regarding pharmaceutical products and services.

Pharmacoeconomic Regulations and Practice at Global Level

Government is the primary payer for health care service including medicines in both developed and non-developed countries. The notable exception is the United States of America. The governments in these countries were using a variety of mechanisms to control the expenditure on health. One of the recent approaches in this line is the adoption of pharmacoeconomic guidelines. From the payers perspective, the use of economic analysis is expected to reduce expenditure as they believe that high prices are responsible for the increased expenditure. The manufacturers use the same economic analysis to justify the price of a product.

Pharmacoeconomic studies come from various sources. However majority of them are either conducted or funded by pharmaceutical firms. From the payers perspective this can cause bias in the findings. Hence they specify pharmaco-economic guidelines and today there are hundreds of guidelines in use by government and private payers like insurance companies.

Currently pharmacoeconomic guidelines are used in many countries **(See Table 16.1)** in different ways. Some countries have published recommendations, while other countries have guidelines. Yet other group of countries have their own submission guidelines for pharmacoeconomics.

Till 2000 only Australia, Cananda and United Kingdom have operational stan-dardized pharmacoeconomic guidelines with explicit criteria for conducting and reporting economic analysis of medicines (Bootman JL, 2005). All the countries shown in the table follow the pharmaco-economic principles though some are lacking standardized explicit guidelines. Non-governmental pharmacoeconomic guide-lines are in operation in USA, covering millions of insured lives and accounting for substantial portion of US drug expenditure.

Australia was the first government to implement pharmacoeconomic guidelines. It has become a reference point for many other countries. In 1992 they published the first guidelines which were revised in 1995, 2000 and 2008. They are very specific on all key elements of a standard economic analysis. It stipulates that the product sponsor must provide as estimate of financial implications for the health budget. Product must be cost effective and affordable to the government. Government will pay most of the cost of the drug through its subsidy.

Table 16.1 Pharmacoeconomic guidelines in countries

	Published PE Recommendations	**PE Guidelines**	**Submission Guidelines**
AFRICA	South Africa	Egypt	
AMERICA-LATIN		Brazil Colombia Cuba Mexico	
AMERICA-NORTH	**USA**	**Canada**	
ASIA	China Mainland	Taiwan South Korea Malaysia	Israel Taiwan Thailand
EUROPE	**Australia** Denmark Hungary Italy Russian Federation Spain Croatia	Baltic (Latvia, Lithuania Estonia) Belgium France Germany Ireland The Netherlands Norway Portugal Slovak Republic Slovenia Sweden	England & Wales Finland Poland Scotland
OCEANIA		New Zealand	Australia

The Canadian guidelines were developed in 1991 and implemented in 1994. They are similar to that of Australia, but more in details. The UK guidelines apply only to England and Wales. Scotland has a similar program known as the Scottish Intercollegiate Guidelines Network (SIGN) which develops clinical guidelines for Scotland.

The US pharmaceutical market is split between a private sector and different government programs. Hence it is not surprising that US is not having a national pharmacoeconomic guideline. However the FDA in US has involved in the pharmacoeconomic assessments.

The United States spends more money on health care, including prescriptions, than any other country, and it continues to grow every year. Pharmacoeconomics plays a pivotal role in the formulary decision-making and has value when assessing biotechnology drugs, therapeutic drug monitoring, and disease management. Pharmacoeconomics is increasingly used by formulary committees to help determine the status of particular medications. Decision regarding whether the drug will be placed on the formulary and what restrictions will be imposed on its use is taken based on the pharmacoeconomic studies (Esmond D, 2005).

As pharmacy services in the US expanded to include programs like medication therapy management (MTM), the need for pharmacoeconomics analyses to measure the value of these services has increased in the recent decades. There is a demand for professionals, particularly pharmacists, who have been trained in pharmacoeconomics.

The Accreditation Council for Pharmacy Education (ACPE) developed standards and guidelines for professional programs in pharmacy leading to a doctor of pharmacy (PharmD) degree.

The 2007 PharmD guidelines included the following topics under the pharmacoeconomics:

Economic principles in relation to pharmacoeconomic analysis

Concepts of pharmacoeconomics in relation to patient care,

Applications of economic theories,

Health-related quality-of-life concepts to improve allocation of limited health care resources.

In addition, the International Society for Pharmacoeconomics and Outcomes Research (ISPOR) Educators' Tool kit Task Force was created to establish useful teaching resources for the pharmacoeconomics educator. The web site includes a list of books and articles that provide an understanding of the field of pharmacoeconomics. Over the last 30 years in the United States, more health care administrators, medical practitioners, and governmental policymakers have turned to pharmacoeconomics analytical tools to assist them in making health care decisions.

During the past 15 years, a substantial international interest has developed in the economic evaluation of healthcare and medical technologies.Globally, the number of colleges and schools of pharmacy providing education in pharmacoeconomics has increased since late 1990s. As pharmacoeconomics continues to emerge as an important field in health outcomes assessment, future research should examine how much of this type of training is theoretical versus practical and how this knowledge is applied. Future research should also assess pharmacoeconomics education in colleges and schools outside of pharmacy (such as medical, nursing, and other health professional schools) and non-academic-based training areas like internships, workshops, and education provided by professional organizations.

In Russia, the Federal Government Standard of Education (FGSE) regulates the professional curriculum of pharmacy. Pharmacoeconomics can be taught either within a base course or as an elective course. However students were trained in Pharmacoeconomics under the elective courses compared to the base courses. Studies found that there is a need for improvement of Pharmacoeconomics education in pharmacy schools by increasing the number of hours dedicated and the development of Pharmacoeconomic textbooks. (Tatiana Makhinova, 2012). There is a large deficit in the availability of courses pharmacoeconomics in Brazil and Egypt at both the undergraduate and graduate and great opportunity for experienced individuals to fill this gap (Soliman AM, 2013). Pharmacoeconomics education is in its infancy stage in these countries.

Pharmacoeconomic Education in India

The discipline of pharmacoeconomics utilizes an evidence-based approach, and overlaps with fields of health economics and clinical or humanistic outcomes. It was first introduced in Indian pharmacy education in the 1990s in the M.Pharm Pharmacy Practice syllabus of certain South Indian Universities which was later adopted by other Indian Universities. In 2008 when the Doctor of Pharmacy (Pharm.D) program was introduced in India, Pharmaco-economics was introduced as a paper along with Pharmaco-epidemiology in the 5th year of the Pharm.D program. By 2013 about 15 thesis were approved by various Indian Universities for the award of PhD degrees in the areas of pharmaco-economics. However, specialized educational program like M. Pharm Pharmacoeconomics or fellowships in pharmacoeconomics are yet to be initiated in Indian Universities. It is interesting to note that there were more than 50 fellowship programs in USA in 2007 (Kane- Gill et al. 2008).

Pharmacoeconomics is the description and analysis of cost of drug therapy to health care systems and society. It is a health care discipline of placing a value on drug therapy.

CHAPTER 17

Cost Analysis and Cost Measurements

Chapter Mission

After learning this chapter you may be able to know:

- The concept of cost in pharmacoeconomics.
- How the costs are categorized in pharmacoeconomics.
- How the cost of therapy is determined.
- Identification of resources used in therapy.
- Assignment of monetary value to resources.
- Determination of costs in Pharmacoeconomic evaluations.

Price and Cost

Two of the most common terms we come across in pharmacoeconomics (as in economics) are price and cost. They seem almost interchangeable, but not to economists. Price should be the same as cost? What exactly is the difference between the terms price and cost in pharmacoeconomics?

In ordinary usage, price is the 'quantity of payment or compensation' given by one party to another in return for goods or services. In modern economies, prices are generally expressed in units of some form of currency like rupees or dollars. In business it is the consideration given in exchange for transfer of ownership of certain items. Price is the basis of all commercial transactions where buyer is willing to pay and the seller is willing to accept the amount. In simple terms we can say that price is the amount a customer pays for a product or service.

Cost is the quantity or amount of rupees or dollars to produce a particular product or service. It is the expense that a business incurs in bringing a product or service to market. Cost refers to what is incurred. Cost is defined as the magnitude of resources consumed (Bootman JL. 2005). The cost of a product or service is the monetary value of resources consumed in its production or delivery. Resources include personnel, plant, equipment and supplies.

In the case of medicines the cost of production is calculated by adding the prices of various materials and process involved in the preparation or manufacture of a particular medicine like active ingredient, diluents, colouring and flavouring agents, containers and packing materials, labels etc. The unit price of a drug product (medicine) is shown as maximum retail price (MRP) on its label. In the case of manufacturing business, generally price is higher than the cost of the item and the difference is the profit. If the MRP of a medicine is 220 INR and its cost of production is 110 INR, the manufacturer makes a gross profit of 110 INR for that medicine unit. Usually price is greater than cost. That's what gives the business a profit. But it's not always the case. The price of a medicine or medicines used is not the same as the cost of the drug therapy.

Concepts of Costs in Therapy or Program

The concept of cost in pharmacoeconomics deals with the resources that are consumed or used or utilised in the production of a good or service. The final products of the health care system are therapies (which are also called programs) that cure, mitigate or prevent disease or ailments affecting health status. In producing these therapies or programs a number of services and items may be used. They are the inputs in the production process that produces therapies as outputs.

Examples of the items used in a therapy are:

Medicines prescribed by physicians and purchased by the patients.

Laboratory tests and investigations.

Physician consultations.

Hospital stay.

Surgical procedures.

These services in turn require a number of essential resources like personnel, utensils, equipment, facilities and logistics. Hence we can consider health care services as intermediary goods as they consume the essential or basic resources and in turn they are consumed in the production of therapies or programs.

In the case of certain pharmacoeconomic analysis, the determination of the basic inputs is very important.

Illustration 1: Take the case of giving insulin injection once daily to a patient. Here the basic inputs of labour and items should be specified.

Illustration 2: Calculate the cost of treating diabetes with drug therapy. Here the services used (intermediate) are sufficient than the basic or essential inputs.

Costs and Consequences

Cost is the total value of resources consumed by a program or drug therapy of interest. It is the input. Costs are more than transactions of money. Costs represent the consumption of a resource that could otherwise be used for another purpose

Consequence is the outcome or benefit. It is the effects, outputs or results of the program of drug therapy of interest. We will discuss it in next chapter in detail. Both the cost and the benefit depend partly on the perspective or the viewpoint chosen for the pharmacoeconomic analysis.

In pharmacoeconomics, consideration is given to both, costs and consequences and it differentiates pharmacoeconomic evaluations from traditional cost containment strategies. Outcome research is defined as studies that attempt to identify, measure and evaluate results of health care services in general. Pharmacoeconomics is not synonymous with outcome research. Pharmacoeconomics is sometimes treated as a division of outcome research that can be used to quantify the value of pharmaceutical care products and services.

Cost Analysis

Cost analysis is an integral part of pharmacoeconomic studies. The first step in any cost analysis is identification of the various costs. Various types of grouping of costs are available. It may be noted that in the 1980s and 1990s costs books on pharmacoeconomics categorized costs into four types namely – direct medical costs, direct non-medical costs, indirect costs and intangible costs. However these terms are not used as such consistently. In another classification, health care costs are grouped into five main categories - direct medical costs, direct non-medical costs, indirect non-medical costs, intangible costs and opportunity costs (Eisenberg J.M., 1989). For all routine practical purposes, direct medical and direct non-medical costs can be clubbed together as Direct costs. Readers need not be confused regarding the sub-classes in direct costs.

In this book we follow a system of categorization of costs as followed by the American College of Clinical Pharmacy for training the PharmD students.(ACCP 2013)

- Direct Cost
- Indirect Cost
- Intangible Cost
- Opportunity Cost
- Incremental Cost

Indicating these categories, when appropriate, will provide a more accurate estimate of the total economic impact of a health care program, or treatment alternative, on a specific population, organization or patient.

Direct Costs

Direct costs are the resources consumed in the prevention, detection or treatment of a disease or illness. Direct costs involve a transfer of money. If money is exchanged for the use of a resource, that is a direct cost. It includes physicians' fees, cost of administering the medication, costs of treating an adverse drug reaction, etc. These costs can be further divided into

Direct Medical Costs

Direct Non Medical Costs

Direct Medical Costs

Direct medical costs are associated with monetary transactions and represents costs that are incurred during the provision of care. It is incurred for medical products and services used for the prevention, detection and treatment of a disease. This includes the cost of drugs, supplies, laboratory tests, payments for doctors' fee, fee or salaries for other health care professionals, time and labour and hospitalisation.

Direct Medical Costs can further be subdivided into Fixed and Variable Costs.

Fixed Costs represent the overhead costs that are relatively constant and not readily influenced at the treatment level. Hence they are often not included in many pharmacoeconomic evaluations. Some examples of fixed costs are those incurred for rent, light, or air conditioner.

Illustration 3: Employees salary is fixed cost. Depreciation of plant and equipment is fixed cost.

Variable Costs are such costs which vary as a function of volume and include drugs, fees for professional service and supplies. When greater number of services are used, more funding would be consumed for these services. Changes in variable costs are important tool to measure cost effectiveness of a treatment alternative.

Illustration 4: Sales commission is a variable cost. Cost of medicines is a variable cost.

Contd...

> Some controversy exists as to whether personnel costs should be considered as fixed or variable costs.
>
> **Illustration 5:** In a hospital setting one might ask whether switching from a treatment that requires administration of medicines three times daily to one administered once daily truly saves time for nursing and pharmacy professionals. One argument is that irrespective of the number of patients or the number of doses, these expenses are constant. Others argue that these activities should be considered as interventions and they can perform other activities when free and hence considered as variable costs.

Direct Non-Medical Costs

These are costs of non-medical services arising due to illness but do not involve purchasing medical services. They include cost of transportation to hospital or doctors' office, cost of special clothing or other items needed, expenses incurred on accommodation needed near the treatment center, on food, family care, clothes, expenses for aids and other related out of pocket expenses.

Indirect Costs

Indirect costs are also known by other names like external costs or indirect medical costs. They are evaluated from the perspective of the society. These are costs of reduced productivity and include wages and salaries lost due to morbidity and income forgone due to premature death or resignation from the job due to inability to work.

Indirect cost is the one borne by the patient and family, e.g. the cost of travel or transportation, loss of family loss of patient income due to absenteeism from work. Indirect costs are less obvious, but important from the perspective of patients. These costs result from morbidity and mortality. Morbidity costs are costs incurred from missing work or lost productivity. Mortality costs are costs incurred due to premature death.

'Indirect benefits' are savings as a result of avoiding indirect costs. They are the increased earnings or productivity gains as a result of medical intervention or product. In the case of chemotherapy and radiation, indirect costs result from the time the patient take off from the work because of the effect of the disease or its treatment. Some indirect benefit will occur at a later period because of the increased productivity by the success of the treatment in decreasing morbidity and mortality.

Estimation of Indirect Costs

Human capital method and Willingness – to- pay method are the two commonly used techniques for estimating the indirect cost in pharmacoeconomics. They are used for the estimation of different types of costs.

Human capital method is used to estimate morbidity and mortality losses based on the person's earning capacity. The value of life is equated with income. The human capital approach utilizes standard labour wage rates or schedules for calculating the earnings lost or gained as a result of illness. There are certain issues with this method. One is that all people are not having same level of income or earnings. Another issue is that certain groups like children, elderly and homeless virtually earn nothing at all. It is suggested to value "imputed" wages for such groups for assigning a value to indirect costs.

In the willingness to pay method, patients are asked how much money they would be willing to spend to reduce the likelihood of illness. There can be high difference in the value given by the patients. Willingness to pay method can be used for both indirect and intangible costs. The human capital method considers only the changes in work loss and productivity due to mortality and morbidity.

Intangible Costs

Intangible costs are the most difficult costs to measure. These are costs incurred, which represent non-financial outcomes of disease and medical care, which cannot be clearly expressed in money value or rupees.

It includes costs of mental agony, pain, suffering, grief, loss of energy, inconvenience etc. These costs can be described as the 'psychic' cost of diseases. Intangible costs result from medical illness itself and from the services used to treat the illness. In the case of chemotherapy and radiation treatments, nausea, alopecia, and fatigue are common intangible costs of treatment.

Intangible costs are difficult to measure or give a monetary value on these types of costs as part of a pharmacoeconomic study. Presently, these costs are often omitted from clinical economic research. Sometimes these intangible costs are included in the indirect costs. It is practicable to incorporate the intangible costs as a part of the quality of life (QOL) assessment programs. Typically intangible costs are identified in economic analysis, but not formally quantified.

Investigators are in the process of developing ways to measure intangible costs.Willingness –to- pay method is sometimes used as a tool to measure intangible costs. In cost utility analysis, the calculation of utility measures is meant to include intangible costs also.

Opportunity Costs

Opportunity costs form an important part of the cost analysis, and should always be ascertained. It can be defined as the benefit forgone when selecting one therapy alternative over the next best alternative. That is, it identifies the value of opportunities, which have been lost by utilizing resources in a particular service or health technology. Opportunity costs assign cost in monetary units to the opportunity foregone. When we have limited money and we spend it on one health care program, we cannot spend the same money on something else. That is, if the money would not have been used for the procedure/drug that is being evaluated then where would it be used.

Opportunity costs are costs of economic benefits forgone when one therapy is used instead of the next best alternative therapy. It includes the cost of lost opportunity or revenue forgone.

> **Illustration 6:** The time one takes to see a cinema is a cost for the viewer because it is time that cannot be used again. The opportunity to use it for another purpose has been forgone.
>
> **Illustration 7:** The time taken for consulting with a particular doctor is another example for opportunity cost as the value of alternative was forgone.

Opportunity cost recognizes that there are limited resources available for utilizing every treatment, and therefore the rationalizing of health care is implicit in such a system. It also allows the cost of the treatment to be evaluated, as its value can be weighed in comparison with other interventions.

> **Illustration 8:** If we spent 'x' % less on the drugs, we would be able to afford 'y' times more on the surgery.

Incremental Costs

Incremental cost is the cost associated with increasing production by one unit. Because some costs are fixed and other variable, the incremental cost will not be the same as the overall average cost per unit. The incremental total is always made up of purely variable costs.

When the medical intervention becomes increasingly intense, typically cost increases. According to the economic principle of decreasing incremental returns, the additional benefit / outcome gained per additional amount (rupees/dollar) spent typically decreases. At some point of increasing expenditures, there may be no additional benefits, or even a reduction in outcome.

Incremental cost can be another way to assess the economic impact of a program or treatment alternative on a population. Incremental costs represent additional cost that a program or therapy alternative imposes over another, compared to the additional effect, benefit or outcome it provides. That is, incremental costs are extra costs required to produce an additional unit of effect.

Other Categories of Costs

Costs are also classified as 'average costs', 'fixed costs', ' variable costs', and 'marginal costs in health care.

Average costs are the simplest way of valuing the consumption of health care resources. It represents the total costs incurred in the delivery of a service of a health care system divided by the units of treatments undergone.

Fixed costs are those that are independent of the number of units of treatments undergone and include rent, heating, lighting, and fixed staffing costs.

Variable costs depend on the number of units of treatment. The cost of the consumption of medicines is an example of variable cost.

Marginal cost is the change in total cost associated with the production of an extra unit (or one less) of a particular service. Because fixed cost remains unchanged as out put increases, marginal cost may be viewed as an average variable cost.

Illustration 9: Treating more patients or treating a patient with more complex pathology requires additional cost known as marginal costs.

Illustration 10: ECG machine is a fixed cost but the paper used in an electrocardiogram machine is a variable cost.

Implications of Definitions of Various Costs

From the definitions and discussions on various categories of costs, the following points become relevant.

1. Cost should not be confused with price or charge in pharmaco-economics. Cost is the magnitude of resources consumed in producing a service or product.
2. Cost is not the same as out –of-pocket payment. Third party payment or charity care or free service are also with components of cost.
3. Cost should not be confused with flow of money. (Illustration 11)

Illustration 11: A new program of Patient Counselling was introduced in the hospital pharmacy services and staffed with the existing pharmacists.

Even though the personnel budget is not increased, there is a labour cost in the new program. The personnel resource is consumed, that is, there is a resource commitment to the program of Patient Counselling. The economic assumption is that the time spent on the new program (Patient Counselling) could have been spent in another productive venture. It is the opportunity cost of a forgone alternative.

Cost of Illness and Cost of Therapy

An illness has a cost because it consumes many resources. The cost of illness (COI) is the sum of all the resources used by the illness. These resources used by the illness can be categorised into three groups namely

Medical Resources

Non Medical Resources

Indirect Costs or Lost Productivity.

Medical resources include the resources used to treat the illness and include hospital care, medicines, supplies and professional services.

Non- medical resources include

(i) All personal out of pocket expenses other than medical care areas. Transportation to the treatment sites and hiring a home nurse or helper are examples of this type of expenses.

(ii) Resources consumed in other sectors due to illness. An illness of a person may cause resources in home department or in education department like police vehicle. Even though they are non- medical in nature, their use is caused because of the illness.

The indirect costs or productivity costs are the costs of morbidity and mortality that we have already seen.

A medical therapy is aimed at prevention, cure or reducing the severity of an illness. Therapy consumes or uses many resources. All the three categories of costs seen for COI are also used here. The net cost of therapy is the sum of the resources used under the three categories like Medical , Non- Medical and Indirect costs. In practice indirect costs are often avoided as they are controversial due to chance for high variation in values.

The total cost of a therapy will include

1. resources used in the therapy
2. resources used in treating adverse effects
3. resources saved if illness is prevented or its severity reduced
4. resources used based on information acquired from the therapy.

Illustration 12: Comparison of cost of dialysis conducted at hospital and home.

The medical resources used in clinical dialysis include equipment, facilities and personnel. Travel expenses to the hospital is direct non-medical cost. If the patient miss the work, the lost productivity is an indirect cost of the treatment. In the case of home dialysis, medical costs will be there as equipment and supplies are used. Non-medical cost are absent as transport and hospital facilities are not used. But home dialysis require a trained helpers service and hence that cost will be included. All these aspects should be considered while comparing the cost of dialysis alternatives.

Illustration 13: Giving injections of antibiotic to patient suffering from infection of prostrate gland. Patient require injection continuously for 3 days two times in a day.

The cost of therapy can be calculated in the same way as in the case of Illustration 13 above. Home care may need the services of a nurse two times a day for three days.

Can Pharmacoeconomic Studies Focus Exclusively on Medical Costs?

Many pharmacoeconomic studies focus exclusively on medical costs. If the scope of analysis is limited to the health care system or if the alternatives do not differ with respect of their effect on non-medical resources, it is appropriate to exclude non-medical costs from the study. Including indirect or productivity costs is often controversial. If they are included in the study, conduct analysis without them. (Bootman JL, 2005).

How to Determine Costs in Pharmacoeconomic Studies?

Determination of costs in pharmaco-economics is a technical and skilled job. It requires the knowledge of the principles of pharmacoeconomics and the various methods used. It also necessitates the understanding of the perspectives used in the study. Fig. 17.1 shows the five steps in the process of determining cost of a therapy or service.

Step 1: Specification of Resources

The first step in the determination of cost of therapy or program is the identification of the resources or inputs consumed by the program. This will help to specify the ingredients used to produce the therapy. The objective of this step is to develop a comprehensive list of inputs or resources used in producing the therapy.

In the case of a therapy, this will help to identify

What medical services are used?

Hospital care? Physician visits?

What are the medicines prescribed?

What non-medical services or indirect costs are involved?

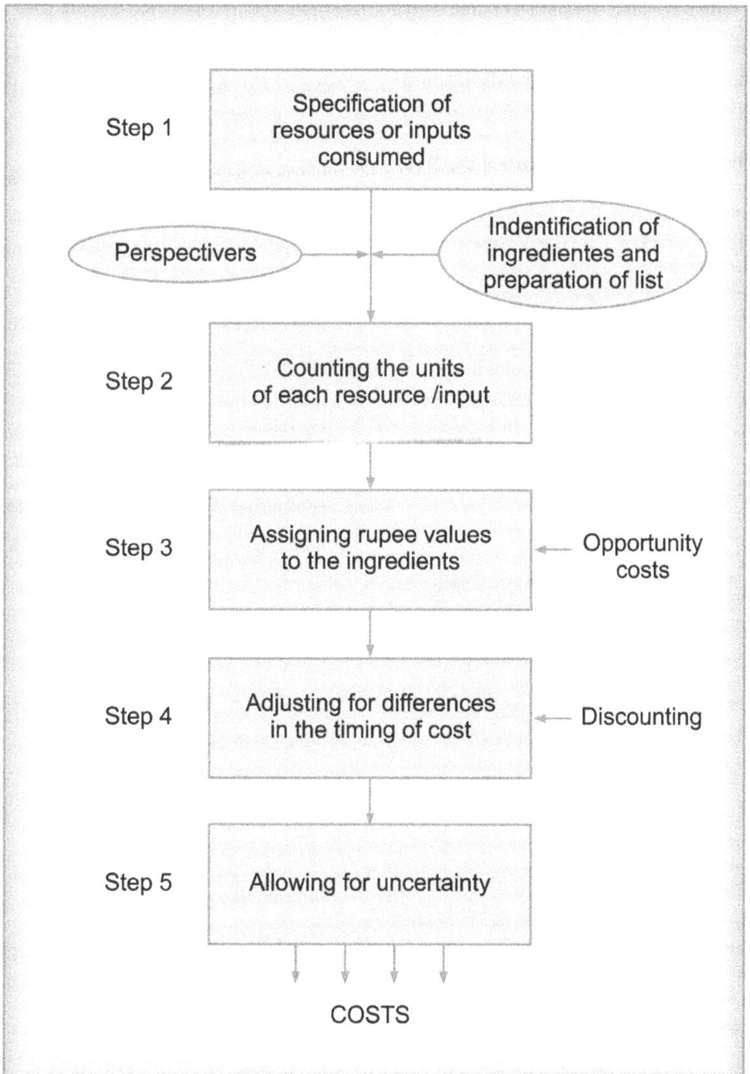

Figure 17.1 Cost determination.

In the case of a service, what types of personnel are required? What equipment? What all supplies are consumable?

An economic evaluation must include all relevant resources. It should not be limited to the ones obvious, easy to measure or identify. Identification of resources can be done independently of assigning a money value in rupees or dollars. Sometimes certain resources may appear to be insignificant, still it is better to list them and drop at the time of analysis. The dropping of ingredients should be done intentionally and consciously after identification and listing.

In determining the relevance of resources we have to specify the scope and perspective of the study. Many perspectives are possible in economics studies. The perspectives are discussed separately. However the Illustration 14 will help to understand the perspective concept at this stage.

Illustration 14: A patient under the coverage of a health insurance scheme in India is admitted in a private tertiary care hospital after being treated as an out- patient for 15 days in some other secondary care hospital. According to the insurance scheme the patient is eligible for hospital expenses, investigations and medicines during the hospital stay. He is also eligible for the medicines and laboratory investigation 2 days prior to admission and 2 days subsequent to discharge. The patient was discharged after 7 days stay and treatment at the tertiary care hospital with a direction to take medicines for 30 days after discharge and take full rest at home for 10 days.

From the perspective of the hospital, relevant costs are those incurred during the hospital stay only.

From the perspective of the insurance company the medicines and investigations two days prior to admission, hospital stay period treatment expenses and the medicines and laboratory investigations for two days after the discharge are relevant.

From the perspective of the patient apart from the earlier noted expenses all other expenses incurred during the 15 days as OP patient in the secondary care hospital prior to admission in the tertiary care hospital, and the expenses after the discharge and rest in the home are relevant. Since the insurance company pays the expenses related to hospital stay they are excluded from his out of pocket expenses.

Step 2: Counting the Units of Each Resources

The resources identified in step No 1 should be subjected to further analysis for identification of units of use or units of consumption. The magnitude of consumption of resources can be measured or counted in that unit.

Illustration 15: Use of medicines can be measured in units of individual doses.

Physician services can be measured in units of procedures.

Contd...

Inpatient services can be measured in number of days.

When the units are counted and reported separately the impact of different monetary values can be easily determined.

Step 3: Assigning Rupee Value to the Units and Resources

After identification of the resources and counting the units, they have to be assigned a monetary value. It is very difficult and complex in nature. The time and effort spent on assigning a monetary value should be proportional to the importance of that resource. More importance should be given to the major resources. The following are the important factors considered for valuation process in USA and many European countries.

(i) Opportunity cost and market price

Opportunity cost is the true cost of consuming a resource. If market price is available that is a good indicator and can be compared with the opportunity cost. Hospital charges are often misleading and they often have limited relationship with the resources consumed. For resources like helpers/ servants, unpaid assistants from a family member etc., which have no price, opportunity cost is the best method.

(ii) Opportunity cost and Average cost

Average cost is often known for various health resources wherever pharmacoeconomics is in practice and use. Hence opportunity cost can be easily compared with the average cost of the resources or its units.

(iii) Opportunity cost and Marginal cost

Marginal cost is the change in total cost as a result of producing one more unit of output. Marginal cost is often considered as a better indicator of opportunity cost than average cost. Fixed expenses included in the average cost are consumed even in the absence of the additional unit. The main problem with marginal cost is that it is often not known, while average cost is often available.

(iv) Allocating Shared resources.

This is based on the concept that if a resource is used by multiple programs or services, the cost of that resource should be allocated among the programs. If a pharmacist starts a new service, the personnel cost is not zero for the reason that he is already working and included in the employees list. Allocation of costs can be made based on many ways like on the basis of square feet/ square meter (cost of space for a program not having own space), time spent (if the personnel are shared among multiple services) or revenue generated (e.g. in allocating administrative expenses for pharmacy) .

Step 4: Adjusting for Differences in the Timing of Costs

We all have a time preference for money. Our preference is to receive rupees or dollars now rather than a future date as they can generate benefits or other returns during the interim period. It is for this reason that we always prefer to pay the rupees later than now. A rupee today is worth more than a rupee tomorrow.

Illustration 16: A lottery ticket winner has the choice of getting one crore INR today or twenty lakh INR per year for the next five years. Which one he will prefer?

In both cases, he will get INR one crore. But in all likelihood he will opt for one crore now. This will help him to invest the money properly and enjoy the benefits.

Discounting of Future Costs

Current and future rupees or costs are not valued equally. When a therapy or program extends over years, the future costs have to be discounted to reflect their current value.

Discounting is the adjusting (reducing) of the costs for differential timing. It should be done if the cost and consequences of a treatment program accrue during different period of at least I year in duration. It will help for a fair and complete comparison.

The present value (PV) is calculated by multiplying the future cost (FC) by the discount factor (DF). Pharmacoeconomic researchers have already arrived at conclusions regarding the DF. The DF is dependent on two factors or variables namely

1. Number of years into the future that expenses is incurred (n)
2. Discount rate (r) .

There is no standard rate or (r) recommended for pharmacoeconomic evaluations. Current bank interest rates are often considered as a bench mark. Researchers recommend that net costs should be discounted to their present value using a rate of 3- 8 % per annum. Model rates used in pharmacoeconomic evaluation appear to be about 5 %.

Illustration 17:

Problem: Given that the DF associated with r = 3 % and 6 % for next 5 years as

Year (n)r = 3 %		r = 6 %
1	0.971	0.943
2	0.943	0.890
3	0.915	0.840
4	0.889	0.792
5	0.863	0.747

Calculate the PV of INR 1000 received a year from now

Answer: If the r = 3%, the PV will be INR 971

If the r = 6%, the PV will be INR 943

Illustration 18:

Problem: A treatment program has costs as follows: 1st year INR 30,000, 2nd year INR 20,000 and 3rd year INR 10,000. With a discount rate of 6 %, what will be the PV of the total cost?

Answer:

The unadjusted cost of three years = INR 60000

PV of 1st year = 30000 x 0.943 = 28290

PV of 2nd year = 20000 x 0.890 = 17800

Contd...

PV of the 3rd year = 10000 x 0.840 = 8400

With a discount rate of 6%, the PV of the costs = 28290 + 17800 + 8400 = INR 54490

Note: In the calculation, we assumed that the expenses were incurred at the end of each period. If it is assumed that the expenses are incurred at the beginning of each year, the PV of first year will the 30000 it self, (no need for discount). PV of 2nd year will be 20000 x 0.943 = 18860. PV of 3rd year will be 10000 x 0.890 = 8900. Hence PV of costs will be 30000 + 18860 + 8900 = 57760.

There is no set rule regarding the best discount rate in economic evaluations. Theoretically, it should reflect the social rate of time preference. Discounting is based on time preference and not on inflation as such. Discounting is done even if inflation rate is zero. Discounting is appropriate when the analysis is longitudinal, following same subjects for more than one year period.

Step 5: Allowing for uncertainty

There are many cases where cost or resource consumption is not known exactly. In such situations we make certain assumptions and estimated figures are derived. A method to compensate for this uncertainty is **"Sensitivity analysis".** In the sensitivity analysis, the economic evaluations are reworked using different estimates or assumptions of the uncertain costs.

Sensitivity analysis is often considered as a "what if" analysis like

What if a price increase (or decrease) for a medicine is assumed?

What if a different hospital rate or fee is used?

What if a different manpower requirement is assumed?

Sensitivity analysis is needed for any cost that is not known with certainty.

Costs of Services in Pharmacy Practice

We should see how the costs are calculated for pharmacy practice service related evaluations like personnel time, medicine costs, physician service and hospital costs.

Personnel time

In the case of specialised pharmacy services like dose adjustments (e.g., paediatric, geriatric, hepatic or renal cases) or preparation of an extemporaneous item, we have to calculate the amount of personnel time. Evaluation of a clinical service also requires the amount of personnel time needed to perform the service.

There are techniques available for work measurements. In engineering time- motion studied are used widely. But in pharmaco-economics, often work sampling and stop watch time studies are used for cost determination.

In work sampling momentary obser-vations are made at selected or predetermined times. After sufficient observations, the percentage of time devoted to each activity including idle time can be determined (number of observations for an activity divided by the total number of observations). In the case of non-repetitive tasks that are not entirely uniform from occurrence to occurrence, the work sampling is widely used.

Stop watch time studies are generally used in repetitive tasks of short durations. This method directly measures the time required to complete a task or activity like dispensing a prescription or calculation of doses for a paediatric patient. Here also we have to conduct the study for a number of persons to find the average time for an ordinary person. After calculating the time, we have to apply the wage rates to find the cost of the labour.

Medicine Costs

One drug say Paracetamol or Ampicillin can have any number of formulations in India. Even a 500 mg paracetamol tab will have different prices for different firms. Even a firm will give the product at varying prices depending on the quantity ordered or purchased at a time. They also offer various discounts and schemes to bulk purchasers. If the number of doses of a medicine used by a patient are known, the appropriate price has to be fixed based on the setting.

In countries where pharmacoeconomics is in practice and applied, average wholesale price (AWP). Since in India the AWP concept is not in application due to the lack of pharmacoeconomic studies we have to find some other realistic methods or comparisons. The prices fixed by Janaushadhi scheme of government of India, selling prices of the fair price community pharmacies like Karunya pharmacies of government of Kerala, the prices of professional community pharmacies etc., can be considered to calculate standard prices for medicines in India. The manufacturers are giving medicines to major hospitals and to government owned agencies like Tamil Nadu Medical Services Corporation, Rajasthan Medical Services Corporation and Kerala Medical Service Corporation at prices very much lower to the open market prices. All these show that there is considerable difference between maximum retail price (MRP) shown on the labels and the standard price of medicines in India.

Physician Services

There are two commonly used methods in pharmacoeconomics for calculating the expenses for physician services. One is to use the actual amount charged and other one is to use the allowable or usual customary charge of a third party payer like insurance companies. The actual amount is also known as the market rate. However it is to be noted that certain corporate speciality hospitals are charging very high rates compared to ordinary hospitals. The Indian health insurance schemes were briefly discussed in the pharmaco-epidemiology chapters of this book. Even if the patient uses the service of a free hospital like government hospital or military hospital, such costs have to be calculated while doing the analysis.

Hospital Services

Assigning values to hospital services is one of the critical and difficult tasks in pharmacoeconomic studies. An error in valuing the hospital services can easily result in misleading conclusions. An important rule in pharmacoeconomics is that if the cost an item is of high value, more time and effort have to be given for such items or expenses. Hospital services being the most expensive of all health care services, they deserve special attention in pharmacoeconomic analysis.

We have already seen the difference between price and cost in earlier chapter. The amount charged for a service is its price. Cost involves the magnitude of resources consumed in producing the services. In pharmacoeconomics, the method for valuing the hospital charges depend on the nature of study and the data available.

Routine Services and Medical Services - Micro costing

In the existence set up it is advisable to follow this system in India for estimating hospital service costs. Here hospital services are grouped into routine services and Medical or ancillary services. Routine services are those that are normal or standard in all patient days in the hospital like room rent (bed rent), food (or dietary), washing (or laundry) and administration. For such services average daily costs apply to each day. It is not equal to marginal costs. If we can do sensitivity analysis, that will be better or more appropriate. Medical or ancillary services include pharmacy services, laboratory and radio-diagnosis. They vary from patient to patient. Hence it can be measured for each patient on daily basis.

This type of costing is considered to be the most precise method of estimating cost. It involves collecting information on resources used for each component of an intervention. Hence it is also known as micro costing.

In countries like USA, Australia and many other European countries the 'per-diem' concept and the rates under 'diagnosis related groups' (DRG) followed by their insurance schemes are widely used in fixing hospital services in pharmaco-economics. However they have very limited application in current Indian set up. We have to be well informed about such concepts in other countries for the conduct of pharmacoeconomic studies in India. Such concepts can be applied with necessary changes in India or other similar countries.

Per-diem Cost

The per diem is simply the average daily cost. It is found by dividing the sum of all costs (routine and ancillary) by the number of patient days. It is an average of all fixed and variable costs. It is not equivalent to the marginal cost. Marginal cost may be less while per diem cost may be high. Per diem cost assumes that all days are equal in terms of resource consumption. But in actual practice we can see that the ancillary resources are intensively used in the initial days and less in the subsequent days. The per diem cost method is considered as the least precise method of estimating hospital costs. According to this concept a by-pass surgery patient and a caesarean delivery patient will have same cost estimate if both of them were in the hospital for 5 days, provided the average cost (per diem) is same. In some countries they have disease specific per diem costs like 1500 dollars per day for appendicitis case or 9000 dollars per day for cardiac by-pass case.

Diagnosis Related Groups (DRG)

A "Diagnosis Related Group" is a payment category that is used to classify patients, especially Medicare patients, for the purpose of reimbursing hospitals for each case in a given category with a fixed fee regardless of the actual costs incurred.

A Diagnosis-Related Group (DRG) is a statistical system of classifying any inpatient stay into groups for the purposes of payment. In US this method is used to classify clinically cohesive diagnosis and treatment procedures that use similar resources. The DRG classification system divides possible diagnoses into more than 20 major body systems and subdivides them into almost 500 groups for the purpose of Medicare reimbursement. Each patient can be assigned one DRG group for reimbursement of cost.

DRGs were first implemented in New Jersey in 1980 with the objective of containing the cost of Medicare. It was started with a small number of hospitals enlisted into three groups according to their budget positions - Surplus, Breakeven, and Deficit - prior to the imposition of DRG payment.The New Jersey experiment continued for three years, with additional cadres of hospitals being added to the number of institutions each year until all hospitals in New Jersey were dealing with this system. The prospective payment system implemented as DRGs had been designed to limit the share of hospital revenues derived from the Medicare program budget and was extended to entire USA in 1983. In 1987, New York state passed legislation instituting DRG-based payments for all non-Medicare patients.

The DRG system was introduced to identify the "products" that a hospital provides. One example of a "product" is an appendectomy. DRGs have been used in the US since early 1980s to determine how much Medicare pays the hospital for each "product", since patients within each category are clinically similar and are expected to use the same level of hospital resources. DRGs may be further grouped into Major Diagnostic Categories (MDCs). DRGs are also standard practice for establishing reimbursements for other Medicare related reimbursements such as to home healthcare providers.

In order to meet the evolving needs in health care, the objective of the DRG system has been expanded and today there are several different DRG systems in the US like. They include

- Medicare DRG-
- Refined DRGs (R-DRG)
- All Patient DRGs (AP-DRG)
- Severity DRGs (S-DRG)
- All Patient, Severity-Adjusted DRGs (APS-DRG)
- All Patient Refined DRGs (APR-DRG)
- International-Refined DRGs (IR-DRG

It may be noted that the DRG system is not having a direct application in India. However the knowledge and awareness of such schemes will help to establish systems for India.

Pharmacoeconomics is the description and analysis of cost of drug therapy to health care systems and society. It is a health care discipline of placing a value on drug therapy.

CHAPTER 18

Outcomes and Perspectives in Pharmacoeconomics

Chapter Mission

After learning this chapter you may be able to know:

- The concept of outcomes or consequences in pharmacoeconomics.
- Categorization of outcomes in pharmacoeconomics.
- Concept of perspectives in pharmacoeconomics.
- Various perspectives in pharmacoeconomics.

In the previous chapter, we have seen the concepts of costs in pharmacoeconomics. Like costs, consequences or outputs of a treatment or program are equally important. Now in this chapter we will discuss the concepts and classes of outcomes or consequences in pharmacoeconomics.

In all full pharmacoeconomic methods or analysis, measurement of outcomes are essential for the assessment of efficacy. For that purpose, efficacy is determined according to the amount of output per unit of input of one program or treatment versus another program or treatment. The assessment of costs in various methods are similar in nature. But the manner in which consequences are assessed varies among the methods or techniques. Good assessments of relative outputs of the competing programs help the researchers to balance the costs of a program with their consequences or benefits.

Classification of Outcomes

Like costs, the outcomes or benefits or consequences can also be grouped into various classes for convenience and analysis. One way of classification is categorizing the outcomes into

- Economic outcomes
- Clinical outcomes and
- Humanistic outcomes.

This method of evaluation is known as Economic, Clinical and Humanistic outcomes (ECHO) model.

Economic outcomes are related to the direct, indirect and intangible costs of medical treatment alternatives. Economic evaluation is the formal process of weighing benefits and costs in an incremental analysis. The economic outcomes can be expressed in terms of money value.

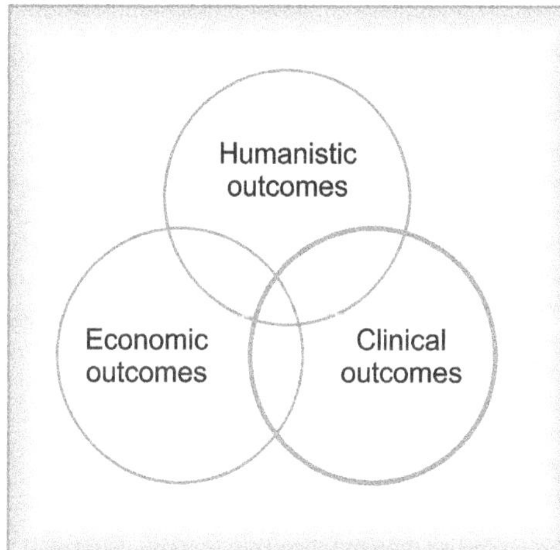

Figure 18.1 Components of clinical decision making.

Clinical outcomes are medical events or results that occur as a result of disease or its treatment, like improvement of the disease condition, cure of the disease, nor worsening the condition or even certain risks like adverse effects or worsening the condition.

Humanistic outcomes are the outcomes of diseases or their treatment on the functions or quality of life of patient (QOL). Factors like healthy life, general well being, social compatibility and physical functions are examples of humanistic outcomes.

Positive versus Negative Outcomes

The benefits of a drug therapy program are often estimated in terms of beneficial effects to the patient. However a comprehensive assessment of benefits will address both positive and negative outcomes of the competing programs.

Sometimes the outcomes are grouped as

Positive outcomes

Negative outcomes

Neutral outcomes

The desired effect of a drug manifested as its efficacy is an example of the positive outcome. Positive outcome can be in the form of

Life years gained,

Cases cured,

Disability days avoided,

Improved functional status or

Improved well being.

We know that modern drugs are useful poisons or double edged weapons. They are not devoid of adverse effects. An undesired effect of a drug manifested as treatment failure or adverse drug reaction is an example of negative outcome. Negative consequences can include

Harmful side effects

Exacerbation of disease condition

Drug toxicity

Treatment failure

Death

The balancing of positive and negative outcomes are critical in pharmacoeconomic studies.

Illustration 1: When an antibiotic like Gentamycin is given to a patient, curing the infection is the positive outcome. Drug toxicity like nephrotoxicity constitute the negative outcomes.

The outcome can also be neutral or 'zero outcome' where neither positive nor negative result is obtained. The administration of placebos in certain patients produce zero outcome.

Intermediate versus Final Outcomes

Intermediate outcomes are also used in programs or therapy. They are more commonly used in clinical trials to demonstrate clinical efficacy because their use helps to reduce the time and cost required to conduct a clinical trial.

Illustration 2: Achieving a decrease in low density cholesterol level with a lipid lowering drug is an intermediate consequence. It serves as an indicator for more relevant final outcomes expressed as a decrease in myocardial infarction rate and an increase in lives saved.

Intermediate effects are used commonly in cost effectiveness analysis as indicators of final consequences of interest. The main problem is in finding reliable intermediate outcome which can predict correctly long term effects.

Contd...

The outcomes or benefits are expressed in terms of units like

Natural units (e.g. years of life saved or peptic ulcers healed),

Utility units (quality adjusted life years (QALYs),

Associated economic benefits (measured in money, which is a common denominator allowing comparisons across different disciplines) and

Money values (formal process of weighing costs and benefits in an incremental analysis).

Economic Evaluation and Development of New Drugs

New drugs are developed in a series of well defined states designated as Phase I through to Phase IV studies. Phase I studies represent the first introduction of a new compound into (usually) healthy people for evaluation of its safety and dosage. Pharmacokinetics, dynamics and ADR are also studied. In the Phase II studies, the new compound is introduced into the patient population, having the disease under study. It is a dose searching study. The safety is evaluated and dosing assessed. Normally 10 to 12 patients are studied at each dose level. It is an exploratory study covering 100–500 patients at 3 to 4 or more centers. The Phase III studies are formal therapeutic trials or confirmatory trials. These are randomized trials evaluating the safety and efficacy of the new compound, compared either with placebo or with a therapy that the new compound could replace. The new drug is given to thousands of patients at this stage and verifies the effect of drug in detail.

In addition of the above three types of study, new drugs are evaluated after they are marketed in what are known as Phase IV or post marketing studies or surveillance. The drug development process allows for timely collection of data that can be used to evaluate the costs and effects (cost and consequences) of pharmaceuticals early in their product life. It also gives opportunity for further data collection and evaluation after the drug is approved and introduced into the market. In certain countries it is mandatory to submit the pharmacoeconomic study results along with the new drug application.

Clinical economics is now being integrated throughout the development process with goals that go parallel with the clinical development stages. Phase I and II are used to develop pilot economy data which gives estimation of the mean and variance of costs, quality of life and utilities for patients with a specific clinical syndrome. They are also used to perform pilot tests of data collection tools including economic case report forms that prospectively capture resources used by patients who will be entered into the Phase III and IV studies. Phase III studies can also include economic assessments of new therapies as a primary or secondary end point (e.g., changes in length of hospital stay or changes in hospitalisation rates). In the Phase IV a wide variety of post-marketing economic studies can also be performed, along with efficiency trials and post-marketing surveillance studies.

Balancing Costs and Consequences

Balancing costs and consequences is the essence of pharmacoeconomic evaluation techniques. The purpose of pharmacoeconomic research is to provide information regarding relative value of treatment of competitive programs through an explicit attempt to balance the costs and consequences of each alternative. Often the results are expressed in terms of a cost per unit of effect.

Perspectives in Pharmacoeconomics

Perspective refers to the point of view from which the economic analysis is performed. Many perspectives are possible in pharmacoeconomic studies focusing on evaluation of medical care. These perspectives can influence the costs and consequences identified, measured and analyzed for a program or treatment. A pharmacoeconomic study can be conducted from a single perspective or a group of perspectives. The generally used perspectives are

- Patient Perspective
- Provider Perspective
- Payer Perspective
- Society Perspective.

The Fig. 18.2 shows some of the perspectives commonly used in pharmacoeconomics.

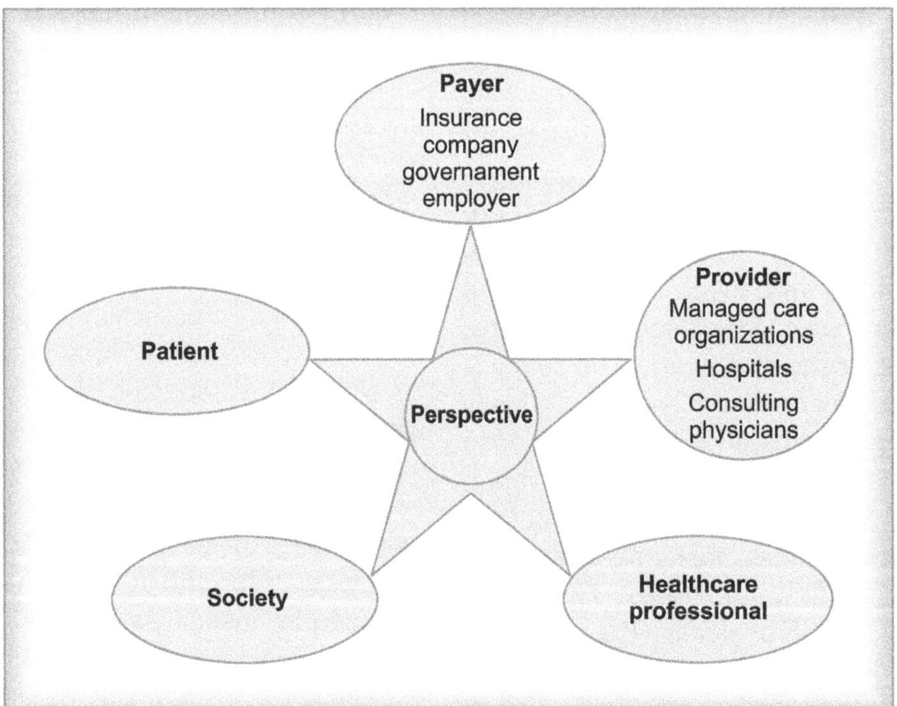

Figure 18.2 Perspectives in Pharmacoeconomics.

Patient Perspective

Patients are the consumers of health care programs and services. What are the costs involved in health care programs from the perspective of patients? All costs incurred to the patient and paid out of pocket are costs from the patient perspective. It includes all costs that are not covered under the health insurance scheme applicable to the patient. Costs incurred due to illness or treatment including morbidity and mortality costs are also included in the costs from the patient perspective. Insurance co-payments, indirect costs in terms of health related work and living limitations are also important from the patient perspective. Consequences from the patient perspective are the clinical aspects of the program or its alternatives. Patients are concerned with the positive and negative outcomes.

Provider Perspective

Providers can be Hospitals, managed care organizations (MCOs) or private practice physicians are the usual providers in health care programs. True expenses of providing the services are costs from the providers perspective. All direct costs like medicines, hospitalization, laboratory investigations and supplies are primary costs from the providers perspective. Salaries of health care professionals may be appropriately identified and measured from the perspective of provider and added to the primary costs.

From the perspective of the provider, indirect costs are not much important as they are not realized from the provider. When making formulary management or drug use policies the view point of the health care organization will dominate.

Payer Perspective

The major payers, other than the patient, in health care programs include Government, Insurance Companies and the Employers. The costs to the payer are those costs of health care programs and services allowed by the payer or reimbursed by the payer. The direct costs are the primary costs from the payers perspective. Indirect costs like lost working days and reduced productivity may also contribute to the total cost of the health care to the payer.

> **Illustration 3:** If an employee has urinary stone disease and treated in the hospital for 7 days and took rest at home for another 7 days, there is an indirect cost to the employer who incurs a loss of 14 productive days for that employee. The payers perspective are used when insurance companies and employers enter into a contract.

Health Insurance in India

Medical care is unbelievably expensive. Medical breakthroughs have resulted in cures for dreadful diseases. These cures, however, are available only to a select few. High operating expenses like therapy for breast cancer costs as much as Rs. 2 lakhs for 3 days, have restricted treatment to the richest. In fact, even among the affluent groups, 20% need to sell their valuable assets in order to accumulate the required amount to meet healthcare costs.

Indirect costs add very much to the financial burden. Indirect sources of expense like travel, boarding and lodging, and even temporary loss of income, account for as much as 30% of the overall cost of treatment.

Health insurance in the form of healthcare financing (Mediclaim) was introduced in India in 1986-1987 by four subsidiaries of General Insurance Company (GIC) to support the ailing healthcare industry. They are,

I. The New India Assurance Company,

II. Oriental Fire and Insurance Co.,

III. National Insurance Co., and

IV. The United India Insurance Co

Later, there has been a liberalization of the Indian healthcare sector to allow for a much-needed private insurance market to emerge. Due to liberalization and a growing middle class with increased spending power, there has been an increase in the number of insurance policies issued in the country.

The development of health insurance in India is a reflection of broader policy changes that are being felt in the Indian economy. As a part of its financial sector reform agenda, the Indian Government liberalized the Indian insurance industry by the enactment of the Insurance Regulatory and Development Authority (IRDA) Act by the Indian Parliament in 1999. This helped for the opening up of the sector for participation of private insurance companies. Prior to liberalization, the insurance sector consisted of the government owned Life Insurance Corporation of India that had a monopoly on life insurance business and the General Insurance Corporation (GIC) of India and its four non-life subsidiaries namely, National Insurance Co., New India Assurance Co., Oriental Insurance Co. and United India Insurance Co.

Since 1999, IRDA has licensed about 30 new private insurance companies, of which more than 20 have foreign equity participation. Major global players like Aegon, Fortis, Future Generali, Principal and Dai-Ichi have tied-up with Indian partners to set up life insurance operations. Health insurance remains vastly underdeveloped in India.

In 2001 various private Insurance companies entered into health care and today the public have choice of buying this insurance from various Insurance companies. The Insurance Regulatory and Development Authority (IRDA) eliminated tariffs on general insurance as of January 1, 2007 which helped to drive additional growth of private insurance products.

Present Players In Health Insurance Industry in India belong to three categories namely:

1. Stand alone Health Insurance Companies
2. Health Insurance from General Insurance Companies
3. Health Insurance from Life Insurance Companies

Society Perspective

Among all perspectives, society is the broadest as it is the only one that considers the benefit to the society as a whole. A good number of researchers in pharmacoeconomics are of opinion that society is the best perspective for pharmacoeconomic studies. All direct and indirect costs are generally included in an economic evaluation performed from the perspective of society. In countries with nationalized medical health care systems, society is the most important and predominant perspective. Costs from the society perspective include patient morbidity and mortality costs and overall costs of providing and receiving medical care.

Controversy in Choosing Perspective

Some controversy exists in the issue of perspective in pharmacoeconomic studies. Majority of researchers are of opinion that society is the best and most relevant perspective from which an economic analysis should be conducted. Regardless of the perspective selected for the study, perspective is very significant and fundamental as all costs and consequences identified, measured and compared will depend on perspective chosen.

Pharmacoeconomics is the description and analysis of cost of drug therapy to health care systems and society. It is a health care discipline of placing a value on drug therapy.

CHAPTER 19

Pharmacoeconomic Methods

Chapter Mission

After learning this chapter you may be able to know:

- The concept of full and partial pharmacoeconomic studies.
- Examples of full pharmacoeconomic methods.
- Examples of partial pharmacoeconomic methods.

Methods of Pharmacoeconomics

The job of economics is to allocate limited resources and distribute output among a large number of agents like individuals, firms, and governments. An economic model is a simplified description of reality, designed to yield hypotheses about economic behaviour that can be tested. An important feature of an economic model is that it is necessarily subjective in design because there are no objective measures of economic outcomes. Different economists will make different judgments about what is needed to explain their interpretations of reality.

One of the purposes of pharmacoeconomics is to help the authorities to allocate the limited resources of medicine and health care facilities among the various stake-holders. The pharmacoeconomic models and methods are helpful tools in that respect. In a pharmacoeconomic model, various inputs (costs) are combined together to produce certain outputs (consequences). Fig. 19.1. shows a simple economic model used in health care and pharmacoeconomics.

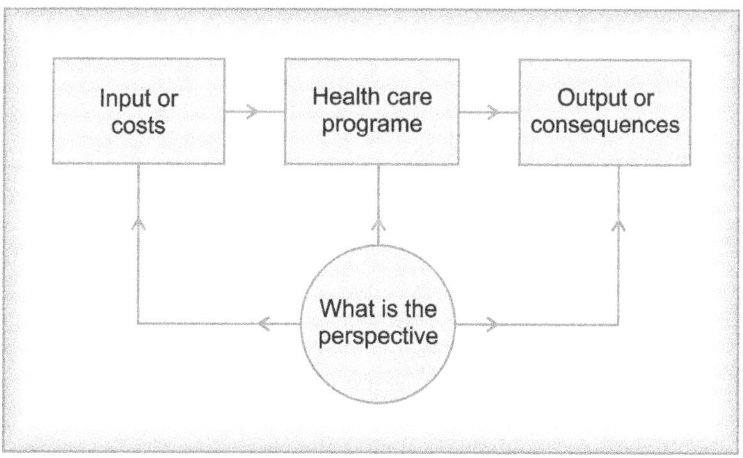

Figure 19.1 Simple model of economic analysis in health care.

There are three important factors for any economic analysis for a rational decision making in health care. They are:

1. Identification and choice among alternatives
2. Assessment of costs and consequences
3. Decision making within the limited / fixed or available budgets.

The choice of the evaluation method depends on the nature of outcomes and the context in which the choices need to be made. The perspective of the analysis is important in the selection of the method.

Various pharmacoeconomic methods are available. These methods can be grouped into two categories - Economic evaluation methods and Humanistic evaluation methods.

The economic evaluation method is focusing on identification, measurement, valuation and comparing of the costs and consequences of the alternatives being considered. It involves a comparison of two or more alternatives comparing their costs and outcomes. Studies have found that the application of economic evaluation methods to health care products like drugs increases their acceptance by both the health care professionals and the public. (McGhan WF,1993).

Commonly used pharmacoeconomic methods are

Cost minimization analysis (CMA)

Cost benefit analysis (CBA)

Cost effectiveness analysis (CEA)

Cost-utility analysis (CUA)

Cost of illness (COI)

Except cost of illness (COI), all other methods are used to compare treatment alternatives. In all the methods, cost is measured in a similar way, but the outcomes are measured in different ways. The commonly used economic evaluation methods including cost of illness are listed in Table 19.1.

Table 19.1 Common Pharmacoeconomic methodologies

Methodology	Cost unit	Outcome Unit
Cost of Illness	Rupees (INR)	Not assessed
Cost Minimization	Rupees (INR)	Assumed to be equal in groups
Cost Benefit	Rupees (INR)	Rupees (INR)
Cost Effectiveness	Rupees (INR)	Natural units/ units of effects
Cost Utility	Rupees (INR)	Utility like QALY

In COI the attempt is to determine the total economic burden of a disease or ailment on the society. All aspects of the disease like prevention, management, morbidity and mortality burdens etc., will be considered in the cost of illness studies.

Apart from economic aspects, pharmacoeconomic evaluations may also focus on humanistic concerns. Today various factors like patient preferences, patient satisfaction, impact of disease and treatment of disease on a patient's health related QOL are applied to pharmacotherapy decisions. Such factors can also be applied in pharmacoeconomic evaluations.

There are cases where only one drug or treatment or program is examined and there is no scope for a complete pharmacoeconomic analysis in such cases. However a descriptive analysis of the individual case is possible. Such studies form part of the partial economic evaluation.

Full and Partial Pharmacoeconomic Evaluations

If the evaluation consists of comparing two or more alternatives and attempts to link both, costs and effects then such evaluations are treated as full economic evaluations. Full economic evaluations comprehensively assess the economic costs and benefits of the program alternatives. Full economic evaluations are needed for evaluation of an intervention as part of a resource allocation decision. They are also useful in the formulary system for determining what drug to be included or excluded in the formulary as part of the disease management program.

Full economic evaluation methods include CMA, CBA, CEA and CUA. Though these methods vary in several aspects, they all can provide a comprehensive analysis of both costs and consequences of the evaluated program alternatives. The quality and usefulness of information is much greater with full economic evaluation, though they may require more time and efforts compared to partial methods. We will have a detailed discussion on each of the methods in upcoming chapters.

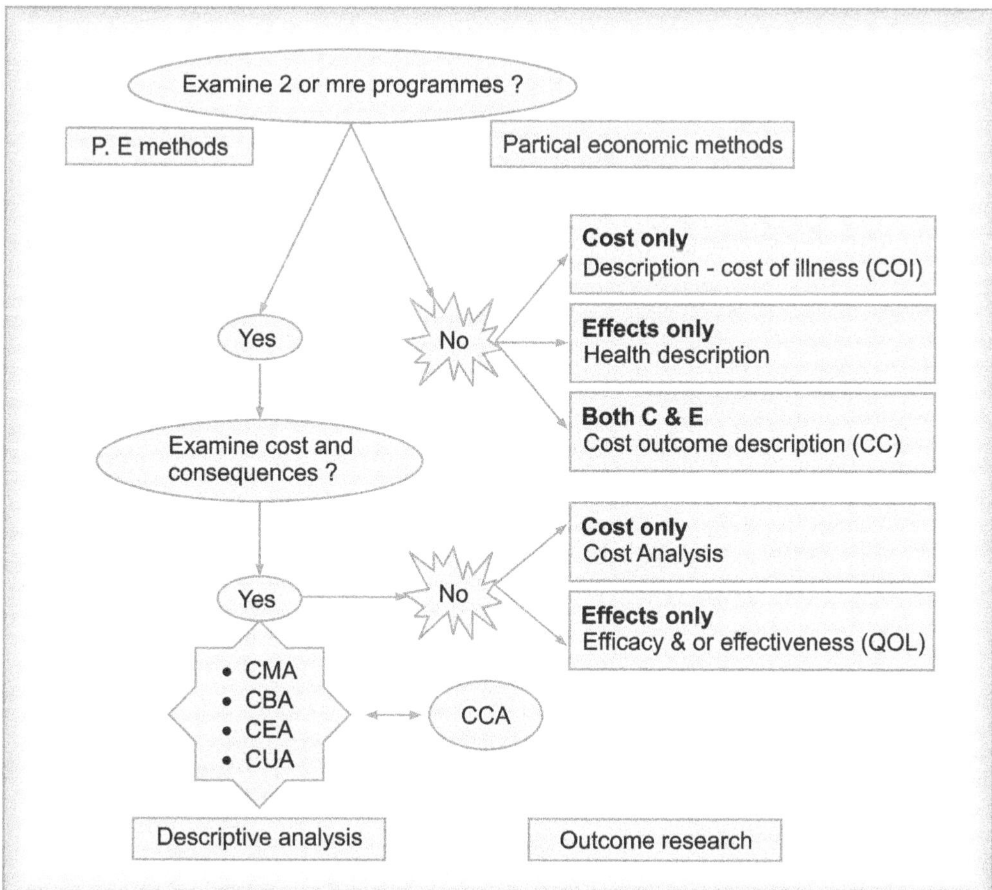

Figure 19.2 Pharmacoeconomic evaluation methods.

Partial Evaluations

Partial economic evaluations measure or examine only a portion of the costs versus consequences issue. They may include only a descriptive tabulation of outcomes or resources consumed. If only consequences or costs of a program are described, then the evaluation is simple outcome or cost description. Partial economic methods include cost analysis, outcome analysis, descriptive analysis and cost consequence analysis.

In cases where only one drug or treatment or program is examined, it becomes a descriptive analysis of that drug or treatment or program. If the program evaluation consists of two or more alternatives and the study is limited to discussions of costs only, or outcomes (consequences) only or discussions on cost and outcomes only , then they are all partial economic evaluation. A study in which the costs and consequences are described, but not compared to alternative options, it is known as a cost- outcome analysis. A cost analysis compares the costs of two or more alternatives without considering the outcomes.

PHARMACOEPIDEMIOLOGY AND PHARMACOECONOMICS

CONCEPTS AND PRACTICE

Pharmacoeconomics is the description and analysis of cost of drug therapy to health care systems and society. It is a health care discipline of placing a value on drug therapy.

CHAPTER 20

Cost Benefit Analysis

Chapter Mission

After learning this chapter you may be able to know:

- The concept of Cost Benefit Analysis in pharmacoeconomic studies.
- How to conduct CBA in pharmacoeconomic studies.
- Methods of measuring benefits in CBA - net benefit and cost benefit ratio.
- Measurement of productivity and intangible costs including human capital and Willingness to Pay (WTP) methods.

Cost benefit analysis (CBA) of medical care compares the cost of a medical intervention to its benefit. It is an economic analysis method that facilitates for the identification, measurement and comparison of the benefits and costs of a program or treatment alternative. In CBA, the benefits realized are compared with the cost of providing it. The costs and benefits are measured in the same units like rupees or dollars. It is easy to do the cost analysis of CBA. However it is a difficult and often controversial task to convert the benefits or outcomes in terms of money value. In CBA the benefits are converted into the equivalent money units in the year in which they occur.

Will the benefits of a program or service exceed the cost of implementing it ? Which program will produce higher net benefit? CBA helps to find answer to such questions. CBA is a basic tool that can be used to improve the decision making process in the allocation of funds to health care and other programs. While the overall concept of CBA is simple, its methodological considerations require a certain degree of technical understanding to apply CBA appropriately. (Bootman JL 2005).

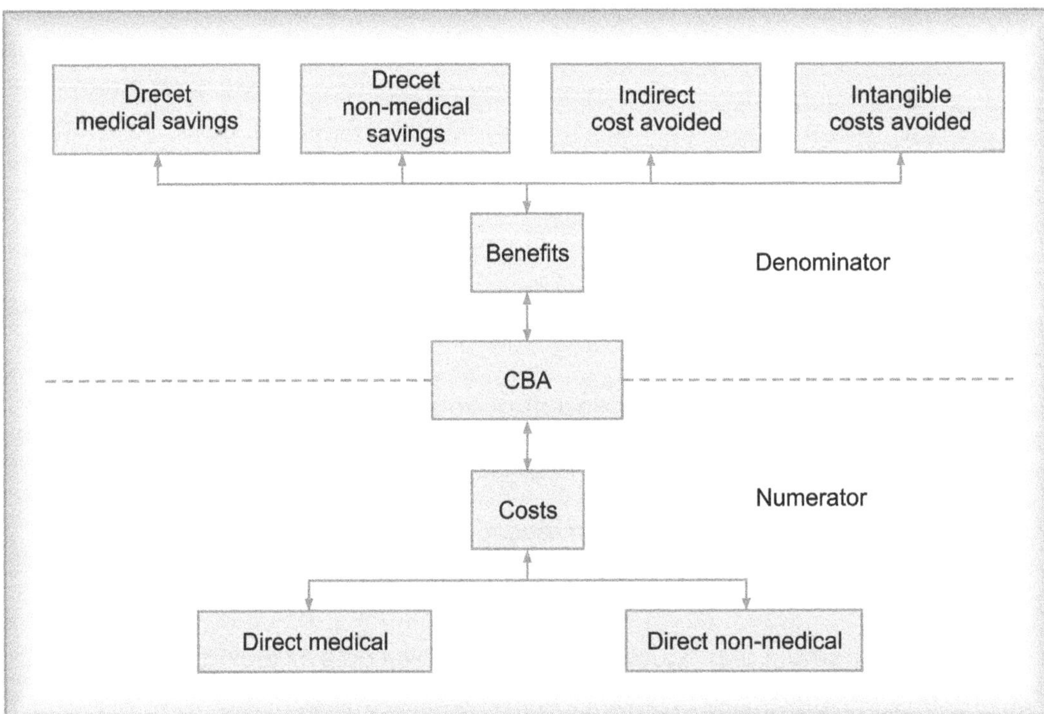

Figure 20.1 Theoretical model of economics of new treatment.

CBA type of pharmacoeconomic analysis is often preferred by economists. However the employment or use of CBA in health care is always a problem. It is not an easy task to give monetary values to the clinical outcomes like relief of pain or improvement of quality of life. It is like evaluating various persons in terms of money. If one is asked to value Mrs. 'Y' of 45 years in terms of Indian rupees, there cannot be uniformity or even acceptance of the value by others. However we can develop certain tools or yardsticks to come to a conclusion. This approach is used in CBA.

CBA compares the total costs of each alternative to the outcomes. Future costs and benefits are discounted or reduced to their current value. In programs and treatment alternatives where costs and benefits are occurring not simultaneously, CBA can be used as the pharmacoeconomic method. It can also be used while comparing programs with different objectives as all benefits are converted into money value like rupees or dollars. The most difficult and challenging part of CBA lies in converting the benefits or outcomes in economic terms. Some benefits are comparatively easy to convert whereas others are difficult and need subjective judgments. CBA quite often ignore intangible benefits (pain, anxiety, stress) that are difficult to express in monetary terms. It may also discriminate against the unproductive population or the dependent population, e.g., the elderly.

Measurement of Benefits

Costs and benefits are considered to be either positive or negative. A cost can be incurred or avoided; a benefit can be gained or lost. Various approaches are suggested for the measurement of benefits in CBA. In CBA, benefits are quite often measured using the concept of contingent valuation. Specific techniques of contingent valuation include methods like willingness to pay (WTP) or the stated preference approach and the human capital approach.

In WTP method, a representative population of the patients are told about the probability of success of a treatment and asked how much each one of them is willing to pay as insurance premium to avail the service, if needed. Alternatively, they can be asked to state how much they would be prepared to pay to avoid a particular event or symptom or a difficulty like pain, nausea, difficulty in walking etc. WTP method measures the person's utility or the desirability of a program or treatment alternative by determining how much money he/she is willing to lose for getting the improved health. In countries with social health care systems funded by the public exchequer or general taxation, it may be difficult to accept or adopt WTP.

Willingness to accept (WTA) is another method of contingent valuation. It is based on the minimum amount a patient or group of patients would accept or receive in order to be prepared to lose or avoid a service. None of the existing methods for measurement of benefits are perfect or ideal.

Cost-Benefit Analysis in Business

A cost-benefit analysis is straight forward when all costs and benefits are measurable in monetary terms.

Case Study 1: M/s Morgan Company have to decide whether to rent an ice cream machine for three summer months from March to May for Rs 5000 from M/s 'Y'. Morgan Company finds that the ice cream machine will produce additional cash inflows of Rs 7500 during the period. The benefit of additional cash in-flows (Rs 7500) exceeds the additional cost (Rs 5000). Morgan Company can take up the project because the cost is Rs 5000 and the benefit is Rs 7500.

All cost-benefit analyses are not simple like this. See cases 2 and 3.

Case Study 2: Cost savings as a benefit. M/s Jupitor is a CRO firm and makes 100,000 (1 lakh) photocopies a year. They do not have their own copy machine and currently pays Rs 0.40 per copy, (total Rs 40,000 a year) to M/s 'Z' Copiers. An offer came to the Jupitor firm so that they can lease a copy machine for Rs 25000 a year. However they have to pay Rs.0.20 per page for paper for the leased machine (Rs 20000).

In this example, the cost of leasing the machine and buying paper (Rs 25000 plus Rs 20000) exceeds the benefit of saving the Rs 40000 normally paid to Z Copiers. Jupitor firm should continue to use Z Copiers for its photocopies. However, Jupitor should take into consideration estimate of the number of copies it needs to be comfortable with its decision. If they need 200000 (2 lakhs) copies this year, instead of 100,000 copies, the cost of the leasing the machine and buying paper for Rs 65,000 (Rs 25000 plus 40000) is cheaper than the Rs 80,000 (2 lakhs x 0.4) savings in fees to Z Copiers.

Case Study 3: M/s Apothecaries is a company engaged in the manufacture of surgical goods required for hospitals. They have to decide whether to give a picnic costing Rs 50,000 for its employees. The company can receive the benefit of increased employee morale and related productivity from the picnic. Better employee morale might cause employees to work harder, increasing profits. However, the link between increased morale and increased monetary profits is quite often tenuous.

Here the decision maker have to use his or her judgment to compare the non-monetary benefit to the monetary cost, possibly deciding that increased employee morale is worth the Rs 50,000 or more cost.

In the preceding cases (Case 1 and Case 2) cost-benefit analysis provided a framework for decision making. The range of objectivity related to measurement of the factors is typical. Techniques used in business as a basis for determining costs and benefits, such

Contd...

as return on investment, are generally quantifiable and thus appear to be objective. However, it is not uncommon for qualitative factors to enter into the decision-making process. Careful decision makers attempt to deal with a difficult-to-quantify factor in as objective a manner as possible. However, cost-benefit analysis in most situations continues to introduce measurement problems.

Cost Benefit Ratios (Benefit to Cost or Cost to Benefit)

The cost benefit analysis used in pharmaco-economics is based on certain basic assumptions like the following:

(i) In health care it is possible to separate one service from the other in a logical and scientific manner.

(ii) There can be opportunity for choice between the different choices.

(iii) The benefits (outcomes) of the various services can be assessed.

(iv) The benefits (outcomes) can be valuated.

(v) The cost of providing each service can be estimated.

(vi) The cost and benefits of the various services can be compared.

(vii) The objective of the analysis is to promote such services in which the benefits outweigh the costs.

$$\text{Cost Benefit Ratio} = \frac{\text{Total Benefit}}{\text{Total Costs}}$$

The cost (C) and benefit (B) are generally expressed as a ratio known as

Benefit to Cost ratio - B/C ratio. That is Benefits divided by Costs

If the B/C ratio is > 1, it shows that the benefit outweighs the cost of providing it and hence such program is of good value.

If the B/C ratio = 1, it shows that the benefit is equivalent to the cost of providing it, that is the benefits equal the cost.

If the B/C ratio < 1, it shows that the cost of providing the treatment of program outweighs the benefit realized by it and hence the program is not economically beneficial.

Net Benefit or Net Cost

In CBA, the costs and benefits are sometimes expressed as a net benefit or a net cost. A program or treatment alternative with the highest net benefit or greatest benefit to cost ratio is considered as the best choice for positive clinical outcome.

If a service costs Rs 10,000 to implement and results in a benefit of Rs 100,000 to the hospital that will have a B/C ratio of 10. Take another service that costs Rs 25 lakhs to implement and results in a benefit of Rs 2.5 crores to the hospital, that too will have a B/C ratio of 10. It shows that caution should be taken when using B/C ratios and CBA as a comparison tool.

Applications of CBA

The overall concept of CBA is simple though it requires certain technical expertise. The major difficulty of CBA is that it requires researchers to express an intervention's costs and outcomes in the same units of money value. As measurement of outcomes in terms of currency is difficult, translating disease and treatment outcomes into monetary measures are always more difficult than translating them into clinical outcome measures. CBA is useful to evaluate an individual program or compare different programs.

Since in CBA, the consequences are measured in terms of the total cost associated with the program, it is not so difficult to do CBA in many situations. CBA can be employed at macro level for policy decisions on health care programs. CBA was evolved from the need to estimate the cost and benefits of public/government sponsored projects and schemes in health care. Expenditure for public projects should be able to produce benefits for the society in large. CBA is useful and helping tool for the judicious allocation of funds or resources for public investments in health care. Cost benefit analysis consists of identifying all the public or social benefits that will result from the program and convert them into rupees or money value in the year in which they occur.

In CBA, the benefits realized are compared with the cost of providing it. The costs of two alternative treatments and the consequences in terms of productivity or sickness benefits may be compared. In the 1980s Fitton et al., determined the total costs to society of three conditions commonly treated in general practice, namely back pain, depression and eczema. In the case of back pain, prescriptions accounted for only 12 percentage of total expenditure and the sickness benefits accounted for 65 percentage. The corresponding percentages for depression were 16 percentage and 63 percentage. But in the case of eczema prescriptions accounted for 70 percentage of costs while sickness benefits accounted for '0' percentage. The reason is clear, in eczema the working capacity is not lost while in back pain and depression it is lost.

Nation wide immunization programs like the Oral Polio vaccine can be subjected to CBA without much difficulty. Such programs can be valued against the reduced mortality or morbidity that can occur as a result of them. In programs and treatment alternatives where costs and benefits are occurring not simultaneously, CBA should be used as the pharmacoeconomic method. It can also be used while comparing programs with different objectives as all benefits which are converted into money value like rupees or dollars. It is useful to evaluate an individual program or compare different programs.

CBA is a best-suited method to justify and document the value of an existing health care service or the feasibility of a new one. It can very well provide data to justify and document that the resources of an institution with clinical pharmacy services can yield high outcomes on investments compared with other institutions competing for the same resources. CBA is useful in examining the values of services like hospital pharmacy prepared intravenous additives and ward preparations by nurses. It will help to demonstrate the value of pharmacy services. The staffing cost and equipment cost can offset against the benefits of reduced morbidity and mortality.

It can also be used to evaluate health care programs like Therapeutic drug monitoring service, Drug Information services, Patient Counselling centers, IV admixture services, Pharmacokinetic services etc., in a hospital set up. In all these cases additional staff like clinical pharmacists and facilities like instruments and equipment are required for which investment in terms of money required. These costs can be compared with the costs of the benefits of reduced morbidity, reduced mortality, reduced medication errors and increased efficiency of the services through the CBA. CBA compares the total costs of each alternatives to the outcomes. Future costs and benefits are discounted or reduced to their current value.

Another virtue of CBA is that it may allow comparisons to be made between totally different areas and not just medical. For example cost benefits of expanding University education (with benefits of improved education and hence productivity) can be compared to back pain clinics (with benefits of making people able to work and enhance productivity). CBA of programs with unrelated outcome is useful when there is shortage of funds and only one program can be implemented. Should the hospital develop a drug information center or establish a cholesterol lowering program for its staff? Through CBA we can find which will generate more benefit compared to cost of implementing each program.

In some countries like United States, CBA are used at all levels of government for allocating resources for the public programs, projects, and schemes that will meet the expectations of people. For example, information from CBA are applied for schemes related to services to the elderly, air pollution or environmental standards. Cost Benefit Analysis is typically used by governments to evaluate the desirability of a given intervention in markets.

The process involves monetary value of initial and ongoing expenses Vs expected return. Constructing plausible measures of the costs and benefits of specific actions is often very difficult. In practice, analysts try to estimate costs and benefits either by using survey methods or by drawing inferences from market behaviour.

Cost-benefit analysis is often used to assess the value for money of very large private and public sector projects. Such projects normally tend to include costs and benefits that are less amenable to being expressed in financial or monetary terms (e.g., environmental damage), as well as those that can be expressed in monetary terms. Private sector organizations tend to make much more use of other project appraisal techniques, such as rate of return, where feasible. The practice of cost-benefit analysis varies between countries. Even in a country, it also varies between sectors (e.g., transport, health). The main differences include the types of impacts that are included as costs and benefits within appraisals, the extent to which impacts are expressed in monetary terms and differences in discount rate between nations.

Illustration 1: Take the case of a hospital where it is intended to establish a hospital pharmacy/ clinical pharmacy based therapeutic drug monitoring (TDM) program. The hypothesis is that the TDM service will help to improve the quality of patient care and save money for the hospital. The scheme prepared and submitted by the head of the hospital pharmacy was approved by the hospital administration in principle; and they agreed to finance it, provided, at the end of the first year, the scheme be evaluated justifying the value of the practice.

The relevant cost and benefit of the program (TDM) should be measured and if appropriate, be converted into rupees using CBA method. Potential benefits will include increased patient compliance, decreased total drug costs and decreased incidence of ADR. Potential costs are primarily the salary and perks for the clinical pharmacist and additional laboratory tests to monitor the patients. The cost benefit (B/C) ratio can be calculated. If the ratio shows a value of 1 or more it can be easily confirmed that the benefit of the pharmacy service (TDM) yields a good return on investment (ROI). This will also help to increase the probability of continuing the financial support from the hospital administration.

In CBA ideally all costs and benefits of the program are to be included for the calculations or analysis. However sometimes it may be difficult to convert certain benefits like improved patient comfort or patient satisfaction etc., in terms of money value. Since valuing health outcomes in terms of money can cause difficulty and controversy, it is suggested that unless outcomes are appropriately expressed in terms of money, CBA should not be selected for pharmacoeconomic analysis.

Conducting Cost Benefit Analysis- *Step Wise Approach*

CBA can be conducted in the following 4 steps.

Step 1: Identification of program and intervention

The first step in conducting CBA is the identification of

- Intervention or Interventions
- Program or Programs
- Therapeutic Regimen or Regimens
- Research Questions to be evaluated

In the first step we determine the type of program and the interventions. This will help to find answers to questions like What impact the program has out side the medicine budget? Whether all patients are involved in the study? Can the program help to reduce the home care costs? Will the patients be able to return to work in next two weeks time? What are the resources needed for the program?

Step 2: Identification and valuation of all resources

The second step is identification and valuation of all resources.

Here resources consumed or cost of providing each intervention or program or regimen have to be identified. Different types of resources should be identified. In certain studies on expenses for training patients for self administration of medicines were also included.

A comprehensive comparison of two drug therapy regimens could include costs for purchasing each medicines, supplies consumed in administering each item, salary and other employee benefit expenses for personnel time consumed in preparing and delivering medicines and hospital resources used to treat an untoward effects of the program alternatives. A hospital or clinical pharmacy could include expenses for personnel time, office space, computers and laptops, telephone and supplies in CBA of Patient counselling services.

Step 3: Identification and valuation of benefits

We have already seen how benefits are evaluated in pharmacoeconomics. Please note that if the benefit of an intervention is lives saved, a money value should be assigned to those lives. If the benefit is fewer days of work missed, actual or estimated patient salary information can be used to give rupee value to those days.

Step 4: Totalling the value of costs and benefits

In the fourth step the sum total of all costs and the sum total of all benefits of each program or intervention or regimen are found. The total cost may be subtracted from the total benefits to find the net benefit.

Net benefit = Total benefits (in Rupees) –
Total Costs (in Rupees)

Some researchers prefer to compute a Cost to Benefit Ratio while others like to use Benefit to Cost Ratio. Since we expect higher value for benefits, it is better to use Benefit to Cost Ratio. If the total benefits exceed the total cost we will get a ratio greater than 1:1.

> **Illustration 2:** If the cost associated with a treatment is 1NR 10,000 and the outcome resulting from the treatment is valued at INR 100,000.
>
> Net benefit is 100,000 – 10,000
> = INR 90,000
>
> The cost benefit ratio would be expressed as Benefit INR 100,000 divided by Cost INR 10,000 or as 10:1. This Ratio should be interpreted as a treatment alternative that produces INR 10 for every INR 1 spent.
>
> The results of a CBA are most commonly expressed as a net benefit as it is often misleading to simply compare ratios. A program that costs INR 10 crores and results in a benefit of INR 100 crores also yields a cost benefit ratio of 10:1. However the relative magnitude of these costs and benefits are dramatically different from the others that yield 10:1.

Perspective of CBA

An important consideration in conducting a CBA or other types of clinical economic evaluations is the perspective of the analysis.

For whom the costs and benefits being assessed? The patient? The Payer? Society? Practitioner?

The money value of the resources may vary depending on the perspective from which the analysis is conducted.

Components of Cost Benefit Analysis

The Fig. 20.2 shows the components of costs and benefits measured while conducting a cost benefit analysis. The cost will generally consist of direct medical and direct non-medical costs.

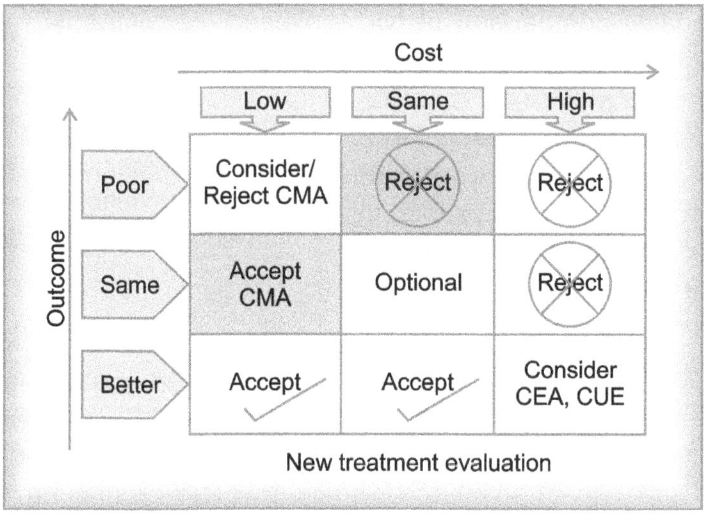

Figure 20.2 Components of CBA.

The benefits of alternative programs can include measures of

- Direct Medical costs saved
- Direct Non- Medical Costs saved
- Indirect costs avoided
- Intangible costs avoided

There are two categories of costs namely Direct Medical and Direct Non-Medical costs. In the case of benefits, there are four categories - namely

(i) direct medical benefits,

(ii) direct non-medical benefits,

(iii) indirect benefits (productivity) and

(iv) Intangible benefits. Often CBA measures only one cost – direct medical costs. However certain researchers of opinion that if only direct costs are measured, then that CBA is not a 'true' CBA.

Indirect costs avoided can be measured by Human Capital (HC) method or by Willingness to Pay (WTP) method. Intangible costs avoided can be measured by Patient Preferences or WTP methods.

Human Capital Method (HC Method)

Human capital approach is one of the methods in use to measure the indirect benefits. It estimates the wages/ salary and productivity loses due to illness, disease, disability or death. Human capital method assumes that the value of health benefits equates the economic productivity they permit. The HC method focus on missed time (in days or weeks or months) and the wage rate due to illness. Wages can be calculated based on the average rate or self-declaration. Missed time can be obtained by self -declaration or verification of the documents.

Contingent Valuation

Contingent Valuation (CV) was originally developed to estimate or predict the value of environmental changes. It is an economic evaluation method currently used in various fields like environmental sciences, traffic safety, value of life and value of health improvements. CV is a method used to determine the value placed or can be placed on a good or service with the help of certain hypothetical (contingent) situations. It is in fact a way of simulating a missing market where the individual expresses his or her valuation for the good contingent on a particular scenario.

Willingness to Pay (WTP) Method

Willingness to pay (WTP) method in pharmacoeconomics is grounded in welfare economic concept. It is a contingent valuation method. It is a direct method that is used to elicit the money values of certain goods or services that is generally not having a prescribed market price. WTP analysis helps to determine the maximum willingness to pay (WTP) of the individual or group with the support of some survey methods using hypothetical statements or questionnaire. It is developed to value certain indirect and intangible aspects of a disease or health condition. It helps to determine how much money people are willing to pay to reduce the chance of an adverse health outcome. WTP is the maximum amount of money prepared to give up by the individual or the group to ensure that the proposed health care measure is undertaken. WTP can be used as a measure of the strength (which can sometimes be weakness?) of an individual preferences.

How to do WTP?

WTP values or estimates can be collected from the person through face to face talk, letters, internet, telephone or through other similar methods. Normally the WTP assessment is preceded by the narration of the benefits of the hypothetical market scenario of the program. The component of narrating the scenario is included with the objective of eliciting the money values. Through this process the respondent is given an accurate explanation of the good or service. The time component (period or days required) as well as the benefit (percentage of improvement) of the program can also be made aware of the respondent at this stage. After the presentation of the benefits, the respondents are asked to value the program in terms of money value, percentage of his/her income or the insurance premium.

Illustration 3: Narration of a hypothetical scenario for the establishment of a new patient counselling centre.

Contd...

Patients on prescribed modern medicines have been found to improve their compliance of the drug therapy through the services of the patient counselling centre. Through the services of qualified and trained clinical pharmacists, the patients get to understand their disease conditions, life style modification required and the various medications prescribed for them by the treating doctors. The patient counselling centre also helps the patients, their care-givers and the public for the following:

1. To know the required information about the prescription and non-prescription (OTC) medicines and get the drug related problems corrected and solved in time.
2. Reduce the occurrence of avoidable or preventable medication errors and adverse drug reactions.
3. Help the patient to manage their illness and diseases as suggested by their treating physicians.
4. Help to recognise and handle situations when the use of medicines occur.
5. Monitor the drug use by keeping records and necessary documents on file.
6. Contact the treating doctor and report the health or drug related issues whenever occur.

The patients can utilise the services of trained and qualified pharmacists in the patient counselling centre without advance booking on a round the clock basis. Generally the time taken for appointment or discussion is about 30 minutes on a visit. An average person can expect a minimum of 50% improvement in his or her drug usage through the patient counselling centre.

The above hypothetical narration of the scenario may help the respondent to value the program in terms of money.

Bidding or Placing of Value

Once the scenario of the program is narrated the persons can be asked to fix their value for the program or intervention - a type of bidding. The bids or the WTP value can be determined in different ways. The commonly used formats for the 'bids' or value include approaches:

(i) ***Open ended questions:*** In open ended questions, the person can expect direct questions from the researcher after the narration of the scenario like "What is the maximum amount you are willing to pay for the 30 minutes consultation with the clinical pharmacist in the patient counselling centre?". The person will then give his or her maximum WTP amount. The main disadvantage of this approach is that most of the people may not be knowing the value of such programs and hence this method is used very rarely.

(ii) ***Closed ended questions:*** The closed ended questions are dichotomous choice (DC) questions. The questions are 'take it or leave it' type. The participants are asked whether or not they are willing to pay a specified amount for the program or intervention. The DC method was accepted by the US Oceanic and Atmospheric administration to assess the contingent valuation method in the environmental field. In recent times, it is popular in health economics and pharmaco-economics.

An example for closed ended questions is "Are you willing to pay rupees 20 for a 30 minute consultation with clinical pharmacist in the patient counselling centre?" Each respondent accepts or rejects only price and the value given to the respondent/ participant may be very much similar to a reasonable or market value for the good or service. It is very much similar to a consumer accepting or rejecting a price fixed by the supplier. The main demerit of the method is one can ask only one question eliciting one WTP value and hence a large sample may be needed to determine the overall WTP value.

(iii) ***Bidding game:*** It is useful method to arrive at the maximum WTP value of a person. Bidding game is almost like an auction where several bids are offered to arrive at the maximum WTP of the individual respondent. The respondent is given the first price that is either accepted or rejected. Then the the second bid is adjusted (raised or reduced) based on the first offer and the third bid based on the second offer and so on. Though the bidding process can go on a number of times, it is ideal to restrict the bids to three or four times. The following is an example for a three times bidding game based on the hypothetical scenario discussed:

Question 1: "Are you willing to pay rupees 20 for a 30 minute consultation with clinical pharmacist in the patient counselling centre?"

Answer : Yes

Question 2: "Are you willing to pay rupees 50 for a 30 minute consultation with clinical pharmacist in the patient counselling centre?"

Answer: No

Question 3: "Are you willing to pay rupees 30 for a 30 minute consultation with clinical pharmacist in the patient counselling centre?"

Answer: Yes

If the bidding game has planned to go up to four stage bidding, the Question 3 would have been "Are you willing to pay rupees 40 for a 30 minute consultation with clinical pharmacist in the patient counselling centre?"

The bidding game is an effective method of finding the respondents maximum WTP. It can be conducted through face to face interaction, telephone or internet. However, it is a time consuming process. Another disadvantage is that it will have a "starting point bias" as the WTP values can be biased depending on the first bid that can be very high or low.

(iv) ***Payment card:*** It is similar to a multiple choice question method in examinations. The payment card method gives the person a list of various WTP values and he or she has to choose one that suits best to him or her.The following is an example for the payment card method based on the hypothetical scenario discussed:

What is the maximum amount you can pay for a 30 minute consultation with clinical pharmacist in the patient counselling centre? Please round your choice.			
Rs 100	Rs 30	Rs 60	Rs 10
Rs 40	Rs 20	Rs 50	Rs 70

The payment card method provides the participant a range of values and he or she has to choose the choice from the given list. It is an easy to practice method. The main dis-advantage of the method is that it can cause bias in the respondents as they are provided with a given range of values. The range provided can 'influence' them in fixing the WTP.

Mail surveys and payment card methods are widely used in developed countries in WTP. In USA, the National Oceanic and Atmospheric Administration (NOAA) based on the recommendations of an expert committee adopted certain guidelines for conducting contingent valuation (CV) studies to finalise WTP. Though NOAA is primarily concerned with environmental issues, its guidelines can advantageously applied in health care sector also. NOAA adopts face-to-face discussions and closed ended (DC) bidding for fixing WTP. Direct face- to- face discussions and interviews can be expensive and time consuming for certain researches. The dichotomous choice (DC) format may require large sample size to accommodate the varying bid levels.

WTP method helps to fix a money value for consequences or benefits which may not have a fixed value as in the case of intangible benefits. It gives due weightage or emphasis to patient preferences and choice and has its ground in welfare economic theory. The main disadvantage of the WTP method is its dependence on a hypothetical scenario of the health care benefit. The criticism is that for hypothetical scenario, one can expect only hypothetical value. It is quite often difficult for people to place a fixed money value on health benefit or improved health-related quality of life or satisfaction. There can be various types of bias like range bias, starting point bias etc., as discussed in the WTP methods. Compliance bias can occur when the participants want to 'please' or 'satisfy' the researcher or interviewer. Strategic bias occur when the respondents over value or understate the WTP value. Research is going on develo-ping a better methodology for fixing valid and reliable WTP values.

Costs and their Timing Adjustments in Pharmacoeconomic Methods

Costs are estimated based on details and information collected over a period of time. This period may vary from a short duration of hours or days to years. Sometimes the costs are estimated based on money spent or saved in future times which too can vary from hours to years. In pharmacoeconomics studies, if the costs are estimated from data collected for more than one year, in retrospective or progressive manner, the costs have to be adjusted to a present value through process like bringing past costs to present (standardization of costs) or bringing future costs to present (discounting of costs).

Standardization of Costs

It is a method for time adjustment for costs where the past costs are brought to the present. The standardization of cost is done when costs are estimated from data obtained for more than one year before. This will help to value the cost at one point in time. As costs increase year by year, patients who received the same treatment in 2005 would have lower costs compared to those who received in 2015. If we compare costs for patients in 2005 with those in 2015, the comparison would not be fair unless both are valued at one point in time. Standardization helps for making a fair and direct comparison the groups in 2005 and 2015.

Method 1: Find the number of units (like dose, tests, visits etc) of each case or resource in 2005. Then multiply the number of units with the current unit cost in 2015 and find total cost in 2015.

Treatment of upper respiratory infection

Item	Units in 2005	Cost per unit in 2015	Total cost in 2015
Doctor	2 consultation	Rs 100	Rs 200
Laboratory	2 investigations	Rs 80	Rs 160
Medicines	40 doses	Rs 12	Rs 480
Visits	10 journeys	Rs 20	Rs 200
Total cost of the treatment in 2015			Rs 1040

Method 2: Another method for standardization of past costs is to find the costs in the respective years and then multiply the amount with inflation rate for that year. In USA the medical consumer price index (CPI) notified on yearly basis is the inflation rate used for adjusting the cost to an year based on this method.

Discounting

Discounting is a method for time adjustment for costs where the future costs are brought to the present. Through this process the money spent or saved in future years can be brought to its present value. Money value is always associated with time. Money received today is valued worth more than the same amount received in future times. In other words money promised or guaranteed in future is valued at a lower rate than money received today. It is the reason why people generally prefer to receive money at the present time rather than tomorrow or a later time. It is more true in business.

In discounting method the cost adjustment is done with the application of a discount rate in calculations. The discount rate is the rate at which future costs and benefits are adjusted to reflect their present values (PV). The discount rate usually varies from 3 % to 8%. With the help of the discount rate, the present value (PV) of a future expenditure can be calculated. In discounting process a discount factor or formula is employed for calculations.

Discount factor (discount formula) =

$$\frac{1}{(1+r)^t}$$

where r = discount rate and t = number of years in the future that the cost occur.

Illustration 4: The treatment cost of rheumatoid arthritis (RA) for the coming four years are as given below:

- 1st year Rs 5000
- 2nd year Rs 3000
- 3rd year Rs 4000
- 4th year Rs 4000

If the discount rate is 5%, calculate the PV (present value) of the total costs for the four years based on discounting. Assume that the costs occur at the beginning of each year.

Answer:

Year	Cost of treatment of RA	Present Value (PV) calculation	PV
Year 1	Rs 5000	$1/(1+r)^t = 5000/1$ =	5000
Year 2	Rs 3000	$1/(1+r)^t = 3000/1.05$ =	2857
Year 3	Rs 4000	$1/(1+r)^t = 4000/(1.05)^2 = 4000/1.1025$ =	3628
Year 4	Rs 4000	$1/(1+r)^t = 4000/(1.05)^3 = 4000/1.157$ =	3455
Total	Rs 16000		Rs 14,940

The total cost of Rs 16000 for the RA treatment for the 4 years becomes Rs 14,940 after the cost adjustment to the present time through discounting.

Illustration 5: In the above example if the expenses occur at the end of the first year (12 months later), instead of at the beginning, what will be the PV of the 4 year expenses?

Contd...

Answer:

Year	Cost of treatment of RA	Present Value (PV) calculation		PV
Year 1	Rs 5000	$1 / (1+r)^t = 5000/ 1.05$	=	4762
Year 2	Rs 3000	$1 / (1+r)^t = 3000/(1.05)^2$	=	2857
Year 3	Rs 4000	$1 / (1+r)^t = 4000/(1.05)^3$	=	3455
Year 4	Rs 4000	$1 / (1+r)^t = 4000/(1.05)^4 = 4000/1.2155$	=	3291
Total	Rs 16000			Rs 14,365

In this case the total cost of Rs 16000 for the RA treatment for the 4 years becomes Rs 14,365 after the cost adjustment to the present time through discounting.

Pharmacoeconomic experts have different views regarding discounting. Some are of opinion that costs and benefits have to be discounted at the same rate, while others feel that outcomes have to be discounted at a different rate.

Pharmacoeconomics is the description and analysis of cost of drug therapy to health care systems and society. It is a health care discipline of placing a value on drug therapy.

CHAPTER 21

Cost Effectiveness Analysis - CEA

Chapter Mission

After learning this chapter you may be able to know:

- Definition and description of Cost Effectiveness Analysis (CEA).
- The concept of CEA in pharmacoeconomic studies.
- Advantages and disadvantages of CEA.
- How to conduct CEA in pharmacoeconomic studies.
- Cost effectiveness grid and cost effectiveness ratios.
- Applications of CEA.

Economic concepts are increasingly used in health care due to the demand to achieve efficiency under the conditions of resource scarcity and constraints. Unlimited needs and wants along with finite resources characterise the health care technology markets. It compels the stake-holders to have proper budgeting and planning process. Optimal benefits are obtained through most efficient allocation of time, money, goods, people and services. Various health care treatment options are available and they have to be evaluated from the perspectives of the numerous economic agents. Cost effectiveness analysis (CEA) has emerged as the pragmatic and powerful pharmacoeconomic method for assessing potential benefits of new programs and methods. Do we receive the greatest benefit for the rupees or money we spend? Economic evaluations are designed to improve the efficiency of the system by attempting to achieve maximum outcomes for the resources consumed.

Definition of CEA

CEA is a pharmacoeconomic method which summarizes the health benefits and resources used by competing health care programs. It measures costs in rupees or money value and benefits in natural health units which are used as indicators of improvement in health.

When the treatment alternatives are not therapeutically equivalent or when it is not desirable to measure the outcomes in terms of rupees or money value, Cost effectiveness (effective) analysis (CEA) is used as a comprehensive pharmacoeconomic method. It helps the policy makers to choose the best from the choices. CEA involves analysis of programs or treatments with different safety and efficacy profiles. The programs will have a common scale of outcome or a common parameter for defining efficacy.

CEA is applied to health programs where the program inputs can be easily measured in terms of rupees or money value and the outcomes are more appropriately described in terms of health improvements (physical or natural units). They are non- rupee units and some of the health improvement units are

- Lives saved,
- Diseases prevented,
- Blood pressure controlled,
- Number of strokes prevented,
- Number of ulcers healed,
- Number of ADR reduced or avoided,
- Free of asthmatic wheezing,
- Life years extended,
- Complications prevented,
- Diseases cured,
- Relief of symptoms like pain, vomiting or nausea,
- Mortality avoided,
- Morbidity reduced,
- Lives saved,
- Increase in life expectancy,
- Side effects reduced,
- Increase in ailment free condition.

It can also be measured in terms of change in an intermediate clinical outcome like

- Cost per night free of pain,
- Night free of wheezing,
- Night provided comfortable sleep,
- Percent change in blood cholesterol level.

CEA is used to summarize the health outcomes of competing health care programs. The results of a CEA are expressed as cost/outcome for both therapies.

Illustration 1: To compare the cost – effectiveness of an H2-receptor blocker and a proton-pump inhibitor, the cost per ulcer healed by each of the two drugs may be calculated and compared.

Advantages and Disadvantages of CEA

It is the most common type of pharmacoeconomic method used in pharmacy and pharmacy practice. Cost can be measured in money value like rupees or dollars. Effectiveness is expressed in natural unit changes in health care. The inputs are measured in rupees and can be done without difficulty. The outputs or the outcomes are measured in natural health units and need not be converted into money value as done in CBA. The health units are commonly used in clinical trials and are hence very much familiar to researchers. It is a helping tool for the policy makers to choose from among the various competing programs or alternatives. CEA compares programs or treatment alternatives with different safety and efficacy profiles. CEA provides an approach to the dilemma of assessing the monetary value of health outcomes as part of the evaluation that we have seen in CBA

The main disadvantage is that the outcomes have to be evaluated in the same clinical units. It means that two anti- diabetic medicines can be compared using CEA, but it cannot be used to compare an anti-hypertensive with an anti- diabetic drug. When several outcomes result from a medical intervention (as in the case of prevention of both death and disability) CEA may consider these two outcomes together only if a common measure of outcome can be developed. Generally, analyses combine different categories of clinical outcome according to their desirability, assigning a weighed utility or value to the overall treatment outcome. In CEA, the effectiveness component of the two comparators should be the same. They should have a common measurable unit. Demonstrations of effectiveness have to be comparative and should measure the outcomes of the control and experimental groups.

The effectiveness should be evidenced by its quantitative estimate. It should be reliable, reproducible and valid. The evidence can be generated by using retrospective data from published studies and rarely through prospective studies which are often expensive.

Cost Effectiveness and Cost Saving Alternatives

The difference between cost effective and cost saving is that cost saving refers to competing alternative that is less expensive. Cost effective alternative need not always mean that the comparator is less expensive. We consider a product or service or a program as cost effective compared to competing alternatives if one of the following three conditions are complied with

1. Cost effective alternative is less expensive or at least as effective as the comparator.
2. Cost effective alternative is more expensive but provide additional benefit which is worth enough for the extra cost.
3. Cost effective alternative is less expensive and less effective where the extra benefit is not worth the extra cost.

Fig. 21.1 shows the cost effectiveness grid. It can be used to illustrate the definition and the concept of CEA.

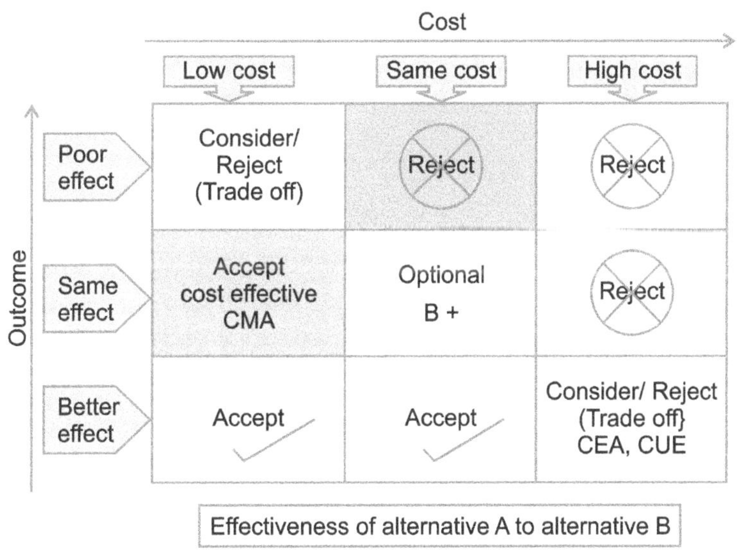

Figure 21.1 Cost effectiveness grid.

The cubes represent possible results when comparing two alternatives with respect to their costs and effectiveness. Options requiring trade off include programs or technologies with higher cost and higher effectiveness or lower cost with lower effectiveness.

[In economics the term trade-off is expressed as opportunity cost, referring to the most preferred alternative given up. A trade- off, then, involves a sacrifice that must be made to obtain a certain product, service or experience, rather than others that could be made or obtained using the same required resources.]

Obtaining data for CEA

Ideally, the pharmacoeconomic analysis can be conducted during the clinical trials. It can be incorporated in the clinical trial and submitted to the authorities along with the NDA. However it is not a practice to insist the conduct of CEA along with the clinical trials in many countries.

Quite often the CEA is conducted on the basis of pre-existing data available in the medical literature. This can lead to uncertainty about both the cost and outcome measures. Moreover, CEA in different countries might have different applications. To validate a study that utilizes such pre-existing data, either a 'risk averse strategy' or a 'sensitivity analysis' needs to be performed.

The risk averse strategy

The risk averse strategy is of special application in CEA studies comparing a new treatment modality with an existing time tested one. The strategy is comparatively simple to load the newer modality with negative assumptions like increased inpatient days, prolonged treatment duration, or similar other assumptions and then compare it with the older one. If the new treatment modality still overshoots the older one, then it can be treated as more cost-effective, in spite of the uncertainties in the data used.

Sensitivity analysis

The sensitivity analysis (SA) does the same function as of the risk averse strategy. It tests for the consistency of the results obtained even when the values of the key variables are changed. It can be a simple SA in which the effect of change is seen in the value of one or more variables on the results analysis. For example if results of a study are based on a seizure relapse rate of 10% at 3 years, what happens to the results if the seizure relapse rate is actually 20%.? It can also be carried out under extremes of conditions of assumptions like being pessimistic (high cost/low efficacy) and optimistic (low cost/high efficacy). Sensitivity analysis can also be done with the help of computer programs. In probabilistic sensitivity analysis, a computer program is used to select different permutations and combinations of variables simultaneously from a large number of variables and a confidence interval can be assigned to the results.

Cost Effectiveness Ratios

Results from a CEA are typically expressed as cost effectiveness ratio - C/E ratio. The numerator of the ratio represents the total costs and the denominator represents the effect or the expression of outcome variable.

Two forms of C/E ratios are generally used

1. Average cost effectiveness ratio (ACER). It is also called simple C/E ratio.
2. Incremental cost effectiveness ratio (ICER).

Average Cost Effectiveness Ratio

Average cost effectiveness ratio represents the total cost of a program or treatment alternative divided by its clinical outcome to yield a ratio representing rupee/ dollar cost per specific clinical outcome gained. This is expressed as

ACER = Health care cost in rupees or dollars ÷ clinical outcome.

(Here the clinical outcome is not based on rupees/ dollars).

It helps to convert the cost and outcome to a single value to allow comparison. With the help of ACER, it is possible to choose the alternative with least cost per outcome obtained. The most cost effective alternative need not be the least costly alternative on all occasions as cost effectiveness need not be solely reduction, but rather cost optimization (Bootman JL, 1993).

Table 21.1 Calculation of ICER using a theoretical model of treatment of hypertension

Alternatives	C	DC	E	DE	ICER =DC/ DE
Diet	50	-	4.8	—	
Drug A	80	30	5.3	0.5	30/.5 = (60)
Drug B	98	18	6.4	1.1	18/1.1= (16.3)
Drug C	120	22	6.7	0.3	22/.3 = 73.3

C = cost, E = effect, DC = difference in cost, DE = difference in effect

Incremental Cost Effectiveness Ratio

In many cases, clinical effectiveness is obtained at an increased cost. Here an additional benefit is obtained for the additional cost. However, we have to ascertain whether this increased cost is justified with its outcome or not. Incremental cost effective ratio (ICER) can be used to determine the additional cost and the effectiveness gained when one treatment alternative is compared with the next best alternative. Instead of comparing the ACER of each treatment alternative, the additional cost that a treatment alternative puts on another treatment is compared with the additional effect or outcome. It is expressed as:

$$\text{ICER} = \frac{[\text{cost in Rs. of (A)} - \text{cost in Rs. of (B)}]}{[\text{effect in \% of (A)} - \text{effet in \% of (B)}]}$$

ICER yields the additional cost required to obtain the additional effect gained by switching from drug A to drug B.

Illustration 2: The Hospital Formulary Committee (Pharmacy and Therapeutic Committee - P&TC) of a hospital has to take a decision regarding Antibiotic A or Antibiotic B has to be included in the Formulary. Antibiotic A has 90% efficacy or cure rate and has a total treatment cost of INR 50,000 for 100 patients. Antibiotic B has 95 % efficacy or cure rate and costs INR 100,000 for 100 patients.

ACER of Antibiotic A = $\frac{50,000}{90}$ = INR 555 per cure

ACER of Antibiotic B = $\frac{1,00,000}{95}$ = INR 1053 per cure

Contd...

$$ICER = \frac{1,00,000 - 50,000}{95 - 90} = \frac{50,000}{5}$$

= INR 10,000

The incremental cost for each additional cure with Antibiotic B is INR 10000.

Using ACER it is found that the additional benefit gained by using Antibiotic B costs INR 498 (1053- 555) per cure.

The costs represents the difference per patient, spread over the 100 patients that were treated. Only the ICER will help us to pose the question of whether one additional cure is worth spending INR 10000 where a cure with Antibiotic A can be achieved for INR 555. The decision to use Antibiotic A or Antibiotic B is often dependent on the severity of the infection. If it is a life threatening infection one may use Antibiotic B where as in a mild or less severe case one may use Antibiotic A only.

Illustration 3: Take a case of the comparison of two drug treatments 'X' and 'Y' in the management of malignancy. Treatment 'X' represents a once a year course treatment, which takes a total of Rs. 4 lakh a year for costs of medicines, anti-emetics, in patient stay, radiology costs, pathology costs, etc. Treatment 'Y' is a new drug treatment for the same condition. Comparative controlled clinical trials have demonstrated an improvement in the average life expectancy from 3.5 years for drug 'X' to 4.5 years for drug 'Y'. The average annual cost for treatment with drug Y is Rs 5 lakhs. Find the ICER.

Ans. Treatment cost for X = Rs 400000.00

Effectiveness for X = 3.5 years

Treatment cost for Y = Rs 500000.00

Effectiveness for Y = 4.5 years

$$ICER = \frac{50,00,000 - 4,00,000}{(4.5 - 3.5)}$$

= Rs. 1,00,000 per life year gained.

Handling of Results in CEA

Consider the four possible results of CEA:

(i) The new treatment is more effective and less expensive. The costs are lowest and the benefits are highest. Here the choice is clear without any ambiguity. It is the choice of preference. Recommend to be selected.

(ii) The new treatment is less effective and more expensive. The costs are high and benefits less. Not to be recommended.

(iii) The new treatment is more effective and more expensive. That is the cost is high and the benefits are more. Here the ICER should be calculated.

A judgement have to be made whether the additional benefits are worth the extra costs of new drug. It is to found whether cost effective or not.

(iv) The new treatment is less effective and less expensive. Here we have answer one question- whether the extra benefits provided by the standard treatment justifies the additional costs of retaining it as a preferred treatment when the option of a new, cheaper but less effective drug exists.

Applications of CEA

The choice of using CEA versus other methods depends on the specific questions identified by the researchers, the types of alternatives investigated, and the information required by the final decision makers. Consideration of the various strengths and weaknesses, limitations, and generalizability are of paramount importance in CEA. It has great use in Formulary system, choosing programs or therapies and comparison of drugs or devices.

The results of a CEA are expressed as cost/outcome for both therapies. Outcome or health benefit is measured in terms of natural units, e.g., number of lives saved, number of strokes prevented, number of ulcers healed, etc. Thus, to compare the cost – effectiveness of an H2-receptor blocker and a proton-pump inhibitor, the cost per ulcer healed by each of the two drugs may be calculated and compared.

CEA is useful in comparing or balancing cost with health outcome for individual patients. It also helps to identify which treatment alternative represents the best outcome for the rupee spent. CEA can provide valuable data to endorse drug policy, formulary system and individual patient treatment decisions. In certain countries (e.g., Canada, New Zealand and Australia) CEA is used to set public policies related to use of drugs. (Langley PC, 1993). CEA is the most commonly applied form of economic analysis in the drug therapy. It does not allow comparisons to be made between two totally different areas of medicine with different outcomes.

Illustration 4:

Pharmacoeconomics in Formulary decision in Australia

In Australia, a drug is included in the Formulary based on the principle that if the new drug is no better than a comparable product, it should not cost more. If the new one is superior to the existing one and is more expensive, and funds are available, any extra expense has to represent 'value for the money'. The Australian federal government subsidizes the use of medicines and pharmaceuticals through a 'formulary' called Pharmaceuticals Benefits Schedule (PBS). If a new drug has to be included in the PBS, the request has to be made by the Pharmaceuticals Benefits Advisory Committee (PBAC) to the health

Contd...

minister. While considering the request, the PBAC will verify the importance of the item, its need for the society, its cost effectiveness and the financial implications of the inclusion.

The PBAC generally consider the request only if the request is accompanied by a pharmaco-economic analysis report. Relative clinical performances and costs of both the new item and comparable items in the list are presented. In the analysis all aspects of costs are considered like lower use of other drugs, fewer consultation and hospital admissions. Then cost effectiveness ratios for both the drugs are developed. To cite examples, in the case of antibiotics the cost of achieving a bacterial cure is considered and in the case of anticonvulsants the cost of achieving a 50 percent reduction in seizure frequency is considered. Once the data has been evaluated, the PBAC will examine and find whether the cost effectiveness ratios represent value for the money. If the PBAC recommends the new item, the file will then go to the pricing authority which uses the drug cost as a basis for negotiation (Managing drug supply 1997).

Comparison of anti-emetics

CEA can be used to compare anti-emetic drugs for developing a policy for the prevention of chemotherapy-induced emesis. Many of the anti-emetic drugs differ with respect to effectiveness, safety and cost. With the help of a CEA these variables can be brought to a single number- the cost-effectiveness ratio. This ratio will allow for a meaningful analysis and comparison. The treatment alternative with a better cost effective ratio or lower cost per unit outcome would be selected for use.

Comparison of lipid lowering drugs

Hakim, et al, conducted a study to evaluate the cost effectiveness of four lipid-lowering agents. The pharmacy department of the hospital initiated the study as it was found that the four drugs were consuming a high percentage of the pharmacy budget but had varying costs and degrees of effectiveness. The alternatives considered in the study were - no drug treatment or diet control alone and four lipid lowering agents. Four measures of effectiveness were - changes in total cholesterol level, high-density lipids (HDL), low-density lipids (LDL) and triglycerides used for the study. It was found that all the four drugs were more effective than the diet alone condition. It was also found that the cost effectiveness ratio was varying. The study suggested that the drug therapy in this case has to be based on the affordability and the clinically relevant target of effectiveness (Hakim Z.1996).

Table 21.2 Comparison of Pharmacoeconomic evaluation methods

Methods being compared	Outcome unit	Type of outcomes	Use
Cost–effectiveness analysis (CEA) (cost in rupees effectiveness in non-money)	Natural unit, e.g. lives saved	Similar	Evaluate new drugs in same class/disease
cost–Minimisation analysis (CMA)	Natural units or clinical effects (equal efficacy, cost in rupees)	Similar	Commonly used in me- too -cases
Cost–utility analysis (CUA)	Quality-adjusted life-years (QALY) (cost in rupee, utility as patient preference)	Different	To measure across therapeutic areas/ diseases
Cost–benefit analysis (CBA) expressed in rupees)	Monetary units (Both cost and benefit	Different	Field of health care economics

General Steps Involved in the Conduct of CEA

The general procedure for the conduct of a CEA can be explained in 5 steps as noted in Fig. 21.2.

Step 1 Define the problem

The research problem that needs to be solved should be identified for conducting an appropriate CEA. The existing alternatives and the perspective needs to be identified for finalizing the research problem. Expert opinion and literature review are needed at this stage. Selection of objectives of the study should also be done at this stage.

In the beginning of the pharmacoeconomics, studies were focusing on specific health problems like morbidity, mortality and disability. Later the researchers started to identify problems related to a variety of preventive and therapeutic modalities with respect to relative cost effectiveness. Later the problems were identified from specific intervention strategies like given drugs, surgical procedure, medical instrument or medical device. If the problem is formulated in terms of specific drug or a specific class of drugs, consideration should be given to the documentation in the medical literature of the acceptability of alternatives to the drug or class of drugs in question.

After the problem is identified, specific objectives have to be developed for comparing the cost and effectiveness of alternative interventions. Decision must be taken concerning how the problem statement cab be quantifiably incorporated into the methodology.

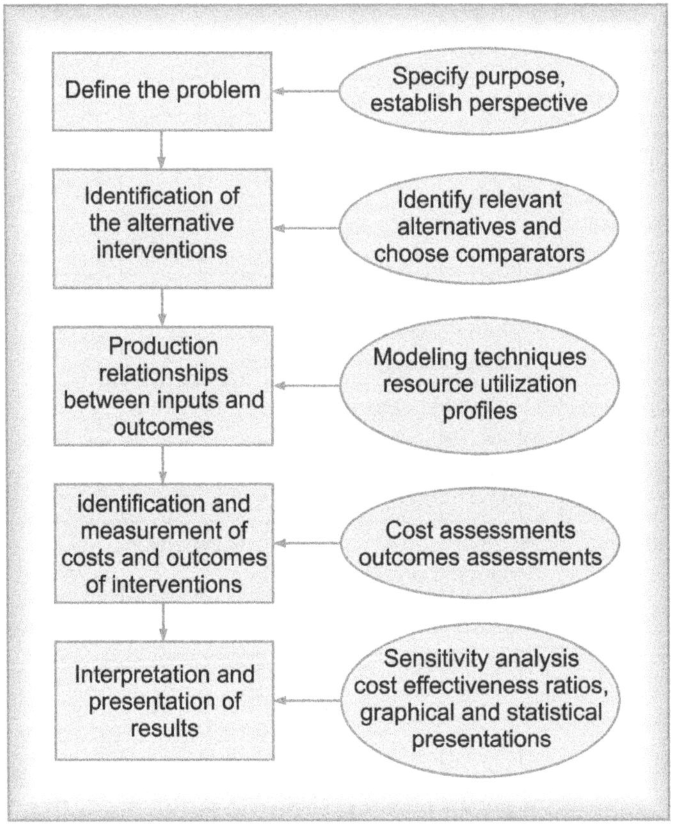

Figure 21.2 General steps in CEA.

Perspective addresses the question "Cost to whom?" The broadest view point is that of the society. The society perspective normally stipulates that all direct and indirect costs and benefits are addressed in addition to the intangible concerns. Narrow perspectives include those of employers, governments, specific providers of care, managed care organizations, hospitals, insurance companies or patients. Establishing the perspective in a CEA is often a challenging job. Conventional economists and pioneers of pharmaco-economics may advocate that a societal perspective be taken as the goals of CEA or CBA. This approach may not really reflect the primary concern of a given patient , payer or provider. Whatever may be the selected perspective, the choice must be taken prior to the starting of CEA.

Step 2: Identification of the Alternative Interventions

Based on the objectives and research question, one has to choose comparators that include the least expensive alternative, a less expensive newly developed regimen, the most widely used drug within the therapeutic class, a preferred agent or choice of drug, a standard therapy from a given class of drugs, or a therapy that provides next highest magnitude of cost effectiveness. In the simplest case individual drugs can be compared with each other for a particular condition. Interventions may also be investigated against multiple disease conditions as required for certain Formulary decisions. To cite an example proton pump inhibitor (PPI) can be compared for both treatment of existing peptic ulcer cases and prophylaxis of recurrent ulcers.

Step 3: Production Relationships between Inputs and Outcomes

After specifying the research problem, objectives, perspective and identification of the alternative interventions, the next step is the description of the relationship between the resource consumption and outcomes. The method to assess the production relationship between inputs and outcomes can be as simple populating a table or flow chart wherein all inputs and their quantities are noted. The quantity of resources consumed would be calculated based upon defined costs in rupees.

Production costs are those associated with providing an intervention and are determined by itemizing the resources used to actually provide the intervention. Health resources consumed for each event would be identified. An important aspect in conducting economic assessments involves the incremental inputs and outputs.

Step 4: Identification and Measurement of Costs and Outcomes of Interventions

Cost analysis in pharmacoeconomics aims at identifying the centers of resource consumption. We have already discussed the concepts of cost analysis in earlier chapters.

Assessment of Outcomes

As in the case of clinical trial investigations, the definition and description of outcomes is important in CEA. Outcome should be clinically relevant and measured in an objective fashion. The outcomes should follow standard criteria for measuring clinical results and should be acceptable within heath care.

The ECHO model (Economic, Clinical and Humanistic Outcome) is one method of classifying the outcomes in pharmaco-economics. It should be kept in mind that these outcomes are often interrelated and inseparable. No single outcome type is more important than another, though clinical outcomes are of particular interest in CEA due to the scope of methodology. Intermediate versus final outcomes, discussed in earlier chapter are relevant and significant in CEA.

Efficacy and Effectiveness in CEA

Often cost estimates used in CEA are obtained from clinical trials or secondary sources. Outcome measures are approximated by data from RCTs. RCTs are also known as cost efficacy studies and are considered as gold standard for assessing the efficacy of medications. In countries like USA and other European union, these studies are essential for approval of medicines by their drugs control department or Food and Drug Administration (FDA).

"Efficacy" data are obtained from RCTs, where conditions are controlled, adherence is almost perfect and the study population is comparatively homogenous. It is important to note that RCTs are used to determine efficacy, that is to find out 'Whether the drug can work under relatively ideal conditions?'

However pharmacoeconomic studies give more focus to the assessment of "Effectiveness", that is to find out ' Whether the drug works in real world naturalistic settings where patient population can be diverse or adherence may be less?'.

If efficacy focus upon the question of "Can it work?", effectiveness address the question "Will it work?". Treatment regimens can be efficacious, but may not necessarily offer the same degree of effectiveness. It means that the therapy may be effective but may not provide the value in certain cases. Efficacy data are easier to obtain than effectiveness data, mainly due to the regulatory requirements of Phase 1 to 3 of clinical trials. Results from RCTs related to efficacy can be used in pharmacoeconomics with necessary adjustments, though these adjustments are often subjective in nature.

Discounting is necessary if the time frame of the study exceeds more than one year, irrespective of whether the inflation rate is zero.

Step 5: Interpretation and Presentation of Results

Results from CEA are often expressed as cost effectiveness ratios. Tables and graphs can also be used in expressing results.

Pharmacoeconomics is the description and analysis of cost of drug therapy to health care systems and society. It is a health care discipline of placing a value on drug therapy.

CHAPTER 22

Cost Utility Analysis - CUA

Chapter Mission

After learning this chapter you may be able to know:

- Definition and description of Cost Utility Analysis (CUA).
- The concept of CUA in pharmacoeconomic studies.
- Advantages and disadvantages of CUA.
- How to conduct CUA in pharmacoeconomic studies.
- Quality Adjusted Life Years (QALY) and its calculations.
- Applications of CEA.

The people or the society always have a love and hate relationship with health care services. The health care services is very much lauded for saving lives and improving the quality of medical care by conquering many diseases and ailments. At the same time the health services are also condemned for the ever increasing costs. In the previous chapters we have discussed the pressing need to maximise the net health benefit out of the utilisation of limited health care resources. Both CBA and CEA were presented as methods for assessing costs and consequences of health care programs, particularly drug therapies. Now we will discuss another method for evaluating the value obtained for the rupees spent on health care - the Cost Utility Analysis or CUA.

Definition of CUA

Cost-utility analysis (CUA) is a formal economic evaluation method of pharmaco-economics which is used for assessing the efficiency of health care programs. Here the measure of effectiveness is utility or preference adjusted outcome.

CUA is very much similar to CEA in certain aspects and hence many are of opinion that CUA is only a type of CEA. We are considering CUA as a separate pharmacoeconomic method for the discussions. In this evaluation method, drugs/ interventions with different out comes can be compared. Hence CUA is used for comparing treatment programs or alternatives with different outcomes. Here outcome is a unit of utility.

Concept of Utility

Utility is the value or worth given on a level of health status, or improvement in health status as measured by the preferences of individuals or society. The concept of 'utility' provides a method for estimating patient preferences for a particular intervention in terms of his/her state of well-being. In CUA outcomes are generally measured in 'utility units' and is expressed as cost / quality adjusted life years (QALY) gained. It is to be noted that there is no true consensus as to the most appropriate measurement approach in CUA. Some prefer to use other terms like 'preference weight' or 'preference value' in place of utility. However the most common outcome unit used in CUA is QALY which incorporates both the quality (morbidity) and quantity (mortality) aspects of life.

Quality Adjusted Life Years (QALY)

The concept of QALY has been discussed in literature for over 40 years.Quality adjusted life years (QALY) represent the number of full years at full health that are valued equivalently to the number of years as experienced. For example a full year of health in a disease free patient may be equal to 1.00 QALY, while a year spent with dialysis would be valued lower as 0.5 QALY. As QALY and other utility measures are very much subjective, there is lack of agreement on which scale should be used for measuring utility. The disagreement among researchers is not only over the QALY concept, but also over how the preferences or utilities for health states between 0.0 and 1.0 are obtained.

Utility is described by an index, which ranges from '0' representing death to '1' representing perfect health. CUA integrates the preferences of patients with health related quality of life (QOL). Cost is measured in rupees or dollars and outcome is measured in patient weighted utilities rather than in physical units. Generally, the utility measure used in CUA is a quality-adjusted life year (QALY) gained. The product of utility and life years gained provides the term quality adjusted life year (that is QALY = QOL x years). It tells us about the quantity and quality of life gained.

QALY is a commonly used measure of health status in CUA, combining morbidity and mortality data. Compared to traditional CEA, it has the advantage that it can combine more than one measure of effectiveness, or both measures of mortality and morbidity into a single measure.

CUA is not disease-specific. By using CUA, the cost/QALY value of various procedures can be calculated and compared. For example, coronary artery bypass graft and the use of erythropoietin in renal failure are totally different procedures; if limited resources need to be allotted to them, this can be done using CUA.

Arranging the cost/QALY values of different programs or interventions in an order (ascending or descending) is called the QALY league table. The QALY league table helps in comparing the utility of different programs. These are useful for resource allocation by policy-makers. The main disadvantage of this type of table is that it can be misleading quite often. Homogeneity of the studies included in the league table is essential. The studies shall have similar data collection techniques, timeframe settings and utility measures.

Cost Utility Ratio

Results of CUA are expressed in a ratio called cost utility ratio (C/U ratio). This ratio is often translated as the cost per QALY obtained. Treatment alternative with lowest cost per QALY is preferred. The CUA is the appropriate method when comparing programs and treatment alternatives that are life extending with major side effects like cancer chemotherapy, which produce reduction in morbidity rather than mortality as in the case of arthritis or when QOL is the important health outcome being analyzed as in the case of use of estrogen for menopausal symptoms.

Compared to other economic evaluation methods, CUA is less frequently used for reasons like absence of agreement in measuring utilities, lack of standards for comparing QALY and problems with the quantification of patient problems. CUA should be reserved for comparing programs and treatment alternatives whose basic goal is improving QOL. It can be used to study the use of ciprofloxacin and co-trimoxazole in the treatment of acute exacerbations of chronic bronchitis (AECB) in adults. The incremental cost utility ratio (ICUR) can be obtained and used in a similar manner as in the case of incremental cost effective ratio (ICER).

Illustration 1: Take a case of the comparison of two drug treatments 'X' and 'Y' in the management of malignancy. Treatment 'X' represents a one year course treatment which takes Rs. 4,00000.00 a year for costs of medicines, anti-emetics, in patient stay, radiological costs, pathological costs, etc. Treatment 'Y' is a new drug treatment for the same condition. The average annual cost for treatment with drug Y is Rs 5, 00000.00. The treatment X provides on average an increase of 3.5 years life expectancy, which is valued at a utility of 0.9. Treatment Y provides on average an increase of 4.5 years life expectancy, which is valued at a utility of 0.8, as it produces more nausea compared to X. Find ICUR

Ans. Treatment cost for X = Rs 400000.00

Effectiveness for X = 3.5 years

Utility of X = 0.9

Hence health gain for X option/ intervention= 3.5 × 0.9 = 3.15 QALY

Treatment cost for Y = Rs 500000.00

Effectiveness for Y = 4.5 years

Utility of Y = 0.8

Health gain for Y option/intervention = 4.5 × 0.8 = 3.6 QALY

ICUR = (Rs 500000- Rs 400000) ÷ [(4.5 × 0.8) – (3.5 × 0.9)]

= Rs 100000 ÷ 3.6 – 3.15

= Rs 100000 ÷ 0.45

= Rs 2,22,222.22 per QALY obtained.

Illustration 2: Take a simple example of two treatments- Z and Y. With treatment Z, the estimated survival is 10 years and the estimated quality of life (relative to perfect health) is 0.7. With treatment Y estimated survival is 5 years and estimated quality of life (related to perfect health) is 0.5. If the cost of treatment of Z is rupees 1,18,000 more to the cost of treatment Y, what will be the cost per QALY?

Ans. Treatment Z

Estimated survival year = 10 years

Estimated quality of life = 0.7

QALY = 10 × 0.7 = 7.00

Treatment Y

Estimated survival year = 5 years

Estimated quality of life = 0.5

QALY = 5 × 0.5 = 2.50

Gain of QALY from treatment Z = 7.00 – 2.5 = 4.50

Total additional cost of 4.5 QALYs = Rs 1,80, 000

Cost per QALY = 1,80,000 divided by 4.50 = Rs 40,000

Advantages and Disadvantages of CUA

CUA has some distinct advantages over CEA and CBA. The advantage of CUA is that it can be applied to the comparison of different types of health outcomes and diseases with multiple outcomes of interest using one common unit like QALY, which is not possible in CEA. Cost effectiveness analysis is limited by the inability to simultaneously incorporate multiple outcomes from the same intervention or to compare interventions with different outcomes. In CEA the outcome measure is in natural units, but no attempt is made to value the consequences in terms of quality or desirability. Cost utility analysis incorporates quality of the health outcomes achieved. As already seen it combines the quality (morbidity) and quantity (mortality) of life outcomes in economic evaluations.

Moreover CUA incorporates both morbidity and mortality into QALY without having the need to give money value to the outcomes as in the case of CBA. Cost benefit analysis suffers from the difficulty of converting all costs and consequences into money values or rupees. It is particularly difficult to convert patient reported outcomes like quality of life into rupees. More over CBA harbours with it the potential for discrimination as it favours treatment for people who are working or those who are rich or wealthy.

The main disadvantageof CUA is that it is often difficult to determine an accurate utility or QALY value. This is very significant to a country like India, where pharmaco-economics is yet in its infancy.

Applications of CUA

When quality of life is the important health care outcome to be measured or evaluated, CUA is having appropriate applications. Researchers have identified several circumstances in which CUA can be used as most appropriate analytical method (Drummond MF 1997). Some of them are noted below

1. When health related quality of life is the important outcome. For example, when comparing interventions that are not expected to have an impact on mortality, but a potential impact on patient function and well being like the treatments for osteoarthritis.
2. When health related quality of life is an important outcome. Evaluation of the outcomes associated with the treatment of acute myocardial infraction is an example. Here both life saved are important outcome measure, so also the quality of lives saved like impact of a treatment induced stroke in a survivor.
3. When the intervention affects both morbidity and mortality and a combined unit of outcome is needed. Evaluation of a therapy where oestrogen use by postmenopausal women is an example. This can improve quality of life. May reduce mortality from certain conditions like heart disease, but may increase mortality from some other conditions like uterine cancer. Another example is the use of statins to reduce cholesterol but may increase the mortality from diabetes as continuous use statins can increase the chances of diabetes.
4. When the interventions being compared have a wide range of potential outcomes and there is a need to have a common unit of outcome for comparison. This is most commonly the case when a decision maker has to allocate limited

resources among interventions that have different objectives and resultant benefits. An example is the choice between providing increased prenatal care or expanding a hypertension screening and treatment program.

5. When the objective is to compare an intervention with others that have already been evaluated in terms of cost per QALY or equivalent gained.

Methods for Assessing Utility

Utility is a quantitative expression of a person's preference for a particular state of health under conditions of uncertainty. Utilities are often expressed in numbers that represent the strength of the individuals preference for different health outcomes. CUA requires an assessment of preferences for health status. A variety of different techniques are being used to assess these preferences. Some analysts measure preferences directly while some others measure preferences indirectly by simply assigning a reasonable value.

Determination of Utilities

The three most common methods of determining the utilities are

Rating Scale (RS)

Standard Gamble (SG)

Time Trade Off (TTO)

In addition to these three methods, Magnitude Estimation and the Person Trade off method are also sometimes used in CUA.

Rating Scales (RS)

Rating scale (RS) require the respondent to give a numerical value to objects. The RS is like a scale or a thermometer with '0' at the bottom and '1' or '100' at the top. The bottom value of '0' represents death and '1' or 100 represents perfect health. Respondents are asked to indicate where the diseases or the health conditions will be put in the scale. The mild diseases or conditions can have a score or place near the 1 or (100) mark at the RS and a severe one near to 0. In developed countries the people are educated enough to read the description of a disease and rate the same in the 10 point or 100 point scale. However in countries like India where literacy is comparatively poor extra effort has to be taken to make the respondent understood about the concept of RS.

Some are of opinion that there are disease conditions worse than death. Hence negative QALYs may be needed to indicate such values. However we follow the 0-1 scale.

Figure 22.1 shows an example of rating symptoms of a disease conditions in a rating scale.

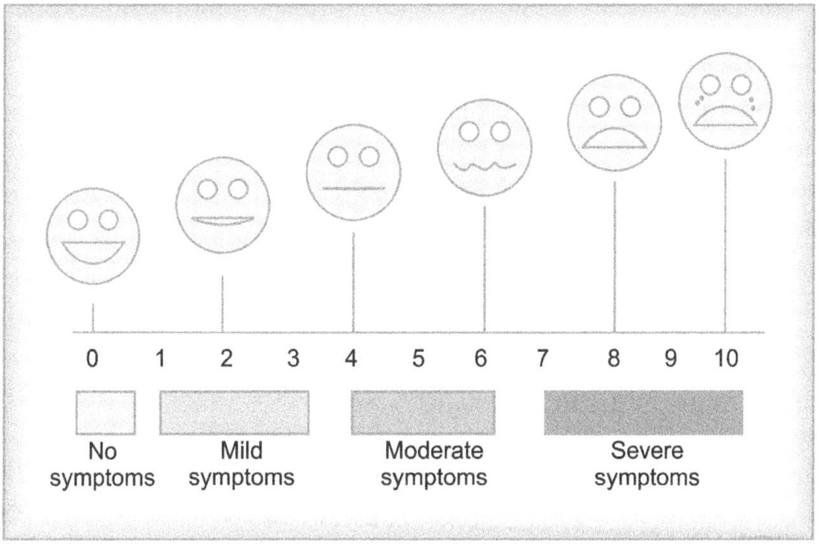

Figure 22.1 Rating Scale

Visual Analogue Scale (VAS) is very much similar to RS but does not have the markings between the values '0' and '1'. The VAS method shows the subject or respondent a line, typically of 10 centimeters in length, with the end points well defined. The task of the respondent is to indicate where his preference rests for the health status in relation to the two poles.

Visual Analogue Scale (VAS)

VAS for itch intensity

No itch 0 ____________________ 10 **Worst imaginable itch**

VAS for sleep disturbance (nocturnal itch)

No sleep loss 0 ____________________ 10 **I cannot sleep at all**

Figure 22.2 Visual Analogue Scale

Rating Scale method can be performed with the support of a questionnaire and does not necessitate a face-to-face interaction. With the help of RS a number of disease conditions can be described to one person. Of the three methods it is comparatively easy and demands less cognitive responses. Generally people may try to distribute their values throughout the range even if some health conditions are very similar in their values. Appropriate applications of rating scales reflect contemporary developments in cognitive sciences.

Standard Gamble (SG) Method

The Standard Gamble (SG) is another commonly used for determining patient preference or utility. The SG offers a choice between two alternatives - Choice A living in the disease condition or state with certainty or Choice B taking a gamble on a new treatment for which the outcome is uncertain. Figure 22.3 shows this trade.

Here the respondents are asked to hypothetically choose between living with the disease or the condition versus taking a serious risk on treatment. Each person is offered two alternatives:

Choice B is treatment with the following two possible outcomes;

(i) Return to normal health. or

(ii) Immediate death.

Choice A is the certain outcome of a chronic disease state for life based on a person's life expectancy.

The probability of normal health is 'p' and immediate death is 1-p for Choice B. The p Vs 1-p for Choice B is varied until the respondent is indifferent between the two alternatives (Choice A and Choice B). At this indifferent stage the respondent may find difficult to choose between the two options as he finds both options almost equal.

> **Illustration 3:** If the respondent or subject is indifferent between Choice A and Choice B when p = 0.65, it means that the utility of the disease state or guaranteed state of disease is 0.65.

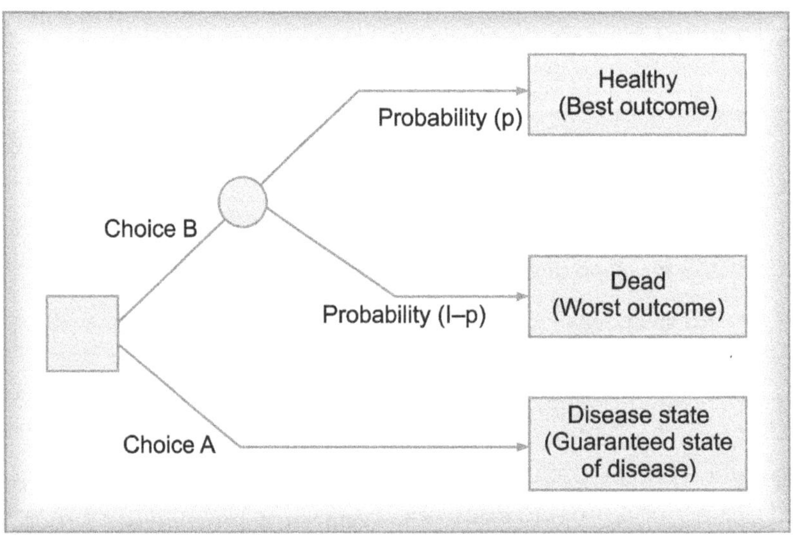

Figure 22.3 Standard Gamble.

Standard Gambling is a comparatively difficult method for the participants. It is based on economic theory. However it is accepted as the best method among the three generally used methods. In SG the subjects need to be asked repeated questions increasing or decreasing the probabilities based on their earlier answers. Face to face setting is more convenient for SG method and questionnaire is less suitable. Also refer Chapter Case study.

Limitations of SG

Treatment of many chronic diseases does not approximate the SG. There is no known product that will cure a patient with arthritis. Similarly there are no known product that is likely to kill a patient with arthritis. Hence the decision making experience of the patient is not likely to include an option that has a realistic gamble. More over the cognitive demands of the task of SG are comparatively high.

Time Trade Off (TTO)

Time-Trade-Off (TTO) is a tool used in health economics to help determine the quality of life of a patient or group. The individual will be presented with a set of directions such as: Imagine that you are told that you have 10 years left to live.

In this method, the person is given two alternatives as in the case of SG method, but in a different manner. Alternative 1 is a specific disease condition for a certain period of time (t). It is the life expectancy for the person with disease. After period of time (t) death is expected. Alternative 2 is a healthy condition for time (x) which is definitely less than time (t). Here time (x) is varied until the respondent is indifferent between the two alternatives. This point is utilised for calculating the utility score which is obtained by dividing (x) by (t).

The TTO method is adaptable to disease conditions and incorporates time factor in it. As in the case of SG, in TTO subjects have to answer repeated questions and necessitates face-to-face interaction.

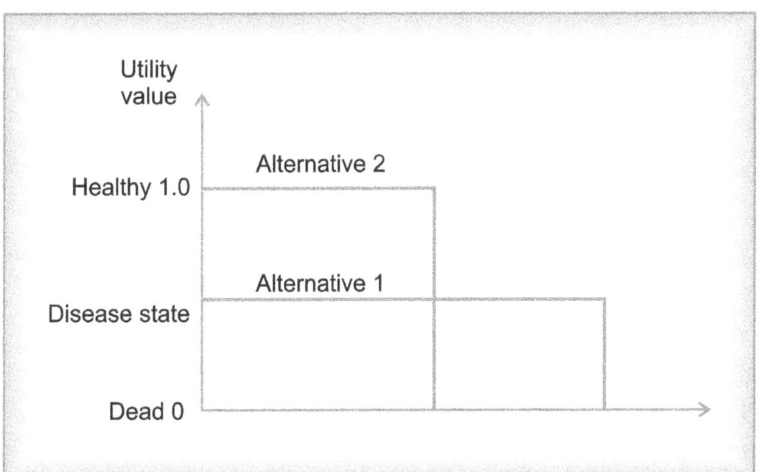

Figure 22.4 Time trade off (TTO)

Illustration 4: Mr Pillai is a 25 year old youth with a further life expectancy of 50 years. He is given two alternatives. Alternative 1 is being impotent for 50 years. Alternative 2 is being healthy and potent for 20 years followed by death. How to find the utility measure using the TTO method?

Ans. Here (t) is 50 years and (x) is originally 20 years. To find the utility value through the TTO method the following procedure is suggested.

First ask Pillai "Do you opt Alternative 1 and be impotent for 50 years rather than choosing Alternative 2 and be healthy and potent for 20 years?". He says "Yes. I choose Alternative 1 option." Now we have to increase the (x) value and continue the questioning as done in the SG method. In this case the second question to Mr Pillai can be "Will you opt Alternative 1 if the Alternative 2 is increased to be being healthy and potent for 30 years?". Pillai replies "Yes". Now the next question can be " Will you opt Alternative 1 if the Alternative 2 is increased to be being healthy and potent for 40 years?" The reply by Mr Pillai is "No. In that case I will opt Alternative 2". The next question can be " Will you opt Alternative 1 if the Alternative 2 is reduced to be being healthy and potent for 35 years?" Now Mr Pillai says " If Alternative 2 is to be healthy and potent for 35 years, I have study it more. I cannot take a decision immediately". At that stage we can state that Mr Pillai is indifferent between the two options of 50 years of impotent and 35years potent life. At this stage (t) value is 50 and (x) value is 35.

The utility score is calculated as (x)/(t) = 35 ÷ 50 or 0.7.

Note: In the above case study, imagine that Mr Pillai replied "No" to the first question. In such a situation he should have been quizzed by lowering (x) time value from 20 to find the indifferent stage and then calculating the utility.

Magnitude Estimation (ME)

Magnitude estimation (ME) is a psycho-physical scaling technique where assessors assign numerical values to the estimated magnitude of an attribute. In ME a specific case is selected as a standard and assigned a particular number. Then other cases are rated in relation to the standard.

Illustration 5: Assume that the standard is given the number 10. If a case is regarded as half as desirable as compared to standard, that will be given a value of 5. If the case is regarded as twice as desirable compared to standard, that will be given a number value of 20.

Person Trade off (PTO)

The Person Trade-Off (PTO) is a methodology aimed at measuring the social value of health status or interventions. The rest of methodologies would measure individual utility and would be less appropriate for taking resource allocation decisions. Basically it consists in asking people how many outcomes of one kind they consider equivalent in social value to X outcomes of another kind. From the public policy perspective, the PTO approach is intended to incorporate social value information.

> **Illustration 6:** Respondents might be asked how many persons in health status B must be helped to provide a benefit equivalent to helping one person in health status A.

Who will determine utilities?

In the utility studies, we generally use the terms like 'respondent' or 'subject' to describe the individual who would be questioned to determine the utility scores. Who is this respondent or subject? He or she can be any person or individual. In pharmacoeconomic studies the patient, health care professional, care giver, relative of patient or persons from the category of general public can become the respondent or subject. Some experts are of opinion that it is better to have patients as respondents while other advocate for healthcare professionals. The former group argue that the patients can understand the effects of the disease better than other people. Those who oppose this view point believe that patients often provide a biased view while comparing their disease with other disease conditions. Again if patients are more qualified to become respondents in utility analysis, then in the case of those who could not value utilities like babies, children and patients with dementia who should do it? Parent? or caregiver?. Some are of opinion that professionals can give good estimates of disease conditions as they understand various disease conditions properly.

Pharmacoeconomics is the description and analysis of cost of drug therapy to health care systems and society. It is a health care discipline of placing a value on drug therapy.

CHAPTER 23

Cost Minimization Analysis - CMA

Chapter Mission

After learning this chapter you may be able to know:

- Definition and description of Cost Minimization Analysis (CMA).
- The concept of CMA in pharmacoeconomic studies.
- Advantages and disadvantages of CMA.
- How to conduct CMA in pharmacoeconomic studies.
- Applications of CMA.

Definition and Description of CMA

Cost minimization analysis (CMA) is a pharmacoeconomic method used to compare two or more treatment (program) alternatives that are equal in efficacy. CMA compares the costs of treatment alternatives in rupees or money value. Outcomes are not compared because of the underlying assumption that the treatment alternatives are therapeutically equivalent. The primary objective of the CMA is to identify the least costly alternative.

CMA is a relatively straightforward and simple method for comparing competing program or treatment alternatives. If no evidence exists to support the therapeutic equivalence of the alternatives being compared, another pharmacoeconomic method should be used. It is to be noted that CMA only shows a cost savings of one program over the other.

Concept of CMA in pharmacoeconomics

CMA involves the determination of the least costly alternative when comparing two or more treatment alternatives. The primary assumption for cost - minimization analysis is that the outcomes of the alternatives are not different, that is the results or benefits of the programs are of equal nature. The alternatives must be therapeutically equivalent, that is, they shall have same benefits/ consequences/ outputs or results. Moreover they shall have an assumed or demonstrated equivalency in safety and efficacy.

After confirming the equivalency in outcome, the cost can be identified, measured and compared in monetary units like rupees or dollars. In the case of certain diseases or ailments the result can be attained in different ways.

> **Illustration 1:** A disease like acidity could be treated in different ways like through surgery or medicines, both are having the same effects of cure of acidity. Hence CMA can be conducted.
>
> **Illustration 2:** The cataract surgery of a patient can be treated in two ways – permitting him to be an out- patient or making him an inpatient. There may not be significant variations in the outcome in both cases. Since clinical efficacy is equal in both programs, they can be compared through CMA.

Applications of CMA

CMA shows a cost savings of one treatment program over another.Here only the input, i.e., the cost, is considered. The cost of drugs should include costs like acquisition costs, cost of preparation, administration cost and storage costs. After considering all these costs, the least expensive agent should be preferred.

CMA is often applied in formulary decision-making where often the available evidence for a new product appears to be no better than for existing products. It is an appropriate method to compare two or more therapeutically equivalent agents or different dosing regimens of same agent. Two drugs 'X' and 'Y' both belonging to the group of anti-ulcer or NSAID or any other identical group could be compared using CMA if they are documented to be equal in efficacy and incidence of adverse effects.

In one study, Carboplatin was compared with Cisplatin for treating ovarian cancer. It was found that, though Carboplatin was expensive per dose as compared to Cisplatin, it was cheaper when the total cost was taken into consideration, as lower toxicity was encountered with the use of Carboplatin. The treatment with Cisplatin always requires a hospital admission because of the need for intensive hydration before and after the procedure. (Tighe M, 1988).

The CMA can be applied in various studies involving generic medicines, medicines with trade or brand names provided they have shown same outcomes. Ciprofloxacin tablets 500 mg manufactured and marketed by different manufacturers can be subjected to CMA if the selected items were reported to have same benefits or outcomes for a specific infection. Similarly if two or more brands of ciprofloxacin tablets 500 mg are having same outputs for a specific purpose, we can do CMA for those branded items. In India it is a practice of the manufacturers to market same medicine under generic name and trade name with same strength and dosage form. In such cases it is easy to do the CMA analysis of those products of the same manufacturer.

Table 23.1 Example of CMA

Category	Cost of X therapy (Antibiotic A) Rs	Cost of Y therapy (Antibiotic B) Rs
Procurement cost	300	320
Storage and maintenance cost	50	50
Administration cost	40	40
Monitoring	100	100
Adverse events	50	00
Total cost	540	510
Out come(effectiveness)	80%	80%
CMA shows that antibiotic B should be selected as both are equally effective to treat the infection		

Again if a hospital decides to introduce compulsory prescribing of generic names of drugs instead of their brand names, then

CMA can be selected as the best pharmacoeconomic evaluation method as it will take into consideration only such items which are having same clinical out comes.

If the therapeutic equivalence of alternatives being compared, has not been established, then more comprehensive methods like cost effectiveness analysis should be adopted.

Advantages and Disadvantages of CMA

The CMA is a simple and straight forward method of evaluation. Since the outcomes are declared as equal, the study need not analyse the outcomes and can focus on inputs only for assessing the costs. It is the best method to compare the various branded products of same drug. It can also be used to study the generic versus branded products. The disadvantage of CMA is that it can be applied to only limited cases.

Cost minimization analysis is a method of calculating drug costs to project the least costly drug or therapeutic modality. Cost minimization also reflects the cost of preparing and administering a dose. This method of cost evaluation is the one used most often in evaluating the cost of a specific drug. Cost minimization can only be used to compare two products that have been shown to be equivalent in dose and therapeutic effect. Therefore, this method is most useful for comparing generic and therapeutic equivalents or "me too" drugs. In many cases, there is no reliable equivalence between two products and if therapeutic equivalence cannot be demonstrated, then cost-minimization analysis is inappropriate.

Is CMA a Full Pharmacoeconomic Method?

In Pharmacoeconomics there is a controversy and debate regarding the status of CMA. Some are of opinion that CMA is only a partial pharmacoeconomic analytical method and not a full pharmacoeconomic method. They are of opinion that the outcomes are not measured in CMA, only the costs are estimated and analysed. Hence it is better to name it as Cost Analysis, they argue. Other who advocate CMA, argue that both costs and clinical outcomes are measured. Clinical outcomes are found to be equivalent.

Pharmacoeconomics is the description and analysis of cost of drug therapy to health care systems and society. It is a health care discipline of placing a value on drug therapy.

CHAPTER 24

Cost of Illness - COI

Chapter Mission

After learning this chapter you may be able to know:

- Definition and description of Cost of Illness (COI).
- The concept of COI in pharmacoeconomic studies.
- Advantages and disadvantages of COI.
- Conduct and applications of COI.

Cost-of-illness (COI) analysis represents the earliest form of economic evaluation in the health care. COI studies have been widely debated and its usefulness as a decision-making tool has been questioned by many health economists. Nevertheless, COIs are among the commonest economic studies in healthcare in many countries (e.g., Italy) COIs are commonly used by organisations, such as World Bank, World Health Organisation and the National Institute of Health (USA).

Definition and Description of Cost of Illness

Cost of illness (COI) evaluation is also known as Burden of disease (BOD) or Burden of Illness (BOI). It is an economic evaluation method used to identify and estimate the overall cost of a particular disease for a defined population. It involves measuring the direct and indirect costs attributable to a specific disease. In many countries like USA, Australia and other European countries, the costs of various diseases like peptic ulcer disease, mental diseases, cancer, etc., have been estimated. COI evaluation is not used to compare competing treatment programs or treatment alternatives. It is used to provide an estimation of the financial burden of a disease.

The COI studies usually include some metric of 'health loss' and try to measure the resource costs incurred in treating the related diseases. The BOD studies measure the 'burden' of years of life lost (YLL) due to premature death, and the years lost due to disability or morbidity (YLD). These two categories make up a measure of 'cost' called total DALYs (disability-adjusted life years), which encompass health care costs and the 'lost economic or societal contribution' resulting from premature death or disability.

Cost of illness measures the economic burden of disease or illness on society. It estimates the maximum amount that could potentially be saved or gained if a disease or a group of diseases were to be eradicated. The first COI studies appeared in the 1950's and since then, thousands of studies have been performed for the U.S. alone. Since 1970s numerous cost-of-illness studies have been conducted throughout the world highlighting the influence of the magnitude of the impact of illness on society. Many of the COI studies were used in public health policy debates at various centers on various occasions.

Basic Concepts of COI Studies

The basic objective of COI study is to evaluate the economic burden that an illness can imposes on society as a whole. The main objective of COI studies is descriptive, that is to itemize, value, and sum the costs of a particular issue or problem with the objective of giving an idea of its economic burden. In conducting COI studies, researchers have to recognize, identify, list, measure and value the costs that a disease and its comorbidities can generate. Analysis of the COI presents useful opportunities for communicating with the public and policy makers on the relative importance of specific diseases and ailments.

Knowledge of the COI helps the policy makers in health care to decide which disease or group of diseases need to be addressed on priority basis. More over the COI studies can indicate for which diseases cures would be valuable in reducing the burden of disease. In the case of specific stake-holders, like the central and state governments, cost-of-illness studies can help show the financial impact a disease has on public programs, like national disease eradication program or starting a medical insurance scheme. For private and corporate employers providing health coverage for their employees. COI studies help to understand which diseases have a serious effect on their costs.

The attributes of COI can range from the incidence or prevalence of disease to its effect on longevity, morbidity, decrease in health status, quality of life (QOL), and financial aspects including direct and indirect expenditures that result from premature death, disability or injury due to corresponding disease and/or its comorbidities. All cost-of-illness studies provide important information for pharmaco-economic studies like cost-effectiveness analysis (CEA) and cost-benefit analysis (CBA) though they can provide only one part of cost analysis. Cost-of-illness studies can provide a framework for the cost estimation in CEA and CBA analyses.

Applications of COI Studies

The cost-of-illness studies are frequently used by policy makers and other government organizations. In some countries (e.g., USA and UK) the published cost of illness repots are used in law suits to recover medical insurance claims. They are also used to estimate the costs of fatal occupational injuries by various countries. The findings of COI would benefit safety and health professionals for promoting education programs aimed at eliminating workplace accidents and fatalities. Cost of illness studies are often cited in disease studies that attempt to highlight the importance of a particular disease like how obesity causes diabetes.

Cost estimates are frequently used to argue that policies on a disease and its related diseases should be given a high priority in a policy agenda setting. COI help authorities to appropriately target specific problems and policies. It is important to know whether a specific disease of interest involves the greater medical and/or social costs. The improvement of cost estimates can be used as a baseline measure to determine the efficacy of health policies and programs. Estimates of COI can also facilitate international comparisons of the disease consequences and various approaches that are available for confronting those consequences.

Limitations of COI Studies

Cost-of-illness studies can demonstrate which diseases may require increased allocation of resources for prevention or treatment. However they are limited in determining how resources are to be allocated because they do not measure benefits. Moreover, these studies use different methods, which can limit the comparability of results and findings. Studies can vary by perspective, sources of data, inclusion of indirect costs, and the time frame of costs. Cost-effectiveness and cost-benefit analyses provide additional information not included in cost-of-illness studies that can be used to determine the best course of action with respect to the disease studied. A clear statement of the study methods can improve cost comparability. Cost-of-illness studies can be used as an important analytic tool in public health policy if conducted with a clear explanation.

Costs in COI

A comprehensive cost-of-illness study includes both direct and indirect costs. The specific focus of a study can make one or the other cost as unnecessary. Direct costs measure the opportunity cost of resources used for treating a particular illness. Indirect costs measure the value of resources lost due to a particular illness.

Direct Costs

When measuring direct costs, studies often measure total direct costs (i.e., the costs of resources used) rather than net direct costs. The net direct costs subtracts future medical costs avoided because of the death of a patient, from total costs. Direct medical costs include hospital inpatient, physician inpatient, physician outpatient, emergency department outpatient, nursing home care, hospice care, rehabilitation care, specialists' and other health professionals' care, diagnostic tests, prescription drugs and drug sundries, and medical supplies.

One challenge with calculating direct medical costs, particularly hospital costs, is that charges are often the only data available. Because of the nature of determining hospital charges, they often do not accurately reflect the underlying costs. Charges are often higher than costs to cover losses from patients who are unable to fully pay their expenses, such as procedures not covered by insurance companies, and to cover the rising costs of replacing and updating medical equipment.

Non-medical direct costs include transportation costs to health care providers; re-location expenses; and costs of making changes to one's food, repair in house or car, or related items. Some non-medical direct costs like research, training, and capital costs (e.g., construction) are generally not included in cost-of-illness studies. It may be difficult to attribute these costs to a particular disease. More over, the capital costs like those required for training health care providers for a particular illness or establishing a new wing or equipment to treat an illness, are also often reflected in the charges of care. Hence they are not included separately in such studies. The specific purpose of the study or the data available may preclude the calculation of non-medical direct costs. The focus is often on direct financial costs as non-monetary costs can be difficult to capture.

Indirect Costs

Indirect costs are those representing the other portion of estimated costs. They include mortality costs; morbidity costs due to absenteeism and presenteeism; informal and other care costs (in terms of the opportunity cost of hiring outside care). In the case of many diseases, indirect costs may be greater than the direct medical costs. Indirect costs include the loss of resources due to morbidity and mortality, which inherently places a monetary value on the value of life. The inclusion of indirect costs in cost-of-illness studies is common and accepted practice.

The idea of placing a value on life can sometimes raise ethical questions. It is mainly due to the availability of wide range of estimates that don't have an agreement on correct method of estimation. Indirect costs inevitably place a lower value on the elderly. It also place a lower value on those who do not work. There is a school of view that such costs should be excluded. Even when indirect costs are included, debate exists about the correct approach.

There are three primary approaches to estimate indirect costs: the human capital method, the friction cost method, and the willingness to pay method.

Human Capital Method

The human capital method measures the lost production, in terms of lost earnings of a patient or caregiver. In the case of mortality or permanent disability the cost is arrived by multiplying the earnings lost at each age by probability of living to that age. The earnings in future years are discounted. Often a one percent real annual growth rate in earnings is assumed. The human capital approach often includes the value of household work, usually valued as the opportunity cost of employing a replacement from the labor market.

The human capital method is the most common and popular method used to calculate the indirect costs of an illness. A criticism of this approach is that certain groups are assigned a higher value than others. The human capital approach utilizes wage rates and employment rates based on the age, sex, or race and hence certain groups that earn less are assigned a lower values.

Friction Cost Method

The friction cost method measures only the production losses during the time it takes to replace a worker. This approach assumes that short-term work losses can be compensated by an employee and the loss of an employee only results in costs in the time it takes a new employee to be hired and trained, known as the friction period.

Proponents of the friction cost method criticize the human capital method for overvaluing the indirect costs, claiming that the productivity losses are often eliminated after a new employee is trained and can replace the former employee. However, the friction cost method is rarely used because it requires extensive data and attempts to estimate only the losses in the friction period. Valuation of the productivity losses is complicated further by firms' use of internal reserves of labour during the friction period, which lowers the estimates of losses even more but can be difficult to calculate.

Willingness to Pay Method

The willingness to pay (WTP) approach measures the amount an individual would pay to reduce the probability of illness or mortality. There are various methods of determining an individual's willingness to pay, including surveys, examining the additional wages for jobs with high risks, examining the demand for products that lead to greater health or safety (e.g., seat belts), and other related methods.

The willingness to pay approach, usually with higher estimates of the value of life than the human capital approach, attempts to ameliorate the problems associated with human capital method. However, this approach is often difficult to implement in cost-of-illness studies. For specific diseases, extensive surveys of people's preferences are needed, although the results rely heavily on people's responses to very specific hypothetical questions about their willingness to avoid certain illnesses.

In the case of communicable diseases, surveys may not help to capture fully the cost of the disease because of externalities. People only take into account the cost to themselves, without taking into account the societal benefit that having fewer people with a communicable disease benefits everybody as the disease is less likely to spread. Thus, the willingness to pay method is often not feasible for a cost-of-illness study.

Perspectives of COI Studies

The COI studies can be conducted from different perspectives, each of which includes slightly different cost items. This will eventually lead to different and wide range of results for the same illness. These perspectives may measure costs to a society, health care system, third-party payers, business sectors, the government, and the patients and their families. Each perspective provides useful information about the costs to the particular group. Table 21.1 gives a general idea regarding the cost categories included in each perspective.

In general, the broader societal perspective is preferred, because the impact of a condition is not solely on the individuals or organizations that are directly involved. Through the societal perspective, we can identify the 'cost shifting' between sectors. It will also account for alternative resources used outside the health care sector. The societal perspective is the most comprehensive because it includes all direct medical costs and indirect costs for all members in a given society where they are involved, and it is often preferred because it allows a complete analysis of all of the opportunity costs attributable to a disease. It is often recommended for possible cost analyses such as CBA, CEA, and CUA.

Table 24.1 Costs included in cost-of-illness studies by Perspective

Perspective Costs	Medical Costs	Morbidity Costs	Mortality	Transportation/ Non-medical cost	Transfer Payments
Societal	All costs	All costs	All costs	All costs	–
Health care System	All cost	–	–	–	–
Third-party Payer	Covered costs	–	Covered costs	–	–
Businesses	Covered costs	Lost productivity	Lost productivity	–	–
Government (Medicare,	Covered Medicaid)	–	–	Criminal justice costs	Attributable to illness
Participants and families costs production	Out-of-pocket House hold production	Lost wages House hold	Lost wages	Out-of-pocket costs	Amount

Types of Studies in COI

There are several approaches in COI like incidence based versus prevalence based, prospective versus retrospective or top down versus bottom up. Epidemiological data used is the criteria for incidence versus prevalence approach. The temporal relationship between the initiation of the study and the data collection is the criteria for retrospective versus prospective studies. Methods chosen to estimate the economic costs is the criteria for top-down versus bottom-up.

Incidence-based Vs Prevalence-based studies

Incidence-based studies estimate lifetime costs. It measure the costs of an illness from onset to conclusion for cases beginning within the period of the study, usually a year. Incidence costs include the discounted, lifetime medical, morbidity, and mortality costs for the incident cohort.

Prevalence-based studies estimate annual costs. It measure the costs of an illness in one period, usually a year, regardless of the date of onset. Prevalence-based studies include all medical care costs and morbidity costs for a disease within the study year. The mortality and permanent disability costs of prevalence-based studies are calculated differently from the other costs. Discounted mortality and permanent disability costs are calculated for all patients who die or become permanently disabled in the study year for that year and each year until the expected age of death.

Prevalence-based studies are more common as they require less data and fewer assumptions than incidence-based studies. Data only need to be collected from one year. Nothing has to be studied or assumed about the survival rate or course of the illness.

Lifetime costs can be calculated from annual costs, assuming a steady state of disease incidence, progression, survival rate, and treatment. However the estimates need not be as accurate as using actual longitudinal data on the full course of the illness due to potential future changes in medical care technology and other assumptions. Despite this limitation, numerous methods provide useful approximations of lifetime costs using annual data and all of them involve the assumption that the structure of future costs is the same as the structure of current costs and then discounting future costs.

Cost-of-illness studies are useful to measure the potential savings of averting a case of an illness. For this purpose, the COI studies can help in cost-effectiveness analysis, cost-benefit analysis, or illness prevention analysis by providing the baseline costs of maintaining the status quo. In the case of an acute illness that has costs only within one year, a prevalence-based or incidence based study would be the same because future costs would not exist. For chronic illnesses with costs that extend past the first year, incidence-based studies provide more information about the costs of averting a case. A prevalence-based study can be performed with a chronic illness. However it has to be interpreted as a snapshot of the costs in one year, rather than the costs that could be saved if all cases of the illness were averted.

Prospective vs. Retrospective Approaches

The COI studies can be conducted in prospective or retrospective ways depending on the relationship between the study kick-off and the data collection. In the retrospective method, all the relevant events have already happened when the study starts. He the researcher collects the data that are already recorded. In the prospective approach the relevant events have not already occurred at the beginning of the study. Here the data collection have be made by following-up the patients over the study time. The prevalence- and incidence-based COI studies can be both performed either in prospective or retrospective way.

The major advantage of retrospective method is that it is less costly and less time consuming than prospective method. The retrospective method can only be possible with sufficient observational datasets. In prospective approach researchers have to design data collection systems they want to adopt. Complete dataset on the illness and the consumption of health care resources at every action and intervention can be made by the analysts from the questionnaires designed and provided to patients or their family members and/or health care providers. In studying a disease with relatively long time span, a prospective and incidence-based approach would be considerably expensive and time consuming.

Bottom Up Versus Top Down Approaches

Bottom-up Approach

In a bottom-up approach, the cost estimation can be stratified into two steps. The first step is to measure and quantify the health inputs employed and the second step is to estimate the unit costs of the inputs used to produce and confer specific medical and health care services. The total costs come out through the multiplication of unit costs by the quantities used. The major difficulty arises here since the data needed and available will vary with the scope of the study. In most cases, national level survey datasets are mainly used because they provide reliable data on medical care utilization so that researchers are relatively easily able to quantify the amount of medical care services along with unit costs or price values.In a more limited study, the investigator has to collect data which may be a disadvantage even though in doing so he may find more reliable estimates of the different cost components than in nationally collected data. An often claimed advantage for comprehensive studies is that by allocating total national expenditures among the major diagnostic categories, one can avoid the risk that the sum of treatment costs of individual diseases – estimated through the bottom-up approach – is greater than total health care expenditure in a given country.

Top-down Approach

The top-down approach, known as the epidemiological or attributable risk approach, measures the proportion of a disease that is due to exposure to the disease or the risk factors. This approach was first developed by Morgenstern et al., and uses aggregated data along with a population-attributable fraction (PAF) known as epidemiological measure to calculate the attributable costs (Morgenstern 1980).

Top-down COIs are likely to present misallocation of costs. The use of national health care expenditures can cause under or overestimates of total direct costs. Similarly the exclusion of cost categories that are not included in national health care expenditures (i.e., transports, informal care) can also affect the estimates of costs by disease category as different disease categories absorb different non-health costs. Another problem with the top- down method is that all costs are attributed to the primary diagnosis, which is a serious problem if we consider that a relevant part of all hospital discharges involve patients with multiple diagnoses.

Econometric Approach

The econometric approach is aimed at estimating the difference in costs between a cohort with the disease and another cohort without the disease. The two cohorts are matched, usually through a series of regression analyses, by various demographic and mediating factors and other chronic conditions. Within the econometric approach, there are two major methods of estimating costs:

(i) a mean differences approach and
(ii) a multiple-stage regression approach.

The mean differences approach compares the mean costs incurred by each of the two cohorts to determine the incremental difference attributable to the disease.

A multiple-stage regression method is typically performed if there are a large number of cases with zero costs and a few cases of very high costs.

> Step wise approach for conduct of COI
>
> 1. Definition of the study perspective.
> 2. Characterization of the unit of analysis.
> 3. Identification of cost items.
> 4. Measurement of cost items.
> 5. Valuation of cost items.
> 6. Uncertainty analyses.

Humanistic Evaluation Methods

Apart from economic aspects, pharmaco-economic evaluations may also focus on humanistic concerns. Today various factors like patient preferences, patient satisfaction, impact of disease and treatment of disease on a patient's health related Quality of Life (QOL) are applied to pharmacotherapy decisions. Such factors can be applied in pharmaco-economic evaluations.

QOL is defined as 'the assessment of functional effects of illness and its consequent therapy as perceived by the patient' (Schipper H, 1990). These effects are expressed as emotional, physical or social impacts on patients. Health related QOL can be measured with the help of structured questionnaires filled by patients. In 1992, Mackeigan published an overview of QOL and its applications in pharmacy (Mackeigan LD, 1992) and it inspired the publication of a variety of other similar views. Since 1980s, efforts were made to include an assessment of economic outcomes of an alternative treatment; and the current trend is to bring the patient back into the decision making process, for which the humanistic outcomes are incorporated in the process.

Pharmacoeconomics is the description and analysis of cost of drug therapy to health care systems and society. It is a health care discipline of placing a value on drug therapy.

CHAPTER 25

Quality of Life and Health Related Quality of Life (QOL & HRQOL)

Chapter Mission

After learning this chapter you may be able to know:

- Definition and description of Quality of life (QOL) and Health Related Quality of life (HRQOL).
- The concept of QOL and HRQOL in pharmacoeconomic studies.
- Challenges in application of HRQOL.
- Measurement of HRQOL.
- Specific instruments for measuring HRQOL and their characteristics.

Introduction

In the present day competitive environment, there is a concern that health care quality is being compromised in the rush to lower costs. This has resulted in the concept to focus the evaluation of health care on the assessment of end results or outcome associated with the health care.

There are different types of outcomes for drug interventions in health care. Rate of disease occurrence, rate of disease recurrence, rate of hospitalization, reduction in mortality are examples of parameters considered as evidence of drug efficacy. Doctors often depend on the manner in which the drugs influence various physiological functions to assess the efficacy of the drugs. Sometimes the physiological status may change without the patient feeling better. Drugs may ameliorate certain symptoms without a measurable change in the physiological function. Sometimes prolonging a life may be achieved at the expense of pain and sufferings. There can be variations in the evaluation of different outcomes.

Other important aspects of usefulness of the drug interventions which encompass the ability to function normally include conditions like be free of pain, have easy physical activities and sexual life, normal psychological thinking, free from social limitations and dysfunctions and other factors like the quality of the environment and contact groups. The recognition and acceptance of many patient oriented and disease oriented parameters of well being or life quality led to the introduction of a technical term in health care called 'health related quality of life' or HRQOL.

Quality of life (QOL) is a broad term that includes attributes such as environment, income, living standards, etc., besides health status. It is an abstract concept, as it relates to ideas or standards and not to real things. QOL, as it is often called, lacks focus and precision. The subjective well being of a patient is influenced by many factors, some of them may be totally unrelated to the disease or treatment process like education, or income.

The aim of measuring QOL is to provide information about the well being of the population at large. The United Nations Human Development Index (HDI) is a typical example (United Nations. 1994.).

Definition of Quality of Life

Illness is lack of health and always affects the quality of life (QOL) of the patient. The relationship between illness and QOL is complex and not symmetrical. QOL is a broad term. It is very difficult to define the term, and even if it is defined, there may not be universal acceptance of the definition. In the literature, the term quality of life has been used in a variety of ways. WHO has defined QOL as 'an individual's perception of their position in life in the context of the culture and value systems in which they live and in relation to their goals, expectations, standards and concerns.' (WHO QOL Group, 1993).

Health Related Quality of Life (HRQOL)

Finding QOL as a very broad term, pharmacoeconomic studies started using another comparatively new but narrow term-health related quality of life (HRQOL) to bring quality of life associated with health related parameters. It has been suggested that studies of health outcomes use the term health related quality of life (HRQOL) to identify effects on health of factors like job satisfaction, environment and other similar ones on the overall quality of life. (Kaplan RM 1982).

It is used exclusively in health care to examine health status alone. However, HRQOL is a multifaceted concept. From the perspective of the patient, HRQOL represents the final common pathway to all physiological, psychological and social influence of the therapeutic process (Schipper H., 1990). Health related quality of life is an appropriate final measure in pharmacoeconomic analysis as it examines health status and allows comparison of treatments of different conditions. Here in this discussion we use only health related outcomes and hence terms QOL and HRQOL are used as interchangeable terms. However readers need not take it as a general rule applicable in all situations.

Definitions of HRQOL both theoretical and practical remain controversial. Often significance is given to the instruments used to measure the ability of patients, in caring for themselves and carrying out their usual roles in life. This is a pragmatic view and has gained ascendancy. There are experts who criticize this approach of HRQOL concept. They argue that unless you are tapping into individual patient's values you cannot measure HRQOL, you can only measure the health status (Gill T.M., 1994).

Schron and Shumaker define Quality of life as 'a multidimensional concept referring to a person's total well being, including his or her psychological, social and physical health status' (Schron E.B., Shumaker S.A., 1992). Another definition given for QOL is 'the value assigned to the duration of life as modified by the impairments, functional states, perceptions, and social opportunities that are influenced by disease, injury, treatment or policy' (Patrick D.L., 1993). The definition of the terminology may vary with the author. However, the commonly measured parameters of HRQOL include the following:

1. **General health.**
   Concepts of general well being
2. **Physical health.**
   Functioning of physical health.
3. **Mental health.**
   Functioning of mental health.
4. **Social health.**
   Functioning of social health.

Health care professionals like physician, pharmacist or nurse view quality of life from the angle of therapeutic outcome. In the case of disease conditions which shorten life expectancy and for which there is no cure, managing symptoms and maintaining functional well-being should be the main objective of the health care. There are four possible QOL standards associated with pharmacotherapy,

(i) QOL is improved.
(ii) QOL is properly maintained.
(iii) QOL is decreased.
(iv) QOL remains unaffected.

These outcomes can be estimated or assessed with the help of biological, physical and other manifestations of the diseases.

Challenges in Application of HRQOL

HRQOL plays an important role in the investigation and documentation of drug effects, both beneficial and harmful. There are many situations where a drug may have an important effect on the HRQOL. The effects of three antihypertensive drugs – methyldopa, propranolol and captopril – on HRQOL were studied long after their introduction in clinical practice by Croog, et al. They came to the conclusion that captopril is having some advantages on HRQOL domains compared to the other two drugs (Croog S.H., 1986). This report had a major impact on the drug prescription pattern at the time of its publication.

As there is no universal agreement on the concept of QOL and HRQOL, researchers engaged in the measurement of HRQOL may face many challenges. They have to define as precisely as possible the aspects of HRQOL in which they are interested. They have to identify the purpose for which HRQOL instrument is to be used. The investigator has to choose the most suitable HRQOL instrument from the available choices. After successfully dealing with the above issues, the researcher has to focus on the measurements, that is, interviews, questionnaires, etc. They have to ensure that the measurements are unbiased, standardised and reproducible. At the final stage of interpreting the data and converting the results into clinically meaningful terms also the investigator may face challenges.

Measurement of HRQOL

The approach of quality adjusted life years (QALYs) occupies a prominent position in the measurement of HRQOL. The QALY approach is based on the assumption that a valid, reliable and acceptable scale can be created for valuing all possible health states and death. It gives full health a value of 1.00 and death a value of 0.00. The life year is treated as the basic unit in this approach. The program or treatment may extend life year. Sometimes the procedure will help to extend life year which is filled with pain. Another procedure may help to extend life year as pain free. No doubt the second one is worth more than the first. Applying a fraction to the number of years of increase in survival, which values these years relative to full healthy years (1.00), makes a 'quality adjustment' and produces a figure for the program's or treatment's impact expressed in QALYs.

A large array of instruments were used by investigators since early 1990s. Researchers have suggested various ways of categorizing these instruments. According to the purpose of their use, instruments are grouped as those designed for screening, for providing health profiles, for measuring preference and for making clinical decisions. Some researchers have categorized instruments into discriminative instruments and evaluative instruments. Guyatt and others have suggested a taxonomy based on the domains of HRQOL which an instrument attempts to cover (Guyatt G.H., 1989). According to this taxonomy, they have broadly grouped HRQOL instruments into two categories- generic instruments and specific instruments.

Generic Instruments for Measuring HRQOL

Generic instruments cover or aim to cover the complete spectrum of function, disability and distress of the patient and are applicable to a variety of populations. Generic instruments are structured to measure HRQOL among various general groups like a particular type of disease group, patient groups like children, elderly or women, group of medical interventions like surgery or general medicine, or range of functions, moods and distress.

Health Profiles

Health profiles are single instruments that measure multiple or different aspects of quality of life that are useful to clinicians and researchers. They normally provide a scoring system that allows aggregation of the results into a small number of scores. Sometimes the aggregation of the results is put into a single score and in that case it is referred to as an index. As generic measures health profiles are designed for use in a variety of conditions.

Some of the commonly used generic instruments of health profiles for measuring HRQOL include Sickness Impact Profile (SIP), Duke - UNC Health Profile, Activities of Daily Living (ADL) and Nottingham Health Policy (NHP). A collection of related instruments from the Medical Outcome Study have become the most popular and widely used generic instruments. It can be self administered or administered by a trained interviewer over the phone or face to face. It is brief, takes 5 to 10 minutes to complete and is reliable. Its validity has been established in clinical situations and disease states.

The Medical Outcome Study Short Form (SF- 36) was originally developed and validated in the US. It is a brief method and the general health profiles provide many advantages to the clinical investigator. Their reproducibility and validity have been established, in different populations. When health profiles are used for discriminative purposes, one can examine and establish areas of dysfunction affecting a particular population. Health profiles used as evaluative instruments allow determination of the effects of an intervention on different aspects of QOL, without necessitating the use of multiple instruments. It helps to save the time of both the patient and the investigator.

Sickness Impact Profile (SIP) examines health status through a descriptive profile of changes in a person's behaviour due to sickness. The SIP contains 12 'categories' which can be aggregated into two dimensions and five independent categories and also into a single overall score. The two dimensions in SIP are physical dimension and psychosocial dimension. The physical dimension has the categories of ambulation, mobility, body care and movement. The SIP has been used in studies of cardiac rehabilitation, total hip joint replacement and treatment of back pain. It is considered as one of the best instruments used to measure HRQOL. The main disadvantage of the SIP is that it has a lengthy questionnaire which makes it difficult for many patients to answer.

The NHP method covers six problem areas - energy, pain, emotional reactions, sleep, social isolation and physical mobility. It is used widely to measure QOL across different countries and for different diseases. It's questionnaire is relatively easy to understand and quick to complete without supervision or interview.

Utility Measurements

The basic elements of utility measurements are, first that it is preference based, and second that the scores are tied to death as an outcome. In clinical studies utility can be measured by the following two methods;

(i) By asking the patient a list of questions about their functional activities; and based on the answers, the patients are classified into certain categories to which a utility value has been assigned.

(ii) By asking the patient to make a single rating which takes into account all aspects of their quality of life.

The most commonly used direct measurement techniques include visual analog scales, time trade off and the standard gamble.

Visual analog scale

HRQOL is measured as a utility measure using single number along a continuum from death of worst imaginable health state (0.00) to full health or best imaginable health state (1.00). The patient is asked to put the mark on the line where he would place one or more health states in relation to the end points. If he rated his health state in a hypothetical scenario at the mid point between 0 and 1 on the scale the value for health state will be 0.5. The use of utility measures in clinical studies involves serial measurement of the utility of the patient's QOL throughout the study. We discussed this in detail in the earlier chapter.

Time trade off

In time trade off technique the patient is asked about the number of years in their present health state they would be willing to 'trade off' for a shorter life span in full health. The patient is offered a choice living for

1. a variable amount of time *x* in perfect health
2. a defined amount of time *t* in health state *i* which is less desirable. We have discussed it in earlier chapter.

Standard gamble technique

Another method is the standard gamble technique where the patient is asked to choose between two alternatives - choice 'A' living in a *sub optimal health state* with certainty or choice 'B' taking a gamble on a new treatment for which the outcome is uncertain. In the choice B he may die immediately or achieve full health for the reminder of life. We have discussed standard gamble in the earlier chapter in detail.

Specific Instruments for Measuring HRQOL

Specific instruments are designed to provide greater detail concerning particular outcomes in terms of functioning and well being associated with a disease condition and its treatment. These instruments focus on disease or treatment issues specifically relevant to the question in hand. They cover specific diseases, specific populations or specific functions. Arthritis Impact Measurement Scale (AIMS), Pediatric Functional Independence Measure (FIM), Asthma Quality of life Questionnaire (AQLQ), Diabetes Quality of Life (DQOL), Kidney Disease Quality of Life (KDQOL) instrument, Quality of Life in Epilepsy (QOLIE) and Hospital Anxiety and Depression Scale (HADS) are examples of specific instruments in use to measure HRQOL.

The rationale for this approach lies in the increased responsiveness that may result from including only those aspects of HRQL, which are relevant and important in a particular disease process or even in a particular patient situation. The researcher can focus the instrument only on the areas that are likely to be affected by a particular drug. Specific instruments can be constructed to reflect the single state. For example how tired have you been? Ans. Very tired, somewhat tired, not at all tired.

Specific instruments are not comprehensive and cannot be used to compare conditions or at times even programs. There is no one group of instruments that will achieve all the potential goals of HRQOL measurement. In studies involving pharmacotherapy, the use of both generic and specific instrument may be the best approach. The generic instrument gives a measurement of general outcome and allows comparability across other disease states or conditions in which it has been used. A specific instrument if selected properly can then provide detailed outcome information regarding anticipated changes in the patients.

Characteristics of Instruments

In most cases, the instruments are used for evaluation of the effects of therapy. The treatment effects are expressed as a change in the score of the instrument over time. However, sometimes the instruments are used to discriminate (categorise into groups) among patients. For example, in the case of evaluating the effect of drug treatment on functional status in patients after myocardial infarction, the patients can be grouped into those with moderate function and those with poor function. This will help the investigator to intervene in the latter group. The purpose for which an instrument is used, often dictates its necessary attributes. There are four characteristics or properties that all instruments for assessment of quality of life must posses:

- validity,
- reliability,
- responsiveness (sensitivity)
- interpretability.

Validity

All instruments used to measure HRQOL must be valid regardless of their particular use. Validity of an instrument refers to its ability to measure what is designed to measure. It is not an absolute property of an instrument. It can be established in different ways and must address several independent aspects of the scale for measuring QOL. Hyland distinguished three major categories of validity based on the study of questionnaires used to assess QOL in patients with respiratory disease. These are criterion validity, content validity and construct validity (Hyland, 1992).

(i) Criterion validity

Criterion validity means that the new test is assessed against an external criterion that is an objective measurement. For example, a psychological assessment of job suitability might be measured against the objective criterion of work output. There is no objective measure that represents health. Hence criterion validity cannot be applied to tests of health related quality of life.

(ii) Content validity

Content validity is an assessment of the extent to which the questionnaire covers the range of topics that it purports to measure. It may cover topics like physical activity, sexual life, emotions, symptoms, etc.

(iii) Construct validity

Construct validity refers to the extent to which results from a given instrument relate to other measures in a manner consistent with theoretical hypothesis. It assumes the existence of a construct or theoretical entity that the questionnaire is measuring. The construct validity of a new test can be assessed in different ways like measurement of impact to treatment (response to treatment) or examination of the internal consistency of the questionnaire. It can be hypothesized that the changes in spirometry (Spirometry is used to diagnose asthma, chronic obstructive pulmonary disease (COPD) and other conditions that affect breathing.) related to use of a new drug in patients with chronic airflow limitation should bear a close correlation with changes in functional status of the patient and a weaker correlation with changes in their emotional condition.

When there is no gold standard, it is often difficult to establish the validity. In cases where there is difficulty in establishing 'criterion validity', the validity of the instrument is established in a stagewise process including examination of the 'face validity' or 'sensibility', 'content validity' and 'construct validity'.

Reliability is necessary but not sufficient for valid measurement.

Reliability

Reliability refers to the extent to which measures give consistent or accurate results. It indicates that the instrument must be reliable in that it measures something in a consistent and reproducible manner. The instrument should have the ability to detect the 'signal' even if there is 'noise' in the measurement process. In the case of discriminative instruments, those that are designed to measure differences among people at a single point in time, this signal comes from differences between patients in HRQOL. Here the way of quantifying the signal: noise ratio is called reliability. If the variability in scores between subjects the signal is much greater than the variability within subjects (the noise) an instrument will be deemed reliable. Reliable instruments will generally demonstrate that stable subjects show more or less the same results on repeated administration.

Responsiveness or Sensitivity

It refers to whether the instrument is capable of detecting a clinically important change, even when the changes are small or nominal. For evaluative instruments, those designed to measure changes within individuals over time, the 'signal' comes from the differences in HRQOL within patients associated with the intervention. The way of determining the signal–to-noise ratio is called 'responsiveness' and refers to an instrument's ability to detect change.

Interpretability

It is another important measurement property of an instrument. Interpretability is the degree to which one can assign qualitative meaning to an instrument's quantitative scores. It is the extent to which one can understand the magnitude of any differences between treatments that a study demonstrates.

Use of Multiple Instruments

In clinical studies often multiple instruments are required to yield all the relevant information. Utility measure contributes a data that is different from the data provided by disease specific measure. However, there are cases where the investigator may want to use both the instruments to get the required data. Sometimes the investigator may administer a battery of specific instruments. Croog, et al, have identified five dimensions of health to measure in a double blind randomized trial of three antihypertensive agents in primary hypertension (Croog SH, 1986). The measures were sense of well-being and satisfaction with life, the physical state, the emotional state and intellectual functioning, ability to perform in social roles and the degree of satisfaction from those roles. The greater the number of instruments used, the greater the probability that one or more will favor one treatment or the other, even if the treatments' true effectiveness is identical.

Conclusions

The topic of quality of life has gained increasing attention in the evaluation of the outcomes associated with health care and pharmacotherapy. Health care providers and administrators have to remember that efforts to improve QOL must not outstrip the ability to maintain or improve QOL. Since HRQOL is a new concept many theoretical and methodological issues remain to be unresolved. Through the discussion in this chapter an attempt is made to sensitize students and health care professionals to the importance of the area and to provide some idea regarding how the concepts of QOL or HRQOL should be related to the practice of health care.

Pharmacoeconomics is the description and analysis of cost of drug therapy to health care systems and society. It is a health care discipline of placing a value on drug therapy.

CHAPTER 26

Construction and Applications of Pharmacoeconomic Studies

Chapter Mission

After learning this chapter you may be able to know:

- Criteria for the conduct of Pharmacoeconomic studies.
- Steps in the conduct of pharmacoeconomic studies.
- Pharmacoeconomics in pharmacotherapy.
- Applications of pharmacoeconomics in pharmacy practice.
- Pharmacoeconomics in drug approval and marketing.
- Relevance of Pharmacoeconomics in India.
- Limitations of pharmacoeconomic methods.

How to conduct of Pharmacoeconomic studies?

There is no formally accepted or generally agreed method for the construction or conduct of pharmacoeconomic studies. However there are a number of acceptable methods. The appropriateness of these methods depends on a number of factors like specific question or objective, perspective of the study, time period for the study and resources like time, money and people available to the researchers. Many researchers and authors specify their own methodology for systematic conductance of pharmacoeconomic studies.

Many countries have also prescribed the guidelines for Pharmacoeconomic evaluations and such aspects were discussed under 'Pharmacoeconomic Regulations and Practice at Global Level' in the earlier chapter.

Criteria for a Pharmacoeconomic Study

The important criteria for the construction or conduct of a pharmacoeconomic study can be listed in 12 steps as noted below

Study objective
Study perspective
Pharmacoeconomic method
Study design
Choice of interventions
Costs and consequences
Discounting
Study results
Sensitivity analysis
Study conclusions
Sponsorship and bias
Use of a comparator

Step 1: Study Objective

There should be a clear statement of the purpose of the study. What is the question being considered? The objective should be clear, concise, well defined and measurable.

Step 2: Study Perspective

The perspective of the study should be selected scientifically. The researcher can select one or more appropriate perspectives like patient, provider, payer or the society. From the selected perspective, analysis should be conducted. An evaluation can be conducted from the single or multiple perspectives, if the costs and consequences identified are relevant to the perspectives selected.

Take the case of a cost-of-illness study. It can be conducted from different perspectives. Based on the perspective there can be variations in the cost. These perspectives may measure costs to society, the health care system, third-party payers, businesses, the government, and participants and their families. Each perspective provides useful information about the costs to the particular group.

The aims or the purpose of the study determines the perspective. A study concerned with the treatment costs of an illness would require the health care system perspective, while a study concerned with how much an illness costs the government would require the government perspective. A study can have more than one perspective. The societal perspective is the most comprehensive and it includes all direct medical costs and indirect costs for the entire members of the society. It does not include transfer payments, such as medicare, health insurance or social security benefits paid to individuals. The societal perspective is often favored because it allows a complete analysis of all of the opportunity costs attributable to a disease. However the societal approach is often difficult as it requires elaborate data. It is very true in the case of diseases which are less common and data are more limited. The societal and health care system perspectives often result in higher cost estimates than the other approaches because of its wide range of costs.

Table 26.1 Costs included in Cost-of-Illness Studies, by Perspective

Perspective Costs	Medical Costs	Morbidity Costs	Mortality	Transportation/ Non-medical cost	Transfer Payments
Societal	All costs	All costs	All costs	All costs	–
Health care System	All cost	–	–	–	–
Third-party Payer	Covered costs	–	Covered costs	–	–
Businesses	Covered costs	Lost productivity	Lost productivity	–	–
Government	Covered (Medicare, Medicaid)	–	–	Criminal justice costs	Attributable to illness
Participants and families costs production	Out-of-pocket House hold production	Lost wages House hold	Lost wages	Out-of-pocket costs	Amount

Step 3: Pharmacoeconomic Method

The method selected for the study should be clearly specified (e.g., CUA, CMA, CBA, CEA, COI). The method should be appropriate to the given problem. If the alternatives differ in their outcome, methods like CMA cannot be selected.

Step 4: Study Design

Pharmacoeconomic evaluation can be retrospective or prospective. Retrospective are capable of reflecting the usual care and can be rich in information. However, prospective studies are always preferred. In the case of pharmacoeconomic studies conducted as part of clinical trials, care should be taken in interpreting the data. In clinical trials, costs need not be reflective of the general practice situation as costs are often protocol driven.

Step 5: Choice of Interventions

All relevant treatment options available should be mentioned and discussed wherever needed. The alternatives compared should be those in practice or use and evidence of their effectiveness should be established.

Step 6: Costs and Consequences

All the important and relevant costs and consequences, for each treatment option selected, should be identified. These costs and consequences identified should be relevant to the perspective of the study and are measurable in appropriate physical units. All costs and consequences must be valued credibly with data sources identified.

Step 7: Discounting

The comparison of treatment alternatives or programs should be made at one point in time. Cost and consequences that occur in the future should be discounted to their present value. Discounting is the adjusting for differential timings. It is the process of reducing any costs and consequences that may occur in the future, back to their present value. If the study is performed over a period of more than one year, discounting should be done using an appropriate discount rate. The rate used typically varies from 3 to 8 percent, representing inflation rate or bank interest.

Discounting is an economic method that captures an individual's preference for income today rather than income in the future. This time preference is often explained by the opportunity cost of interest. Income earned today can earn interest through investment. For example, given an interest rate of 3 percent, a payment of Rs100 lakhs today is worth more than the same payment in one year because Rs 0.30 lakhs of interest can be earned if the payment is received today. Discounting allows us to calculate the present value of payments (or costs) that occur in the future.

Discounting is relevant for direct and indirect costs that accrue past the first year. Numerous possible discount rates can be used to discount future costs, with each representing a slightly different approach.

Step 8: Study Results

A detailed discussion of the study assumptions and the limitations of the study should be specified. How to interpret the results in the context of different practice settings should be mentioned. The results should reflect that appropriate statistical analyses were performed. It may often be appropriate to express the study results in terms of increases; that is, to use incremental cost analysis.

Step 9: Sensitivity Analysis

In the case of pharmacoeconomic studies, it is imperative that researchers test the sensitivity of the study results using sensitivity analysis (SA). Sensitivity analysis is the process of testing the robustness of an economic evaluation with the help of changes in the results. Variables like, per cent effectiveness and incidence of ADRs can be varied over a range of values and hence results are recalculated. SA is important because of the very common need for investigators to use assumptions and estimates for unknown variables.

Step 10: Study Conclusions

The conclusions of the study should be justified properly. Researchers should assist the reader in extrapolating study conclusions to clinical practice. Both internal validation and external validation should be performed. Internal validation involves justification of the conclusions from the study. External validation involves the generalization of the conclusions. In certain cases, conclusions from the study may be statistically significant, but it may or may not be clinically relevant. Sometimes it may be vice versa.

Step 11: Sponsorship and Bias

At the time of evaluating the quality and usefulness of a study, the aspect of sponsorship should be considered properly. Many studies are conducted or sponsored by companies or organizations. The potential for bias should not be ignored or assumed.

Step 12: Use of a Comparator

A 'comparator' becomes essential for certain pharmacoeconomic studies which compare the new drug or procedure or program with an older drug or existing intervention. The comparator can either be the 'gold standard' drug / intervention in that condition or the most commonly used drug, dosage or procedure. The choice of the comparator can in certain cases lead to considerable bias as in the case of using an older-generation drug (in spite of the availability of better options) or a sub-optimal dose as a comparator.

Pharmacoeconomics in Pharmacotherapy

Though a variety of strategies are available to incorporate pharmacoeconomics into pharmacotherapy or drug therapy, the widely used strategies for applying pharmaco-economics to assess the value of pharmaceutical products and services are the following:

(i) Using the results of published pharmacoeconomic studies.

(ii) Building economic models.

(iii) Conducting pharmacoeconomic research.

Use of Published Studies

Pharmacoeconomic studies are published in many primary sources like pharmacy, medical and nursing journals, though considerable variations are seen in the quality of such studies. Variations in practice settings and patterns, patient populations and costs among the different health care systems and different countries, make generalization of the study findings difficult. Moreover, the variations in the study perspectives, data sources and analytical styles may also present a challenge for the practitioners.

If these studies are scientifically evaluated and critically analyzed to identify the limitations and recognition of their merits, that will be useful and helpful for clinical decision making in drug therapy. Questions like "are the findings of the study applicable to the local situation?", "do the results apply in other situations and have a general utility?", "what are the merits of the study?", etc., will help to find the utility of the published study in the present situation.

Building Economic Models

Modeling studies use existing clinical and / epidemiologic data to project future outcomes. Use of economic models can provide support for various clinical decisions. Studies can use data from various sources available within (internal) and from outside (external) a health care organization. The general approach to modeling involves modification and adaptation of existing models. Sometimes a distinct model is developed to answer a specific question. Clinical decision analysis is widely used in modeling in practice settings. Clinical decision analysis is an explicit, quantitative and prescriptive approach to choosing among various alternative outcomes. Building an economic model can help to forecast the impact of medication use in various settings.

Conducting Pharmacoeconomic Research

In the absence of literature and incapability to build a model, pharmacoeconomic research or evaluation is the only alternative. Both time and money are consumed in the evaluation. This strategy should be reserved for pharmacy decisions that may have a significant impact on cost or quality of care. The various criteria discussed earlier under literature usage, are applicable to conduct pharmacoeconomic analysis. Development of a policy or an intervention, its implementation and educating health care professionals and follow up are also important in pharmacoeconomic research.

Applications of Pharmacoeconomics

Pharmacoeconomics identifies, measures, and compares the costs and consequences of drug therapy to healthcare systems and society. 'Applied pharmacoeconomics' is defined as putting pharmacoeconomic principles, methods, and theories into practice settings with the objective of quantifying the value of pharmacy products and pharmaceutical care services used in real-world environments. Healthcare practitioners and professionals can benefit from applying the principles and methods of pharmacoeconomics to their daily practice settings. In modern health care the practitioners are increasingly required to justify the value of the products and services they provide.

One of the primary applications of pharmacoeconomics in clinical practice today is to aid clinical and policy decision making. Through the selection and application of suitable methods of pharmacoeconomics, practitioners and administrators can make better, more informed decisions regarding the products and services they provide.

Complete pharmacotherapy decisions should contain assessments of three basic outcome areas whenever appropriate:

> Economic,
>
> Clinical, and
>
> Humanistic outcomes
>
> This concept is known as Economic Clinical and Humanistic Outcome (ECHO) model.

Traditionally, most drug therapy decisions were based solely on the clinical outcomes (e.g., safety and efficacy) associated with a treatment alternative. During the past 30 years, it has become quite popular or necessary to include an assessment of the economic outcomes associated with a treatment alternative. The recent trend also incorporates the humanistic outcomes associated with a treatment alternative, that is, to bring the patient back into this decision-making equation. The ECHO model for medical decision making has become prevalent in current healthcare settings.

Pharmacoeconomic studies will also help to, compare drugs in the same therapeutic class or drugs with similar mechanism of action, and in establishing accountability and responsibility. Practicing pharmacists in community, hospital, and clinical settings in India can benefit considerably from the application of the principles of pharmacoeconomic into their normal practice settings. Proper application of pharmacoeconomics will empower the pharmacy practitioners and administrators to make better and more informed decisions regarding products and services they provide.

Historically, the principles of pharmacoeconomics were applied in the field of hospital pharmacy activities.In the healthcare settings, pharmacoeconomic methods can be applied for effective formulary management, individual patient treatment, medication policy determination, and resource allocation. The cost effectiveness data was used to support the addition or deletion of a drug to or from a hospital formulary.

Pharmacoeconomics can provide critical cost-effectiveness data to support the addition or deletion of a drug to or from a hospital formulary, with or without restriction. Pharmacoeconomic assessment of formulary actions is becoming a standardized part of many pharmacy and therapeutic committees in recent times. The formulary system right from the national level to the institutional level can be strengthened with the help of studies in the areas. It will also help for the rationalization of the drug procurement system in the country and for the practical implementation of the standard treatment protocols and policies related to medicines.

Development and implementation of protocols and guidelines based on sound pharmacoeconomic data can have a great impact on influencing prescribing patterns and will help to promote appropriate and cost effective use of medicines throughout the health care system in the country. Implementation of sound drug-use guidelines / policies will ensure the most appropriate and cost-effective use of drugs and pharmaceuticals in the healthcare system.

In a country like India, which is having limited budget for health care, pharmaco-economics can provide the data required to justify certain specific services like establishment of Drug Information centers, Patient Counselling services, therapeutic drug monitoring, hospital formulary system and other patient oriented clinical pharmacy activities and allocating resources for such programs.

Fig. 26.1 shows various decisions that can be endorsed and supported using pharmacoeconomics.

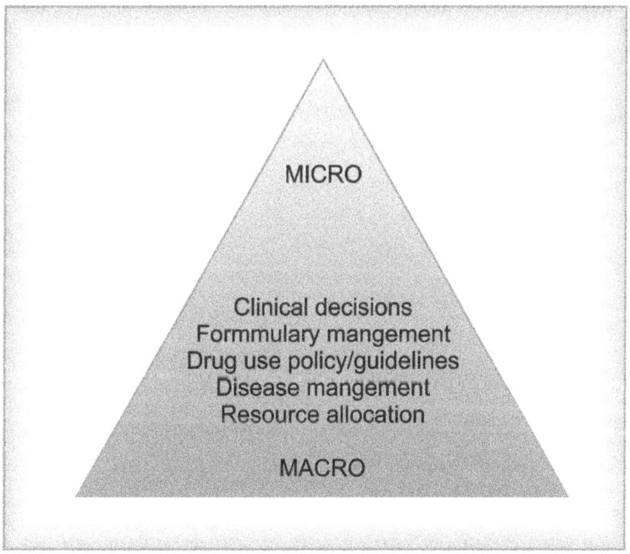

Source: DiPiro JT, Tablert RL, Yee GC, Matzke GR, Wells BG, Posey LM: Pharmacotherapy: A Pathophysiologic approach, 8th Edition: www.accesspharmacy.com

Fig. 26.1 Applications of pharmacoeconomics in health care

The pharmacoeconomic studies find value in :

Fixing the price of a new drug;

Re-fixing the price of an existing drug;

Finalizing a drug formulary;

Creating data for promotional materials of medicines.

Compliance of requirement for drug license

Including a drug in the medical/ insurance reimbursement schemes.

Introduction of new schemes and programs in hospital pharmacy, Clinical pharmacy, Hospital Pharmacy and Community Pharamcy.

The application of pharmacoeconomics also can be useful for making a decision about an individual patient's therapy. The impact a drug on a patient's HRQOL can be evaluated with the help of pharmaco-economics.

In 1990, the UK Department of Health issued advise to the pharmaceutical industry, encouraging it to provide economic data for its new products. After four years, the Department of Health issued guidelines for conducting economic evaluations of drugs. The important aspect of the UK guidelines was that they were drawn up by a joint working group from the Department of Health and the Association of the British Pharmaceutical Industry. The government has addressed the issue of quality of health care through promotion of clinical governance. In 1998, National Institute for Clinical Excellence (NICE) was established in UK, with the objective of improving standards of patient care and to reduce inequities in access to innovative treatment. In 2001, the Department of Health prescribed a target of a 40 per cent reduction in the number of serious errors in the use of prescribed medicines by 2005, through its publication 'Building a safer NHS for patients'.

Pharmacoeconomics in Drug Approval and Marketing

Evidence about quality, efficacy, and safety of the drug is an essential requirement for drug licensing and approval . Given the ever-increasing healthcare costs, this evidence needs to be backed by evidence of cost-effectiveness as well. Evidence comparing the effectiveness of available treatments for a particular disease condition and their related costs need to be presented to the licensing authority before they are introduced in the market.

Australia was the first country tointroduce evidence based pharmacoeconomic guidelines for medication reimbursement in 1992. Since 1993, the Australian Pharmaceutical Benefit Scheme enforces the production of evidence about economic evaluation of the drug before its introduction in the market.

The drug manufacturer provides the submission form to the Pharmaceutical Benefits Advisory Committee for inclusion of the drug in the reimbursement list who then verify the evidence provided by the manufacturer. The committee provides recommendations to the health ministry about drug inclusion in the reimbursement list on the basis of evidence about its cost effectiveness. The final decision making by the policy makers about the cost-effectiveness of the drug is determined by the following factors:

1. The importance of the clinical area
2. The availability of alternative treatments
3. The likely effect of listing on the healthcare system and other therapeutic activities
4. The investment of the sponsor in primary research.

Many other countries like UK, Belgium, Finland, Norway, Portugal, Sweden and Hungary also follow a similar process such as Australia. The Netherlands also introduced the pharmacoeconomic evaluation in 2005. Germany has an institution for economic evaluation research and Spain has regional centers that perform health technology assessment. In Denmark, France, and Italy, pharmaceutical companies provide data about economic evaluation on a voluntary basis. The Central Drug Standard Control Organization (CDSCO) in India is yet to make economic analysis compulsory for Drug approval.

Relevance of Pharmacoeconomics in India

India is a thickly populated country with 1/6th of the world's population. The number of medicines is very large, perhaps the largest in the world. Being the third largest producer of medicines by volume in the world, Indian pharmaceutical industry has a strong position at the global level. Given the issues prevalent in the Indian healthcare system, pharmacoeconomics has many applications. Pharmacoeconomics can aid in decision making when evaluating the affordability of and access to the right medication to the needy.

Brand name prescriptions are the rule of the day. Formulary system is very weak. Treatment protocols exist only in theory. The resources are scarce and competing programs are plenty in health care. The concept of health care insurance is yet to be popularized in the country. Pharmaceutical companies encourage practitioners to prescribe branded products, often in exchange for favours. Studies on prescriptions patterns of medical practitioners in India have reported that very few prescriptions have generic names. By the use of brand names, patients are denied the opportunity to choose the cheapest alternative.

Formulary system involves preparing, updating, and using a list of essential medications with their detailed information and standard treatment guidelines (STGs). A formulary list is an indicator of good pharmaceutical practice and rational drug usage. The formulary consists of appropriate therapies and cost-effective medications which are of a good quality. It is a precise list which makes the process of procuring, storing, distributing, and using the drugs very easy.

Pharmacoeconomics can be used as a tool to study various issues in the drug therapy program in the country. Practicing pharmacists in community, hospital and clinical settings in India can benefit considerably from the application of the principles of pharmacoeconomics into their normal practice settings. Globally the contemporary practicing pharmacists are increasingly required to justify the value of the pharmaceutical products and services they provide in the health care.

Proper application of pharmacoeconomics will empower the pharmacy practitioners and administrators to make better and more informed decisions regarding products and services they provide. Pharmacotherapy decisions were traditionally depending solely on clinical outcomes like safety and efficacy; and pharmacoeconomics teaches us that there are three basic outcomes to be considered – clinical, economic and humanistic – in drug therapy. It is accepted by all, that appropriate drug selection decisions could not be made today based on acquisition costs only.

Applied pharmacoeconomics plays a very significant role in this aspect. There are numerous occasions wherein decision making between alternative drugs, requires the application of the principles of pharmacoeconomics by the pharmacists. Pharmacoeconomics as a tool, aids in the decision making process involving the combination of cost and outcomes.

Pharmacoeconomic data is a strong weapon and powerful tool to endorse or reject various clinically oriented decisions ranging from the level of the patient (micro level) to the level of resource allocation (macro level) in health care system. It is an effective tool in the formulary system, drug use policy (including antibiotic policies) and disease management (treatment protocols).

Applied pharmacoeconomics can also help in decision making in assessing the affordability of medicines to the patients, access to the medicines when needed and comparing various products for treatment of a disease. It will help to introduce accountability for those who promote certain type of high cost medicines and services.

Pharmacoeconomic evaluations have to be used as a basis for resource allocation and utilization in the country. It is particularly important for health policy decision-making. It is important that this concept be understood not only by policy-makers, health administrators and health managers, but also by primary care providers.

Take the case of epilepsy. Ninety percent of the world's 40 million people with epilepsy live in developing countries including India. Still there are only meager facilities for the care of epilepsy diseases. There is fierce competition for resources, the allocation of which is primarily in the hands of health policy-makers. A large multi-centre study conducted in the 1990s in India, addressed for the first time the utilization of medical services by patients with epilepsy in India. (Thomas SV 1999)

The study also examined some direct costs of epilepsy care in India, and brought out some interesting aspects of pharmaco-economics. It was found that newer antiepileptic drugs like lamotrigine, if administered without any selection criteria, would increase the costs of treatment many times over conventional treatment. The new drugs have certain economic advantages in cases of intractable epilepsy due to the decrease in hospital visits, admissions, fever, adverse drug reactions, and a better quality of life for the patient.

Table 26.2 Examples of countries that have national economic guidelines

Examples of countries that have national guidelines for pharmacoeconomic studies	
Australia	Italy
Belgium	Netherlands
Canada	New Zealand
Denmark	Norway
England	Poland

In India, primary care providers are also provided with many new drugs of same category in addition to the existing old drugs. Often the new drugs are available in large quantities. It can confuse the doctors and administrators for the judicious selection and rational use of medicines. A new drug has to be approved for a program based on pharmacoeconomic analysis. It should be equal or more effective compared to the existing drug and shall have some economic or related advantage. Primary care providers too have to understand and appreciate the concept of pharmacoeconomics. In some countries (e.g., Australia, Canada and New Zealand) pharmacoeconomic evaluation is a mandatory part of the dossier for new drug applications, and also for the drug to be considered for reimbursement by health care or insurance companies. (Walley T 1997).

Limitations of Pharmacoeconomic Studies

As most of the Pharmacoeconomic evaluations are conducted by pharmaceutical companies with a commercial interest in ensuring that their products are viewed in a favourable line, the chance for bias cannot be overruled. This would be a confounding variable in the interpretation of the results of such trials. As we have already seen, the economic implications of a study would differ depending upon the perspective being evaluated.

If the clinical trial is conducted in a well designed manner, the results of the study conducted in one country can be applied to a certain extent in other countries also. However in the case of pharmacoeconomic studies, it is not at all possible. Always there are basic differences in the money value, exchange rates of money, cost and outcome approaches and social, cultural and other aspects of the society. Hence the pharmacoeconomic analysis conducted in one country cannot be expected to have application in another country as such. Another fundamental difference between pharmacoeconomic and clinical trial research is the extrapolation of results.

Currently there is no uniformity in the design and analysis of pharmacoeconomic studies. Published studies follow different approaches and often help to create confusion among the readers. In the case of new drugs, it is difficult to justify a separate and independent pharmacoeconomic study due to the increase in costs. However the evaluation can be done at any time during the clinical trials. Pharmacoeconomics gives importance to the social benefits rather than the individual aspects. Hence one can say that

Pharmacoeconomics does not come in the way of Hippocratic ethics of what is best for the person or individual and is based on a broader utilitarian ethics of what is best for the society.

Conclusions

Pharmacoeconomics is comparatively a young science in health care which is still in the trial test of its methodologies. In the era of rising medical costs, Pharmacoeconomics focuses on 'value for money' and educate about its importance. It focuses on the costs and benefits of drug therapy. The pharmacoeconomic evaluations provide a basis for resource allocation and utilization. Pharmacoeconomic analysis can be conducted as an economic assessment incorporated into clinical trials. Such trials should compare the new drug / procedure with an older drug or existing intervention.

Pharmacoeconomic evaluations provide a basis for resource allocation and utilization, and are increasingly becoming important for health policy decision-making. It is important that this concept be understood not only by policy-makers, health administrators and health managers, but also by primary care providers. Pharmacoeconomics is improving with its applications.

Its need is undeniable, more so in a developing country like India. Its potential value in improving patient care is like 'icing on the cake'. The PE study results will help to improve the patient care with the social perspective. Efforts are needed to improve the validity, reliability and robustness of the PE studies to make them more acceptable and reproducible. An important limit of PE is that the whole process is open for bias. If the studies are conducted or sponsored by pharmaceutical firms the chances for bias may be more.

By understanding the principles, methods and application of pharmacoeconomics, pharmacists will be more equipped to make better and more informed decisions regarding the use of medicines and services in health care. There is much scope and potential for pharmacoeconomic studies in India.

Pharmacoeconomics is the description and analysis of cost of drug therapy to health care systems and society. It is a health care discipline of placing a value on drug therapy.

CHAPTER 27

Case Studies in Pharmacoeconomics

Chapter Mission

After learning this chapter you may be able to know:

- Background and implications of selected pharmacoeconomic methods.
- Understand the theory and practice of selected pharmacoeconomic designs.
- How to answer simple case studies in pharmacoeconomics.

Case 27.1: Provider Perspective Direct Cost

Problem

From the perspective of a provider, which one of the following is a direct cost of health care

A. The rupees paid out of pocket by patients directly to their physicians for consultation.
B. The fee for the CT scan conducted.
C. The cost of medicines paid to the hospital pharmacy.
D. The salary of the nurse who supervise the therapy.

Answer

The amount paid out of pocket by patients directly to their physicians (A) is a direct expense to the patient. Fee for CT scan (B) and cost of medicines (C) are direct expenses to the third party payers (Insurance company) and to the patient for co-payment. Salaries of nurses or pharmacists who monitor or supervise the therapy are direct expenses from the perspective of the provider. Hence option D is the answer to the problem.

Case 27.2: Pharmaco-economic Method

Problem

Drug A and Drug B are two antibiotics belonging to the group Aminoglycosides. Literature review of published studies prove that they are therapeutically equivalent with respect to safety and efficacy. Both have to be used for the same duration (No of days). How ever these two drugs differ in the following respects

Cost category	Drug A	Drug B
Unit cost	Rs 80	Rs 170
Dose regimen	3 times a day	Once daily
Expensesto buy drugs	Rs 30	Rs 80

You area clinical pharmacist in the ward round team and asked to recommend the best treatment alternative to the patient. It is public Indian hospital where treatment is free but some medicines like drug A and Drug B have to be purchased by the patient. Our patient is from a very poor family and has to pay out of pocket for the medicines. Which drug would you recommend?

Solution

Both the drugs belong to the same class with equal efficacy. The primary focus is to determine which drug is least expensive for the patient. If both are equal with respect to safety and efficacy, CEA or CUA are not needed. As there are documentary evidence for therapeutic equivalence, CMA is the most appropriate and simple method to apply in this case. The three costs are quantified and becomes Rs 270 for drug A and Rs 250 for drug B. Hence in this case drug B is the obvious choice.

Case 27.3: Treatment of Epilepsy

Problem

Perform the CEA of any two types of treatment programs of epilepsy practiced in Indian hospital set ups.

Solution

Step 1. Define the objective

The purpose is to identity which drug regimen should be the therapy of choice for the treatment of epilepsy based on CEA ?

Step 2. Enumerate the different ways to achieve the objective.

The treatment choices are

1. Conventional AEDs monotherapy (Option 1)
2. Multiple therapy with newer AEDs (Option 2)

Step 3. Identify and measure the cost of each option.

All the inputs required for each option should be identified and the costs determined. When there are joint inputs and outputs, cost allocation methods must be used to determine the share of costs of the relevant options.

Step 4. Identify and measure the benefits of each option.

Benefits can be measured in DALYs (disability adjusted life years) or other units. In the case of epilepsy the seizure free weeks/ months/ years can be taken as the units of measure.

Step 5. Calculate and interpret the cost effectiveness of each option.

The cost effectiveness ratio is total cost divided by number of units of output. Better overall efficiency is indicated by a lower cost per unit of output.

Step 6. Perform sensitivity analysis on the conclusions.

Sensitivity analysis measures how different assumptions made in the course of estimating costs and outputs affect the conclusions. Sensitivity analysis identifies the values or assumptions about which there is uncertainty and determines their likely range of values and recalculates study results based on a combination of the 'best guess' and estimates of key values.

Case 27.4: Partial Economic Evaluation

Problem

Which one of the following is an example of a partial pharmacoeconomic evaluation?

A. A comparison of the costs and consequences of two alternatives

B. A cost utility analysis

C. A comparison of the costs of two equally effective alternatives

D. A quality of life (QOL) comparison of multiple treatment alternatives.

Answer

Partial economic evaluation provides a descriptive assessment of resource used or outcome. It does not provide a comprehensive assessment of both costs and consequences of competing alternatives. The first option (A) is CBA, second (B) is CUA and third (C) is CMA. They are all full pharmacoeconomic methods hence not the answer to the problem. The last option (D) compares the consequences (QOL) only of multiple programs without considering the costs. Hence that is a partial pharmacoeconomic evaluation. It makes option "D" as the correct answer to the problem.

Case 27.5: Treatment of Childhood Pneumonia

Problem

Perform the CEA of any two types of treatment programs of childhood pneumonia practiced in Indian hospital set ups.

Solution

Step 1. Define the objective

The purpose is to identity which drug regimen should be the therapy of choice for the treatment of childhood pneumonia based on CEA ?

Step 2. Enumerate the different ways to achieve the objective.

The treatment choices are

1. Short course therapy with expensive drugs (Option 1)
2. Traditional long course with cheaper drugs (Option 2)

Step 3. Identify and measure the cost of each option.

All the inputs required for each option should be identified and the costs determined. When there are joint inputs and outputs, cost allocation methods must be used to determine the share of costs of the relevant options.

Step 4. Identify and measure the benefits of each option.

Benefits can be measured in DALYs (disability adjusted life years) or other units.

Step 5. Calculate and interpret the cost effectiveness of each option.

The cost effectiveness ratio is total cost divided by number of units of output. Better overall efficiency is indicated by a lower cost per unit of output.

Step 6. Perform sensitivity analysis on the findings.

Sensitivity analysis measures how different assumptions made in the course of estimating costs and outputs affect the conclusions. Sensitivity analysis identifies the values or assumptions about which there is uncertainty and determines their likely range of values and recalculates study results based on a combination of the 'best guess' and estimates of key values.

Case 27.6: Intermediate Outcome

Problem

The Economic, Clinical and Humanistic outcome (ECHO) model recognises the existence of intermediate outcomes. Which one of the following is an example of an intermediate outcome?

A. A patient's physical functioning and mental well being.

B. Clinical laboratory investigation results.

C. Total cost of hospitalization.

D. Adherence to the prescription

Solution

Each of the endpoints of ECHO model (Economic, Clinical and Humanistic) involves intermediate outcomes. Humanistic intermediaries can include specific behaviours of a group of people or an individual. Adherence to the drug regiment or prescription is an example of intermediate outcome. Compliance can be affected by non-behavioural factors like cost of the drug or patients belief system or attitude towards taking drugs. All will have an impact on the outcome. In a statistical model, adherence to prescription or drug regiment is considered both as dependent and independent variable. As an independent variable, adherence can be evaluated for its effect on the dependent variable of humanistic outcomes. In this way adherence to the prescription or drug regimen is an example of intermediate outcome. Hence choice D is the answer.

Case 27.7: Transport of Medicines in Govt. Set Up.

Problem

Perform the CEA of any two types of transport systems available in the country for the transporting of medicines from the state head quarter to the peripheral centers like the primary health centers (PHC).

Solution

Step 1. Define the objective

The purpose is to identity which transport system should be chosen for the transport of medicines from the state head quarters to the peripheral centers based on CEA ?

Step 2. Enumerate the different ways to achieve the objective.

1. Purchase of a vehicle for delivery of medicines (Option 1)
2. Contract with a private party for delivery of medicines (Option 2)

Step 3. Identify and measure the cost of each option.

All the inputs required for each option should be identified and the costs determined. When there are joint inputs and outputs, cost allocation methods must be used to determine the share of costs of the relevant options.

Step 4. Identify and measure the benefits of each option.

In this case indicators like timely performance, safety, absence of damage to the drug consignments etc., can be the benefits.

Step 5. Calculate and interpret the cost effectiveness of each option.

The cost effectiveness ratio is total cost divided by number of units of output. Better overall efficiency is indicated by a lower cost per unit of output.

Step 6. Perform sensitivity analysis on the conclusions.

Sensitivity analysis measures how different assumptions made in the course of estimating costs and outputs affect the conclusions. Sensitivity analysis identifies the values or assumptions about which there is uncertainty and determines their likely range of values and recalculates study results based on a combination of the 'best guess' and estimates of key values.

Case 27.8: Economic Outcome

Problem

Which one of the following options best describes Economic Outcome.?

A. The direct, indirect and intangible costs compared with the consequences of medical treatment alternatives.

B. The medical events that occur as a result of a disease or treatment.

C. The consequences of a disease or treatment on a patient's functional status or QOL.

D. Drug effects on the patient functioning. .

Answer

Clinical outcomes are defined as medical events that occur as a result of a disease or treatment. The drug effects on the patient functioning (D) and the medical events that occur as a result of a disease or treatment (B) are examples of Clinical out comes. Humanistic outcomes are the consequences of a disease or treatment on patient functional status or quality of life (C). Economic outcomes are the total costs of medical care associated with treatment alternatives balanced against clinical or humanistic outcomes. Hence choice " A" is the answer to the problem.

Case 27.9: Utility Measuremet

Problem

Mary is a 45 year old working women suffering from rheumatoid arthritis (RA) for quite some time. Now she is given two alternatives by her treating doctor:

Alternative 1. Knee replacement surgery with probabilities for normal health and death.This option will have a 70% p value of returning to normal health and (1-p) value of 30% of dying.

Alternative 2. Continue the oral and external medicines and employ a care giver cum attendant with a walking stick for the rest of her life.

How will you determine the utility with the help of SG method?

Solution

Arrange a face to face discussion with Mrs Mary. Ask her "Will you prefer to have the Alternative 1 (knee replacement surgery) if the chance of successful operation is 70% (p = 70%).?" Mary says "Yes". That is she prefers Alternative 1 to Alternative 2 when the chance of success is 70% and immediate death is 30%. Now she will be asked the next question "Will you prefer to have the knee replacement surgery if the chance of success is 65%?" Mary says "Yes". The third question can be "Will you like to have the knee replacement surgery if the chance of success is 55%?" Mary says "No". To the final "Will you prefer to have the knee replacement surgery if the chance of success is 60%?". Mary says "I have think about it as I give equal value to both the Alternatives". At this point we can conclude that Mary is at her point of indifference. The two options are nearly equal to her and she may not be able to decide between the two as done in other cases.

The utility measure for Mary for her RA disease condition can be calculated as:

(i) probability (p) of 60 % or

(ii) 0.6.

The utility shows living a normal life after the knee replacement surgery. This calculation hold good for chronic type of disease or condition and may not have much application in other cases.

Pharmacoeconomics is the description and analysis of cost of drug therapy to health care systems and society. It is a health care discipline of placing a value on drug therapy.

CHAPTER 28

References used in Pharmacoeconomic Chapters

Chapter Mission

After learning this chapter you may be able to know:

- Important references used in various Chapters of this book.
- References for further reading.

For Further Reading

ACCP Updates in Therapeutics – The Ambulatory Care Pharmacy Preparative Review and Rectification Course. Volume 2 American College of Clinical Pharmacy Lenexa, Kansas. 2013.

Bootman JL, Werheimer A, ZaskeD, Rowland C. Individualizing gentamicin dosage regimen on burn patients with gram negative septicemia a cost benefit analysis. J Pharm Sci 1979; 68: 267-72.

Bootman JL. The basics of pharmaco-economic analysis. Pharm Rep 1993; 23: 14-15.

Bootman JL Townsend RJ, McGhan WF. Principles of Pharmacoeconomics, Third Edn. Harvey Whitney Books Company 2005. USA.

Clemens K, Garrison Jr LP, Jones A et al. Strategic use of pharmacoeconomic research in early drug development and global pricing. Pharmacoeconomics. 1993; 4: 315-322.

Cooper MH, Culyer AJ. Health economics. London: Penguin, 1973.

Croog SH, Levine S, Testa MA et al. The effects of antihypertensive therapy on the quality of life New Engl J Med 1986; 314: 1657-1664.

Detsky AS, Naglie IG; A clinician's guide to cost effectiveness analysis; Ann Intern Med. 1990; 113: 147-54.

Drummond M. Principles of economic appraisal in health care. New York: Oxford University Press, 1980.

Drummond MF, Smith GT, Wells N.; Economic evaluation in the development of medicines; London, Office of Health Economics, 1988 : 33.

Drummond MF, O'Brien B, Stoddart GL, Torrance GW. Methods for the economic evaluation of health care programmes. 2nd ed. New York Oxford University Press, 1997.

Eddy DM. Cost-effectiveness analysis: is it up to the task?. J Am Med Assoc 1992: 267: 3342-3348.

Eisenberg JM. Clinical economics: a guide to the economic analysis of clinical practices. J Am Med Assoc 1989; 262: 2879-2886.

Esmond D. Nwokeji, and Karen L. Rascati, Pharmacoeconomic Education in Colleges of Pharmacy Outside of the United States-American Journal of Pharmaceutical Education 2005; 69 (3) Article 52.

Gill TM, Feinstein AR. A critical appraisal of quality-of-life measurements. J Am Med Assoc, 1994; 272: 619-626.

Guyatt GH, Veldhuyzen Van Zanten SJO, Feeny DH, Patrick DL. Measuring quality of life in clinical trials: a taxonomy and review. Can Med Assoc J 1989; 140: 1441-1447.

Hakim Z, Pierson JF, Pathak DS. A proposed model for conducting institutional specific cost-effectiveness analysis : a case study of lipid lowering agents. Pharm Practice Mgt. 1996; 16(1) 79-97.

Hepler CD, Strand LM. Opportunities and responsibilities in pharmaceutical care. Am J Hosp Pharm 1990; 47: 533-543.

Hyland ME. Quality-of-life assessment in respiratory disease: an examination of the content and validity of four questionnaires. Pharmaco Economics 1992; 2: 43-53.

Kane-Gill S, Reddy P, Gupta S, Bakst A. Guidelines for Pharmacoeconomic and outcomes research fellowship training programs. Pharmacotherapy 2008; 28 (12): 1552-55.

Kaplan RM, Bush JW. Health related quality of life measurement for evaluation, research and policy analysis. Health Psychol 1982; 1: 61-80.

Kozma CM, Reeder CE, Schulz RM, Economic, clinical and humanistic outcomes: A planning model for pharmacoeconomic research. ClinTher 1993; 15: 1121-1132.

Langley PC. The role of pharmacoeconomic guidelines for formulary approval: The Australian experience. ClinTher 1993; 15: 1154-1176.

Mackeigan LD, Pathak DS. Overview of health related quality of life measures. Am J Hosp Pharm 1992; 49: 2236-2245.

Managing drug supply: The selection, procurement, distribution and use of pharmaceuticals. 2ndEdn. 1997. Kumarian Press, IncUSA.)

McGhan W, Rowland C, Bootman JL. Cost-benefit and cost-effectiveness: Methodologies for evaluating innovative pharmaceutical services. Am J Hosp Pharm. 1978; 35: 133-140.

McGhan WF. Pharmacoeconomics and the evaluation of drugs and services. HospFormul 1993; 28:365-378.

Morgenstern H, Kleinbaum DG, Kupper LL. Department of Epidemiology and Public Health, School of Medicine, Yale University, New Haven, CT. Int J Epidemiol 1980; 9: 97-104.

Pashos CL, Klein EG, Wanke LA, ISPOR Lexicon.1stEdn. International Society for Pharmacoeconomics and Outcome Research. 1998. Princeton, NJ.

Patrick DL, Erickson P. Health status and health policy. Allocating resources to health care. New York, Oxford University Press. 1993: 22.

Pooja Desai, Karen Rascati. Training Pharmacists to use pharmacoeconomics and outcomes research tools in practice. Pharma Times 2013; 45(5) 9-12.

Samuelson PA. Economics. New York: McGraw Hill, 1976.

Sanchez LA, Lee TJ. Use and misuse of pharmacoeconomic terms. Top Hosp Pharm Manage 1994; 13: 11-22.

Schipper H, Clinch J, Powell V. Definitions and conceptual issues. In: Spilker B, ed. Quality of Life Assessments in Clinical Trials. New York, Raven 1990. 11-24.

Schumock GT, Meek PD, Ploetz PA, Vermeulen LC. Economic evaluations of clinical pharmacy services-1988-1995. Pharmacotherapy 1996; 16: 1188-1208.

Schron EB, Shumaker SA. The integration of health quality of life in clinical research: Experience from cardiovascular clinical trials. Prog Cardiovasc Nurs, 1992; 7(2): 21.

Soliman AM, Hussein M, Abdulhalim AM; Pharmacoeconomic education in Egyptian schools of pharmacy. Am J Pharm Educ. 2013 Apr 12: 77 (3): 57.

Spilker B. Quality of Life Assessments in Clinical Trials. New York, Raven 1990.

Tatiana Makhinova, Elena V. Makhinova, Karen Rascati, Pharmacoeconomic Education for Pharmacy Students in the Russian Federation. College of Pharmacy University of Texas at Austin. 2012.

Thomas SV, Abraham PA, Alexander M. Utilization of services for epilepsy and its economic burden in India: A multi-center study. *Epilepsia* 1999;40, 2:198.

Tighe M, Goodman S. Carboplatin versus Cisplatin. Lancet. 1988; 1372-1373.

Townsend RJ. Post marketing drug research and development: An industry clinical pharmacist's perspective. Am J Pharm Educ. 1986; 50: 480-482.

United Nations. The human development report. Oxford: OxfordUniversity Press. London. 1994.

Walley T, Haycox A. Pharmaco-economics: Basic concepts and terminology. Br J ClinPharmacol 1997; 43: 343-8.

Warner KE, Luce BR. Cost benefit and cost effectiveness analysis in health care: WHO QOL Group. Study protocol for the World Health Organization Project to develop a quality of life assessment instrument (WHO QOL). Quality of life research 1993; 2: 153-159.

INDEX

www.ingramcontent.com/pod-product-compliance
Ingram Content Group UK Ltd.
Pitfield, Milton Keynes, MK11 3LW, UK
UKHW061533190726
13845UKWH00005B/92

9 789352 301324